Understanding Nursing Research

Understanding Nursing Research

SECOND EDITION

Nancy Burns, PhD, RN, FAAN

Jenkins Garrett Professor
School of Nursing
University of Texas at Arlington
Arlington, Texas

Susan K. Grove, PhD, RN, CS, ANP, GNP

Professor of Nursing
Assistant Dean, Graduate Nursing Program
School of Nursing
University of Texas at Arlington
Arlington, Texas

W.B. SAUNDERS COMPANY
A Division of Harcourt Brace & Company
Philadelphia London Toronto
Montreal Sydney Tokyo

W.B. Saunders Company

A Division of Harcourt Brace & Company

The Curtis Center
Independence Square West
Philadelphia, Pennsylvania 19106

Library of Congress Cataloging-in-Publication Data

Burns, Nancy, Ph.D.
  Understanding nursing research / Nancy Burns, Susan K. Grove. —
2nd ed.
     p.   cm.
  Includes index.
  ISBN 0-7216-8106-9
  1. Nursing—Research—Philosophy.   I. Grove, Susan K.   II. Title.
  [DNLM: 1. Nursing Research—methods.   WY 20.5 B967u 1999]
RT81.5.B863   1999
610.73′072—dc21
DNLM/DLC   98-43924

UNDERSTANDING NURSING RESEARCH   ISBN 0-7216-8106-9

Printed in the United States of America

Last digit is the print number: 9   8   7   6   5   4   3   2   1

To my family:
My husband Jerry Burns, for his tolerance of long hours
glued to a computer when he would rather have me
nearer to him in his retirement years;
Our daughters, Robin Hardin and Melody Davidson,
whose striving to develop their potential delights me;
Our grandsons, Brady Bell, Layton Davidson, and Skylar Davidson,
whose endless enthusiasm for learning
continually refreshes my own.
NANCY

To my parents, Virginia and Delbert Grove,
who provided me with a strong work ethic, a desire to accomplish my goals,
and a wish to make a contribution to my profession.
To my husband, Jay Suggs, who is the light of my life.
SUSAN

Preface

*R*esearch is a major force in nursing, and the knowledge generated from research is changing practice, education, and health policy. Our aim in developing this essentials book, *Understanding Nursing Research,* is to create an excitement about research in undergraduate students. This text emphasizes the importance of baccalaureate-educated nurses being able to critique research and use the findings in practice. Thus, a major strand throughout the text is critiquing the steps of the research process with the goal of utilizing research findings in clinical practice. By making nursing research an integral part of baccalaureate education, we hope to facilitate the movement of research into the mainstream of nursing. We also hope this text increases students' awareness of the knowledge that has been generated through nursing research that is relevant to their practice. Only through research can nursing truly be recognized as a profession with a unique body of knowledge.

Developing a second edition of *Understanding Nursing Research* has provided us an opportunity to clarify, reorganize, and condense the essential content for an undergraduate text. Revisions in the text for the second edition are based on our own experiences with the text and input from dedicated reviewers and inquisitive students who provided us with many helpful suggestions. The chapters in the second edition have been reordered with some essential changes in their content. This presentation of content assists undergraduate students in overcoming the barriers they frequently experience in understanding the language used in nursing research.

Chapter 1 introduces the reader to nursing research, the history of research, and the significance of research for nursing practice. As with the first edition, the reader is provided information on quantitative and qualitative research, but the second edition also introduces outcomes research. Chapter 2 introduces the steps of the quantitative research process and describes the different types of quantitative research (descriptive, correlational, quasi-experimental, and experimental). The content of Chapter 4 in the first edition—problems, purposes, and hypotheses—is now Chapter 3, which is more consistent with the steps of the research process. The first edition lacks a separate chapter on literature review, which is now Chapter 4 of this text. This chapter provides a background for reading, critiquing, and summarizing research literature to determine the current knowledge in a selected area for use in nursing practice. Chapter 5 stresses the importance of frameworks in research and provides guidelines for critiquing frameworks in published studies.

A discussion of ethics, Chapter 10 in the first edition, has been moved to Chapter 6 at the request of reviewers and to promote clarity in understanding the use of ethics in research. New content in this chapter includes scientific misconduct and the use of animals in research, which will facilitate students' critique of the ethical aspects of studies. The content on validity and reliability in Chapter 7, on design, has been reduced to a level more appropriate to an undergraduate learner to promote clarity and conciseness. Content related to outcomes research has also been added to this chapter. Chapter 8, on population and sample, and Chapter 9, on measurement and data collection in research, have been updated to reflect current knowledge in the literature. Chapter 10 introduces the student to statistical concepts and provides a background for examining statistical results in research reports.

Chapter 11, on qualitative research, has been completely rewritten to provide the reader with a better understanding of the process of conducting qualitative research. Opportunities for students to have simple group experiences in collecting and analyzing qualitative data have been suggested within the text of the chapter. Chapter 12 summarizes and builds upon critique content provided in previous chapters and gives direction for conducting critiques of quantitative and qualitative studies. The text concludes in Chapter 13 with a discussion of the importance of research utilization in nursing and provides specific guidelines for using research findings in practice.

A variety of changes were made throughout the second edition of this text. We increased strategies to assist the learner in linking research findings to practice, such as selecting study examples to which students can easily relate as beginning clinicians. Research examples in the second edition have been updated to include recently published nursing studies. Critical thinking is promoted in the reader by generating relevant questions when presenting new ideas and by expanding the critique sections throughout the text. An important new feature of this second edition is an appendix that provides guidance to the students in using Internet resources to facilitate their learning and to provide opportunities to go beyond the content provided in text and classroom.

The second edition of *Understanding Nursing Research* is appropriate for use in a variety of undergraduate research courses for generic and RN students since it provides an introduction to many research methodologies such as quantitative, qualitative, and outcomes research. This text assists students in reading research literature, critiquing published studies, and summarizing research findings for use in practice. This book is also a valuable resource for practicing nurses in critiquing and using research findings in their clinical settings.

The *Instructor's Manual* for the second edition is now on a CD-ROM, rather than in printed form. The transparencies from the first *Instructor's Manual* have been developed into PowerPoint Presentations with the extensive addition of new slides. Reviewers requested that the critique questions be placed on slides as well as other key ideas, which has been done. The CD and the use of PowerPoint also make it possible to include a variety of visuals on the slides. The PowerPoint Presentations are viewable in Win 3.x and Win 95/98. The Manual includes test items, syllabi, and classroom activities that are provided in both rich text format and ASCII, making it easy for the faculty member to access and print them through most word processing software.

The *Study Guide,* available as a companion to the text, includes three recently published nursing studies that can be used in classroom discussions as well as to address the study guide questions. The *Study Guide* provides exercises that target comprehension of the meaning of concepts used in each chapter. Exercises, such as fill-in-the-blank and matching, allow the students to check their understanding of the chapter content. Exercises in critique allow the students to apply their new knowledge to critiquing the three articles provided in the back of the *Study Guide.* For students who enjoy a little fun with their learning, crossword puzzles related to chapter content are provided. A computer disk with multiple-choice questions that provide feedback to the student about how well he or she has comprehended the content in each chapter accompanies the *Study Guide.* When a student selects a wrong answer, the computer program provides a rationale for why the answer is wrong, and directs the learner back to a relevant section of the textbook.

Acknowledgments

Developing this essentials research book was a two-year project and there are many people we would like to thank. We would like to express our appreciation to Dean Elizabeth Poster, Associate Dean Carolyn Cason, Assistant Dean Mary Lou Bond, and the faculty of the School of Nursing at the University of Texas at Arlington for their endless support and encouragement. We also would like to thank other nursing faculty across the country who have used our book to teach research and have taken some of their valuable time to send us ideas and to identify errors in the text. A special thanks to the students who have read our book and provided us honest feedback on its clarity and usefulness to them.

We would like to recognize the excellent reviews of colleagues who suggested many of the revisions in this text: Wendy Budin, PhD, RNC, College of Nursing, Seton Hall University, South Orange, New Jersey; Anne Fish, PhD, RN, College of Nursing, Ohio State University, Columbus, Ohio; Erika Madrid, DNSc, RN, CS, Holy Names College, Oakland, California; Dr. Cora Newell-Withrow, Associate Professor of Nursing, Eastern Kentucky University, Richmond, Kentucky; Penny Powers, PhD, RN, Department Head and Professor, College of Nursing, South Dakota University, Rapid City, South Dakota; and Barbara Rogers, PhD, RN, School of Nursing, University of Mississippi Medical Center, Jackson, Mississippi.

In addition, we would like to thank the people at W. B. Saunders Company who helped produce this book: We would like to extend a special thanks to Thomas Eoyang, Vice President & Editor-in-Chief, who has been a wonderful editor for our research texts. Thomas is very supportive of us personally, provides us with essential resources, and most importantly is focused on excellence in textbook production. We would also like to thank the following individuals who have devoted extensive time to the development of the second edition, instructor's manual, study guide, and computer disk: Elizabeth Byrd,

Assistant Developmental Editor; Gina Hopf, Editorial Assistant; Nancy Lombardi, Production Editor; and David Murphy, Production Manager of Electronic Products.

Nancy Burns, PhD, RN, FAAN
Susan K. Grove, PhD, RN, CS, ANP, GNP

Contents

Discovering Nursing Research

OBJECTIVES

Completing this chapter should enable you to:

1. *Define research and nursing research.*
2. *Compare and contrast nursing research with research in other disciplines.*
3. *Discuss the importance of research in nursing.*
4. *Discuss the current participation of nurses in research.*
5. *Describe your role in research as a professional nurse.*
6. *Describe the development of nursing research from the time of Florence Nightingale to the present.*
7. *Discuss the following ways of acquiring knowledge in nursing: tradition, authority, borrowing, trial and error, personal experience, role-modeling, intuition, reasoning, and research.*
8. *Identify the different types of quantitative and qualitative research conducted in nursing.*
9. *Discuss the contribution of quantitative, qualitative, and outcomes research to the development of nursing knowledge.*
10. *Discuss the importance of critiquing research reports and summarizing findings for use in practice.*

RELEVANT TERMS

Authority
Borrowing
Case study
Control
Critique
Deductive reasoning
Description
Explanation
Inductive reasoning
Intuition
Knowledge
Mentorship

Nursing research
Personal experience
Prediction
Premise
Outcomes research
Qualitative research
Quantitative research
Reasoning
Research
Role-modeling
Traditions
Trial and error

*W*elcome to the world of nursing research. You might think it strange to consider research a "world," but it is truly a new way of experiencing reality. Entering a new world requires learning a unique language, incorporating new rules, and using new experiences to learn how to interact effectively within that world. As you become a part of this new world, your perceptions and methods of reasoning will be modified and expanded. For example, research involves questioning, and you will be encouraged to ask questions such as: Why is this nursing intervention being used? What is the effect of this intervention? Would another intervention be more effective? What research has been done in this area? What is the quality of the studies conducted in this area? Are the findings from the studies conducted on a nursing intervention ready for use in practice? How can research findings be used in practice?

Because research is a new world to many of you, we have developed this textbook to facilitate your entry into and understanding of this world and its contribution to the delivery of quality nursing care. The purpose of this chapter is to explain broadly the world of nursing research. The importance of nursing research to practice and your role in research are addressed. The history of research in nursing is explored, with a presentation of the scientific accomplishments in the profession over the last 150 years. The ways of acquiring knowledge in nursing are discussed, including the significance of research in developing nursing knowledge. The chapter concludes with an introduction to the different types of research methodologies that are implemented in nursing: quantitative, qualitative, and outcomes research.

What Is Nursing Research?

The word *research* means "to search again" or "to examine carefully." More specifically, research is diligent, systemic inquiry or study to validate and refine existing knowledge and develop new knowledge. Diligent, systematic study indicates planning, organization, and persistence. The ultimate goal of research is the development of a body of knowledge for a discipline or profession, such as nursing.

Defining nursing research requires determining what is relevant knowledge for nursing. Because nursing is a practice profession, research is essential to develop and refine knowledge that can be used to improve clinical practice. Practicing nurses, such as yourself, need to be able to read research reports to identify effective interventions for practice and to implement these interventions to promote positive outcomes for patients and families (Omery, Kasper, & Page, 1995). For example, extensive research has been done to determine the most effective technique for administering medications through an intramuscular (IM) injection. Beyea and Nicoll (1995) summarized this research and developed a procedure for administering IM injections. The procedure identifies the best needle size and length to use, the safest injection site (ventrogluteal site), and the best injection technique to deliver medication and decrease patient discomfort. This is essential information for you to know in giving IM injections so that the outcomes are accurate delivery of medication, minimal discomfort for the patient, and no physical damage to the patient. This procedure for administration of IM injections is presented in Chapter 13.

Nursing research can have an impact on your individual practice and also can be used to change practice for an entire hospital or corporation of hospitals. For example, Shoaf and Oliver (1992) studied "the effectiveness of normal saline versus normal saline containing 10 U per 1 mL heparin for preventing loss of an intermittent intravenous site (heparin lock)" (p. 9). The results of this study "indicated that heparinized saline is not needed to maintain the patency of an intermittent intravenous site, and the use of saline solution alone is less irritating, causes less phlebitis, is less expensive to patients, and saves nursing time" (Shoaf & Oliver, 1992, p. 9). This study and several others have produced similar results, so this knowledge is ready for use in practice (Goode et al., 1991). Nurses in several hospitals have changed their practice and are using normal saline to irrigate patients' heparin locks because nursing research has shown that this intervention provides high-quality, cost-effective outcomes for patients and the hospitals (Shively et al., 1997).

Nursing research is also needed to generate knowledge about nursing education, nursing administration, health care services, characteristics of nurses, and nursing roles. The findings from these studies indirectly influence nursing practice and thus add to nursing's body of knowledge. Educational research is needed to provide high-quality learning experiences for nursing students. Nursing administration and health services studies are needed to improve the quality of the health care delivery system. Studies of nurses and nursing roles can influence nurses' productivity and job satisfaction. For example, Gardner (1992) studied the job conflict, satisfaction, and retention of new graduate nurses employed by hospitals. She found that as job conflict increased, job satisfaction decreased and that decreased job satisfaction resulted in decreased retention. Gardner recommended that "job conflict management should be included in any comprehensive retention effort" and that hospitals should create a "work environment capable of empowering and retaining nurses" (p. 84). These research findings are important because job conflict, job satisfaction, and retention of new graduates influence their productivity and patient care, which, in turn, affect the costs of health care agencies.

In summary, nursing research is needed to develop and refine knowledge that directly and indirectly influences nursing practice. Therefore, in this textbook, *nursing research* is defined as a scientific process that validates and refines existing knowledge and generates new knowledge that directly and indirectly influences nursing practice.

Why Is Research Important in Nursing?

The nursing profession is accountable to society for providing high-quality care for patients and families. The health care provided by nurses must be constantly evaluated and improved based on new information. Through nursing research, scientific knowledge can be developed to improve nursing care, patient outcomes, and the health care delivery system. Nurses need scientific knowledge to improve their decision-making regarding what care to provide patients and how to implement that care. A solid research base is needed to document the effectiveness of selected nursing interventions in treating particular patient problems and promoting positive patient outcomes. In addition, nurses need to use research findings to determine the best way to deliver health care services so that the greatest number of people receive care.

Nursing's scientific knowledge base is expanding rapidly with the generation of new findings by nurses and other health professionals using a variety of research methods. You can learn about these relevant research findings by reading research and clinical journals, attending professional conferences and meetings, and examining the extensive health care information that is provided on the Internet. The knowledge generated through research is essential to provide a scientific basis for description, explanation, prediction, and control of nursing practice.

Description

Description involves identifying the nature and attributes of nursing phenomena and sometimes the relationships among these phenomena (Chinn & Kramer, 1995). Through selected research methods, nurses are able to describe what exists in nursing practice, discover new information, or classify information for use in the discipline. For example, Gates and Lackey (1998) determined that no studies had been conducted to examine the role of youngsters in providing care for adults with cancer, so they conducted a descriptive study in this area. The study findings indicated that children and adolescents were expected to be caregivers as part of their family role and that they found the caregiving to be hard but gratifying. This knowledge is important because nurses have a prominent role in working with caregivers, and it is important to understand and support the young caregivers in a family. This descriptive research is essential groundwork for studies that will focus on explanation, prediction, and control of nursing phenomena.

Explanation

In *explanation*, the relationships among variables are clarified, and the reasons why certain events occur are identified. For example, research has indicated that elderly patients' risk of developing pressure ulcers is significantly related to their level of mobility and the type of support surface (bed) on which they are placed (Kemp et al., 1993; Vyhlidal et al., 1997). This information about mobility and support surfaces can be used to explain the incidence of pressure ulcers in elderly patients. You could also use this knowledge in selecting nursing interventions to prevent pressure ulcers. Determining relationships among variables provides a basis for conducting studies for the purpose of predicting and controlling patient outcomes.

Prediction

Through *prediction*, one can estimate the probability of a specific outcome in a given situation (Chinn & Kramer, 1995). However, predicting an outcome does not necessarily enable you to modify or control the outcome. With predictive knowledge, nurses could anticipate the effects nursing interventions would have on patients and families. Health promotion research is being conducted to predict the effects of healthy behaviors such as exercising regularly, eating a balanced diet, and not smoking on health status and longevity. For example, Topp and Stevenson (1994) studied the effects of a long-term exercise program on the cognitive and physical functioning of older adults. They found that the attendance rate and amount of effort expended during the exercise program significantly promoted a positive health attitude and maximum physical functioning in this population. Nurses working with the elderly can use this knowledge to encourage them to participate in health promotion activities to improve their quality of life.

Control

If one can predict the outcome of a situation, the next step is to control or manipulate the situation to produce the desired outcome. *Control* can be described as the ability to write a prescription to produce the desired results. Nurses could prescribe certain interventions to help patients and families achieve high-quality outcomes. Based on the research of Meek (1993), nurses could prescribe slow stroke back massage to promote comfort and relaxation in hospice patients. Using the research findings of Hastings-Tolsma et al. (1993), you could prescribe the use of warm (not cold) applications for the resolution of intravenous (IV) infiltrations. Using the research of Hansell et al. (1998), a social support intervention could be implemented to reduce the stress and promote the coping of parents caring for their children with human immunodeficiency virus/acquired immunodeficiency syndrome (HIV/AIDS). Studies that document the effectiveness of specific nursing interventions make it possible to provide care that will produce the best outcomes for patients and their families. The quality of research conducted in nursing impacts not only the quality of care delivered but also the power of nurses in making decisions about the health care delivery system.

What Is Your Role in Nursing Research?

Now that you have been introduced to the world of nursing research, what do you think will be your research role? You might think that you have no role in research, that research is the responsibility of other nurses. However, generating a scientific knowledge base and using this knowledge in practice requires the participation of all nurses in a variety of research activities. Some nurses are producers of research and conduct studies to generate and refine the knowledge needed for nursing practice. Others are consumers of research and use research findings to improve nursing practice.

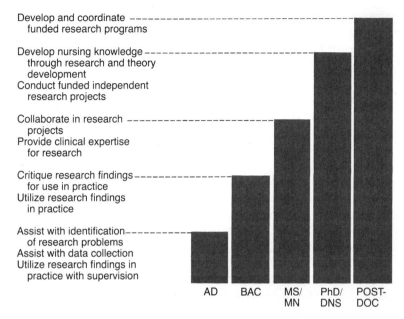

Develop and coordinate
   funded research programs

Develop nursing knowledge
   through research and theory
   development
Conduct funded independent
   research projects

Collaborate in research
   projects
Provide clinical expertise
   for research

Critique research findings
   for use in practice
Utilize research findings
   in practice

Assist with identification
   of research problems
Assist with data collection
Utilize research findings in
   practice with supervision

AD   BAC   MS/   PhD/   POST-
            MN   DNS   DOC

FIGURE 1-1
Research participation at various levels of education preparation. (American Nurses Association
[1989]. *Education for participation in nursing research.* Kansas City, MO: American Nurses Association, with permission.)

Participation in research can occur at all levels of educational preparation.
As indicated in Figure 1-1, nurses with an associate degree in nursing (ADN),
a bachelor of science in nursing (BSN), a master of science in nursing (MSN),
a doctorate degree, and postdoctorate education have a role in research (American Nurses Association, 1989). The researcher role expands with advanced
education and expertise. Thus, the nurse with a BSN has a significant role in
critiquing research findings for use in practice. Nurses with a BSN also provide
valuable assistance in identifying research problems and collecting data for
studies. The maximum preparation of postdoctorate education provides a background for doing all the research activities identified for the other levels of
educational preparation and for the development and coordination of funded
research programs (see Fig. 1-1).

   This textbook was developed to encourage you to be a consumer of research. It provides content to assist you in reading research reports, critiquing
these reports, and summarizing the findings for use in practice. Reading research reports requires an understanding of the research process that is detailed
throughout this text. A *critique* of research involves careful examination of all
aspects of a study to judge its strengths, limitations, meaning, and significance.
Critiquing is a major focus of this textbook and is discussed in several chapters.
The findings from research reports need to be summarized to determine their

potential use in practice. Chapters 4 and 13 provide direction for reading and summarizing the research literature and using research knowledge to change practice. We hope that this text will increase your understanding of research and facilitate your use of study findings in practice.

Nurses' Participation in Research: Past to Present

Nurses' participation in research has changed drastically over the last 150 years. Initially, nursing research evolved slowly, from the investigations of Nightingale in the nineteenth century to the studies of nursing education in the 1930s and 1940s and the research of nurses and nursing roles in the 1950s and 1960s. In the 1970s and 1980s, an increasing number of nursing studies focused on clinical problems and produced findings that had a direct impact on practice. Clinical research continues to be a major focus for the 1990s, with the goal of developing a research-based practice. Reviewing the history of nursing research enables you to identify the accomplishments and understand the need for further research. Table 1-1 outlines the key historical events that have influenced the development of research in nursing.

Florence Nightingale

Nightingale's (1859) initial research focused on the importance of a healthy environment in promoting patients' physical and mental well-being. She studied aspects of the environment such as ventilation, cleanliness, purity of water, and diet to determine the influence on patients' health (Herbert, 1981). However, Nightingale is most noted for her collection and analysis of soldier morbidity and mortality data during the Crimean War. This research enabled her to change the attitudes of the military and society toward the care of the sick. The military began to view the sick as having the right to adequate food, suitable quarters, and appropriate medical treatment. These interventions drastically reduced mortality from 43% to 2% in the Crimean War (Cook, 1913). Nightingale made a major impact on people's health. She used research knowledge to make significant changes in society, such as testing public water, improving sanitation, preventing starvation, and decreasing morbidity and mortality (Palmer, 1977).

Nursing Research from 1900 to the 1960s

The *American Journal of Nursing* was first published in 1900, and late in the 1920s and 1930s, case studies began appearing in this journal. A *case study* involves an in-depth analysis and systematic description of one patient or a group of similar patients to promote understanding of nursing interventions. Case studies are one example of the practice-related research that has been conducted in nursing over the last century.

In 1950 the American Nurses Association (ANA) initiated a 5-year study on nursing functions and activities. The findings from this study were used to de-

TABLE 1-1.	Historical Events Influencing Research in Nursing
Year	*Historical Event*
1850	Nightingale, first nurse researcher
1900	*American Journal of Nursing* (first published)
1950	American Nurses Association (ANA) study of nursing functions and activities
1952	*Nursing Research* (first published)
1953	Institute of Research and Service in Nursing Education
1963	*International Journal of Nursing Studies* (first published)
1965	ANA sponsored nursing research conferences
1967	*Image* (Sigma Theta Tau publication) (first published)
1970	ANA Commission on Nursing Research
1978	*Research in Nursing & Health* (first published)
	Advances in Nursing Science (first published)
1979	*Western Journal of Nursing Research* (first published)
1982–83	Conduct and Utilization of Research in Nursing Project (published)
1983	*Annual Review of Nursing Research* (first published)
1985	National Center for Nursing Research (NCNR) established within the National Institutes of Health
1987	*Scholarly Inquiry for Nursing Practice* (first published)
1988	*Applied Nursing Research* (first published)
	Nursing Science Quarterly (first published)
1989	Agency for Health Care Policy and Research (AHCPR) was established
	Clinical practice guidelines were first published by the AHCPR
1992	*Healthy People 2000* was published by Department of Health and Human Services (DHHS)
	Clinical Practice Guidelines: *Urinary Incontinence in Adults, Acute Pain Management*, and *Pressure Ulcers in Adults* were published by AHCPR
	Clinical Nursing Research was first published.
1993	NCNR was renamed the National Institute of Nursing Research (NINR)

velop statements on functions, standards, and qualifications for professional nurses in 1959. Also during this time, clinical research began expanding as nursing specialty groups, such as community health, psychiatric-mental health, medical-surgical, pediatrics, and obstetrics nursing, developed standards of care. The research conducted by the ANA and the specialty groups provided the basis for the nursing practice standards that guide professional practice (Gortner & Nahm, 1977). The increase in research activity during the 1940s prompted the publication of the first research journal, *Nursing Research,* in 1952.

In the 1950s and 1960s, nursing schools began introducing research and the steps of the research process at the baccalaureate level, and master's-level nurses were provided a background for conducting research. In 1953 the Institute for Research and Service in Nursing Education was established at Teacher's College, Columbia University, New York, which provided learning experiences in research for doctoral students (Gortner & Nahm, 1977).

In the 1960s an increasing number of clinical studies focused on quality care and the development of criteria to measure patient outcomes. Intensive care units were being developed, which promoted the investigation of nursing interventions, staffing patterns, and the cost effectiveness of care (Gortner & Nahm, 1977). An additional research journal, the *International Journal of Nursing Studies,* was published in 1963. In 1965, the ANA sponsored the first of a series of nursing research conferences to promote the communication of research findings and the use of these findings in practice.

Nursing Research in the 1970s

In the late 1960s and 1970s, nurses were involved in the development of models, conceptual frameworks, and theories to guide nursing practice. The nursing theorists' works provided direction for future nursing research. In 1978, Chinn began publishing the journal *Advances in Nursing Science,* which included nursing theorists' works and related research.

Another event influencing research during this decade was the establishment of the ANA Commission on Nursing Research in 1970. In 1972 the commission established the Council of Nurse Researchers to advance research activities, provide an exchange of ideas, and recognize excellence in research. The commission also influenced the development of federal guidelines concerning research and human subjects and sponsored research programs nationally and internationally (See, 1977).

The communication of research findings was a major issue in the 1970s (Barnard, 1980). Sigma Theta Tau, the international honor society for nursing, sponsored national and international research conferences, and the chapters of this organization sponsored many local conferences to communicate research findings. *Image,* first published in 1967 by Sigma Theta Tau, includes research articles and summaries of research conducted on selected topics. Two additional research journals were first published in the 1970s: *Research in Nursing & Health* in 1978 and *Western Journal of Nursing Research* in 1979.

Nursing Research in the 1980s and 1990s

The conduct of clinical research was the focus of the 1980s, and clinical journals began publishing more studies. One new research journal was published in 1987, *Scholarly Inquiry for Nursing Practice,* and two in 1988, *Applied Nursing Research* and *Nursing Science Quarterly.* Even though the body of empirical knowledge generated through clinical research increased rapidly in the 1980s, little of this knowledge was used in practice. During 1982 and 1983, the materials from a federally funded project, Conduct and Utilization of Research in Nursing (CURN), were published to facilitate the use of research to improve nursing practice (Horsley, Crane, Crabtree, & Wood, 1983). In 1983, the first volume of the *Annual Review of Nursing Research* was published (Werley & Fitzpatrick, 1983). These volumes include experts' reviews of research in selected areas of nursing practice, nursing care delivery, nursing education, and the nursing profession. These summaries of current research knowledge encourage the use of research findings in practice and provide direction for future research.

Another priority of the 1980s was to obtain increased funding for nursing research. Most of the federal funds in the 1980s were designated for medical studies involving the diagnosis and cure of diseases. However, the ANA achieved a major political victory for nursing research with the creation of the National Center for Nursing Research (NCNR) in 1985. The purpose of this center is "the conduct, support, and dissemination of information regarding basic and clinical nursing research, training and other programs in patient care research" (Bauknecht, 1985, p. 2). Under the direction of Dr. Ada Sue Hinshaw, the NCNR became the National Institute of Nursing Research (NINR) in 1993. NINR (1993) has selected five research priorities for 1995 through 1999: community-based nursing models, effectiveness of nursing interventions in HIV/AIDS, cognitive impairment, living with chronic illness, and biobehavioral factors related to immunocompetence.

Outcomes research is emerging as important methodology for documenting the effectiveness of health care services in the 1990s. This effectiveness research evolved from the quality assessment and quality assurance functions that originated with professional standards review organizations (PSROs) in 1972 and, more recently, peer review organizations (PROs). In 1989, the Agency for Health Care Policy and Research (AHCPR) was established to facilitate the conduct of outcomes research and the communication of the findings to health care practitioners. The AHCPR produced clinical practice guidelines that are useful for your practice, such as pain management in children, pressure ulcer prevention, and management of incontinence. During the last decade, nurses have conducted a large number of studies that have advanced the development of nursing knowledge for use in practice.

Acquiring Knowledge in Nursing

Some key questions one might ask about knowledge are: What is knowledge? How is knowledge acquired in nursing? Is most of nursing's knowledge based on research? *Knowledge* is essential information that is acquired in a variety of ways, is expected to be an accurate reflection of reality, and is incorporated and used to direct a person's actions (Kaplan, 1964). During your nursing education, you have acquired an extensive amount of knowledge from classroom and clinical experiences. You have had to learn, synthesize, incorporate, and apply this knowledge so that you could practice as a nurse.

The quality of your nursing practice depends on the quality of the knowledge that you learned. Thus, you need to question the quality and credibility of new information that you hear or read. For example, what were the sources of the knowledge that you acquired during your nursing education? Were the nursing interventions you were taught based on research or tradition? Which interventions are based on research, and which need further study to determine their effectiveness? Nursing has historically acquired knowledge through tradition, authority, borrowing, trial and error, personal experience, role-modeling, intuition, and reasoning. Only recently have many of the research findings been included in nursing textbooks or instructors' lectures. This section introduces you to different ways of acquiring knowledge in nursing. Some nursing actions are based on sound scientific knowledge, but others need to be questioned, studied, and revised to reflect current research findings.

Tradition

Traditions include "truths" or beliefs that are based on customs and past trends. Nursing traditions from the past have been transferred to the present by written and verbal communication and role-modeling and continue to influence the practice of nursing. For example, many of the policy and procedure manuals in hospitals contain traditional ideas. Traditions can positively influence nursing practice because they were developed from effective past experiences.

However, traditions can also narrow and limit the knowledge sought for nursing practice. For example, nursing units are frequently organized and run according to set rules or traditions that might not be efficient or effective. Often these traditions are neither questioned nor changed because they have existed for long periods and are frequently supported by people with power and authority. Many traditions have not been tested for accuracy or efficiency through research, and even those not supported through research tend to persist. For example, many cardiac patients are required to take basin baths throughout their hospitalization despite the findings from nursing research that "the physiologic costs of the three types of baths (basin, tub, and shower) are similar; differences in responses to bathing seem more a function of subject variability than bath types; and many cardiac patients can take a tub bath or shower earlier in their hospitalization" (Winslow, Lane, & Gaffney, 1985, p. 164). Nursing's body of knowledge needs to have an empirical rather than a traditional base if nurses are to have a powerful impact on health care and patient outcomes.

Authority

An *authority* is a person with expertise and power who is able to influence opinion and behavior. A person is given authority because it is thought that she or he knows more in a given area than others do. Knowledge acquired from authority is illustrated when one person credits another as the source of information. Nurses who publish articles and books or develop theories are frequently considered authorities. Students usually view their instructors as authorities, and clinical nursing experts are considered authorities within their clinical settings. Many customs or traditional ways of knowing are maintained by authorities; but, like tradition, much of the knowledge acquired from authorities has not been validated by research. Although the knowledge may be useful, it needs to be questioned and verified through research.

Borrowing

Some nursing leaders have described part of nursing's knowledge as information borrowed from disciplines such as medicine, sociology, psychology, physiology, and education (McMurrey, 1982). *Borrowing* in nursing involves the appropriation and use of knowledge from other fields or disciplines to guide nursing practice. Nursing has borrowed in two ways. For years, some nurses have taken information from other disciplines and applied it directly to nursing practice. This information was not integrated within the unique focus of nursing. For example, some nurses have used the medical model to guide their nursing practice, thus focusing on the diagnosis and treatment of disease. This type of borrowing continues today as nurses use advances in technology to become highly specialized and focused on the detection and treatment of disease.

Another way of borrowing, which is more useful in nursing, involves integrating information from other disciplines within the focus of nursing. Because disciplines share knowledge, it is sometimes difficult to know where the boundaries exist between nursing's knowledge base and that of other disciplines. However, borrowed knowledge has not been adequate for answering many questions generated in nursing practice.

Trial and Error

Trial and error is an approach with unknown outcomes that is used in a situation of uncertainty in which other sources of knowledge are unavailable. Because each patient responds uniquely to a situation, there is uncertainty in nursing practice. Hence, nurses must use trial and error in providing nursing care. However, trial and error frequently involves no formal documentation of effective and ineffective nursing actions. With this strategy, knowledge is gained from experience but often is not shared with others. The trial-and-error approach to acquiring knowledge can also be time-consuming because multiple interventions might be implemented before one is found to be effective. There is also a risk of implementing nursing actions that are detrimental to patients' health. If research were conducted on nursing interventions, one could select and implement interventions based on scientific knowledge rather than chance.

Personal Experience

Personal experience involves gaining knowledge by being personally involved in an event, a situation, or a circumstance. In nursing, personal experience enables you to gain skills and expertise by providing care to patients and families in clinical settings. Learning that occurs from personal experience enables you to cluster ideas into a meaningful whole. For example, you may read about giving an injection or be told how to give an injection in a classroom setting, but you do not "know" how to give an injection until you observe other nurses giving injections to patients and actually give several injections yourself.

The amount of personal experience affects the complexity of a nurse's knowledge base. Benner (1984) described five levels of experience in the development of clinical knowledge and expertise: (1) novice, (2) advanced beginner, (3) competent, (4) proficient, and (5) expert. Novice nurses have no personal experience in the work they are to perform, but they have preconceived notions and expectations about clinical practice that they obtained during their education. These notions and expectations are challenged, refined, confirmed, or disconfirmed by personal experience in a clinical setting. The advanced beginner nurse has just enough experience to recognize and intervene in recurrent situations. For example, the advanced beginner is able to recognize and intervene in managing patients' pain.

Competent nurses are able to generate and achieve long-range goals and plans because of their years of personal experience. The competent nurse also is able to use personal knowledge to take conscious, deliberate actions that are efficient and organized. From a more complex knowledge base, the proficient nurse views the patient as a whole and as a member of a family and community. The proficient nurse recognizes that each patient and family responds differently to illness and health. The expert nurse has an extensive background of experience and is able to identify accurately and intervene skillfully in a situation. Personal experience increases an expert nurse's ability to grasp a situation intuitively with accuracy and speed. Through Benner's (1984) research, one gains an increased understanding of the knowledge that is acquired through personal experience. Additional research is needed to clarify the dynamics of expert nursing practice and to determine methods that will facilitate meaningful personal experiences for nursing students and new graduates.

Role-modeling

Role-modeling is learning by imitating the behaviors of an expert. In nursing, role-modeling enables the novice nurse to learn through interactions with or examples set by highly competent, expert nurses. Role models include admired teachers, expert clinicians, researchers, or individuals who inspire students through their examples (Rempusheski, 1992). An intense form of role-modeling is *mentorship,* in which the expert nurse serves as a teacher, sponsor, guide, and counselor for the novice nurse. The knowledge gained through personal experience is greatly enhanced by a high-quality relationship with a role model or mentor. Some new graduates enter internship programs provided by clinical agencies so that they can be mentored by expert nurses during their first few months of employment.

Intuition

Intuition is an insight or understanding of a situation or event as a whole that usually cannot be explained logically (Rew & Barrow, 1987). Because intuition is a type of knowing that seems to come unbidden, it may also be described as a "gut feeling" or a "hunch." Because intuition cannot be explained scientifically with ease, many people are uncomfortable with it. Some even say that it does not exist. However, intuition is not the lack of knowing; rather, it is a result of "deep" knowledge (Benner, 1984). The knowledge is so deeply incorporated that it is difficult to bring it to the surface consciously and express it in a logical manner. Some nurses can recognize intuitively when a patient is experiencing a health crisis. Using this intuitive knowledge, they can assess the patient's condition and contact the physician for medical intervention.

Reasoning

Reasoning is the processing and organizing of ideas in order to reach conclusions. Through reasoning, people are able to make sense of both their thoughts and their experiences. This type of thinking is often evident in the verbal presentation of a logical argument in which each part is linked to reach a logical conclusion. The science of logic includes inductive and deductive reasoning. *Inductive reasoning* moves from the specific to the general; particular instances are observed and then combined into a larger whole or a general statement (Chinn & Kramer, 1995). An example of inductive reasoning follows.

Particular Instances

A headache is an altered level of health that is stressful.

A terminal illness is an altered level of health that is stressful.

General Statement

Therefore, it can be induced that all altered levels of health are stressful.

Deductive reasoning moves from the general to the specific or from a general premise to a particular situation or conclusion (Chinn & Kramer, 1995). A *premise* or proposition is a statement of the proposed relationship between two or more concepts. An example of deductive reasoning follows.

> **Premises**
>
> All human beings experience loss.
> All adolescents are human beings.
>
> **Conclusion**
>
> Therefore, it can be deduced that all adolescents experience loss.

In this example, deductive reasoning is used to move from the two general premises about human beings and adolescents to the conclusion that "All adolescents experience loss." However, the conclusions generated from deductive reasoning are valid only if they are based on valid premises. Research is a means to test and confirm or refute a premise so that valid premises can be used as a basis for reasoning in nursing practice.

Acquiring Knowledge Through Nursing Research

Acquiring knowledge through tradition, authority, borrowing, trial and error, personal experience, role-modeling, intuition, and reasoning is important in nursing. However, these ways of acquiring knowledge are inadequate in providing a scientific knowledge base for nursing practice. The knowledge needed for practice is both specific and holistic, as well as process oriented and outcomes focused; thus, a variety of research methods are needed to generate this knowledge. This section provides an introduction to quantitative, qualitative, and outcomes research methods that have been used to generate knowledge for nursing practice.

Introduction to Quantitative and Qualitative Research

The majority of the studies conducted in nursing from 1930 to 1980 used quantitative research methods. *Quantitative research* is a formal, objective, systematic process in which numerical data are used to obtain information about the world. This research method is used to describe variables, examine relationships among variables, and determine cause-and-effect interactions between variables (Burns & Grove, 1997).

Qualitative research is a systematic, subjective approach used to describe life experiences and give them meaning (Munhall & Oiler, 1993). Nurses' interest in conducting qualitative research began in the late 1970s; today, an extensive number of qualitative studies are conducted using a variety of qualitative research methods. This type of research is conducted to describe and promote understanding of human experiences such as pain, caring, powerlessness, and

TABLE 1-2. Classification System for Nursing Research Methods

I. Types of Quantitative Research
Descriptive research
Correlational research
Quasi-experimental research
Experimental research

II. Types of Qualitative Research
Phenomenological research
Grounded theory research
Ethnographic research
Historical research

III. Outcomes Research

comfort. Because human emotions are difficult to quantify (assign a numerical value), qualitative research seems to be a more effective method of investigating emotional responses than quantitative research. In addition, qualitative research focuses on understanding the whole, which is consistent with the holistic philosophy of nursing (Munhall, 1989).

Quantitative and qualitative research are two general categories of research. Several types of quantitative and qualitative research have been conducted to generate nursing knowledge for practice. These types of research can be classified in a variety of ways. The classification system for this textbook (Table 1-2) includes the most common types of quantitative and qualitative research conducted in nursing. The quantitative research methods are classified into four categories: descriptive, correlational, quasi-experimental, and experimental. Descriptive research is conducted to explore new areas of research and to describe situations as they exist in the world. Correlational research is conducted to examine relationships and to develop and refine explanatory knowledge for nursing practice. Quasi-experimental and experimental studies are conducted to determine the effectiveness of nursing interventions in producing positive outcomes for patients and families. These types of research are discussed in Chapter 2.

The qualitative research methods included in this textbook are phenomenological, grounded theory, ethnographic, and historical research. Phenomenological research is an inductive descriptive approach used to describe an experience as it is lived by a person, such as the lived experience of chronic pain. Grounded theory is an inductive research technique that is used to formulate, test, and refine a theory about a particular phenomenon. Grounded theory was initially developed by Glaser and Strauss (1967) and was used to formulate a theory about the grieving process. Ethnographic research was developed by the discipline of anthropology for investigating cultures through an in-depth study of the members of the culture. Health practices vary among cultures, and these practices need to be recognized in delivering care to patients, families, and communities. Historical research is a narrative description or analysis of events that occurred in the remote or recent past. Through historical research, past mistakes are examined to facilitate an understanding of and an effective response to present situations. Qualitative research methods are the focus of Chapter 11.

Introduction to Outcomes Research

The spiraling cost of health care has generated many questions about the quality and effectiveness of health care services and the patient's outcomes related to these services. Consumers want to know what services they are purchasing and if these services will improve their health. Health care policymakers want to know if the care is cost-effective and high-quality. These concerns have promoted the conduct of *outcomes research* that is focused on examining the end result of care or determining the changes in health status for the patient (Rettig, 1991). Four essential areas that require examination through outcomes research are: (1) the patient's responses to medical and nursing interventions; (2) functional maintenance or improvement of physical functioning for the patient; (3) financial outcomes achieved with the provision of health care services; and (4) the patient's satisfaction with the health outcomes, care received, and the health care providers (Jones, 1993). Nurses are taking an active role in conducting outcomes research by participating in multidisciplinary research teams that are examining the outcomes of health care services. This knowledge provides a basis for improving the quality of care nurses deliver in practice.

SUMMARY

The purpose of this chapter is to introduce you to the world of nursing research. Research is defined as diligent, systematic inquiry to validate and refine existing knowledge and generate new knowledge. Nursing research is defined as a scientific process that validates and refines existing knowledge and generates new knowledge that directly and indirectly influences nursing practice. Through nursing research, scientific knowledge can be developed to improve nursing care, patient outcomes, and the health care delivery system. The knowledge generated from research is used to describe, explain, predict, and control aspects of nursing practice.

Nurses' participation in research over the past 150 years has changed drastically. Initially, research evolved slowly from the investigations of Nightingale in the nineteenth century to the studies of nursing education in the 1930s and 1940s and the research of nurses and nursing roles in the 1950s and 1960s. However, in the 1970s and 1980s, an increasing number of nursing studies focused on clinical problems. The conduct of clinical research continues to be a major focus for the 1990s, with the goal of developing a research-based practice. A recent major accomplishment for nursing was the development of the NINR, which provides essential funding to further nursing research. The historical review of nursing research activities clearly indicates the gains that have been made in developing nursing knowledge.

Nursing has historically acquired knowledge mainly through tradition, authority, borrowing, trial and error, personal experience, role-modeling, intuition, and reasoning. However, these ways of acquiring knowledge are inadequate in providing a scientific knowledge base for nursing. Research is needed to develop and refine scientific knowledge for use in practice. The knowledge nurses need is not only narrow and specific but also broad and holistic. Thus, a variety of research methods are needed to generate nursing knowledge. Nurses conduct both quantitative and qualitative research to address nursing problems. Quantitative research is a formal, objective, systematic process using numerical data to obtain information about the world. This research method is used to describe, examine relationships, and determine cause and effect. Qualitative research is a systematic, subjective approach used to describe life experiences and give them meaning. Knowledge generated from qualitative research will provide meaning and understanding of specific emotions, values, and life experiences. Quantitative and qualitative research complement each other because they generate different kinds of knowledge that are useful in nursing practice.

Different research methods can be classified in a variety of ways. In this textbook, quantitative research is classified into four types: descriptive, correlational, quasi-experimental, and experimental. Four types of qualitative research included are phenomenological, grounded theory, ethnographic, and historical. A third research method presented in this text is outcomes research, which is focused on examining the end result of care or in determining the changes in health status for the patient. The spiraling cost of health care has generated many questions about the quality and effectiveness of health care services and the patient's outcomes related to these services; these questions are often best addressed by conducting outcomes research.

In conclusion, this textbook was developed to encourage you to be a consumer of research. You are provided content to assist you in reading research reports, critiquing the reports, and summarizing the findings for use in practice. We hope that you will come to value research and to recognize the impact it can have on your practice, the nursing profession, and the health care system.

REFERENCES

American Nurses Association (ANA). (1989). *Education for participation in nursing research.* Kansas City, MO: American Nurses Association.

Barnard, K. E. (1980). Knowledge for practice: Directions for the future. *Nursing Research, 29*(4), 208–212.

Bauknecht, V. L. (1985). Capital commentary: NIH bill passes, includes nursing research center. *American Nurse, 17*(10), 2.

Benner, P. (1984). *From novice to expert: Excellence and power in clinical nursing practice.* Menlo Park, CA: Addison-Wesley.

Beyea, S. C., & Nicoll, L. H. (1995). Administration of medications via the intramuscular route: An integrative review of the literature and research-based protocol for the procedure. *Applied Nursing Research, 8*(1), 23–33.

Burns, N., & Grove, S. K. (1997). *The practice of nursing research: Conduct, critique, and utilization* (3rd ed.). Philadelphia: Saunders.

Chinn, P. L., & Kramer, M. K. (1995). *Theory and nursing: A systematic approach* (4th ed.). St. Louis: Mosby.

Cook, E. (1913). *The life of Florence Nightingale* (Vol. 1). London: Macmillan.

Gardner, D. L. (1992). Conflict and retention of new graduate nurses. *Western Journal of Nursing Research, 14*(1), 76–85.

Gates, M. F., & Lackey, N. R. (1998). Youngsters caring for adults with cancer. *Image: Journal of Nursing Scholarship, 30*(1), 11–15.

Glaser, B. G., & Strauss, A. L. (1967). *The discovery of grounded theory: Strategies for qualitative research.* Chicago: Aldine.

Goode, C. J., Titler, M., Rakel, B., Ones, D. S., Kleiber, C., Small, S., & Triolo, P. K. (1991). A meta-analysis of effects of heparin flush and saline flush: Quality and cost implications. *Nursing Research, 40*(6), 324–330.

Gortner, S. R., & Nahm, H. (1977). An overview of nursing

research in the United States. *Nursing Research, 26*(1), 10–33.

Hansell, P. S., Hughes, C. B., Caliandro, G., Russo, P., Budin, W. C., Hartman, B., & Hernandez, O. C. (1998). The effect of a social support boosting intervention on stress, coping, and social support in caregivers of children with HIV/AIDS. *Nursing Research, 47*(2), 79–86.

Hastings-Tolsma, M. T., Yucha, C. B., Tompkins, J., Robson, L., & Szeverenyi, N. (1993). Effect of warm and cold applications on the resolution of IV infiltrations. *Research in Nursing & Health, 16*(3), 171–178.

Herbert, R. G. (1981). *Florence Nightingale: Saint, reformer or rebel?* Malabar, FL: Robert E. Krieger.

Horsley, J. A., Crane, J., Crabtree, M. K., & Wood, D. J. (1983). *Using research to improve nursing practice: A guide, CURN Project.* New York: Grune & Stratton.

Jones, K. R. (1993). Outcomes analysis: Methods and issues. *Nursing Economics, 11*(3), 145–152.

Kaplan, A. (1964). *The conduct of inquiry.* New York: Harper & Row.

Kemp, M. G., Kopanke, D., Tordecilla, L., Fogg, L., Shott, S., Matthiesen, V., & Johnson, B. (1993). The role of support surfaces and patient attributes in preventing pressure ulcers in elderly patients. *Research in Nursing & Health, 16*(2), 89–96.

McMurrey, P. H. (1982). Toward a unique knowledge base in nursing. *Image, 14*(1), 12–15.

Meek, S. S. (1993). Effects of slow stroke back massage on relaxation in hospice clients. *Image: Journal of Nursing Scholarship, 25*(1), 17–21.

Munhall, P. L. (1989). Philosophical ponderings on qualitative research methods in nursing. *Nursing Science Quarterly, 2*(1), 20–28.

Munhall, P. L., & Oiler, C. J. (1993). *Nursing research: A qualitative perspective* (2nd ed.). Norwalk, CT: Appleton-Century-Crofts.

National Institute of Nursing Research (NINR) (September, 23, 1993). *National nursing research agenda: Setting nursing research priorities.* Bethesda, MD: National Institutes of Health.

Nightingale, F. (1859). *Notes on Nursing: What it is, and what it is not.* Philadelphia: Lippincott.

Omery, A., Kasper, C. E., & Page, G. G. (1995). *In search of nursing science.* Thousand Oaks, CA: Sage.

Palmer, I. S. (1977). Florence Nightingale: Reformer, reactionary, researcher. *Nursing Research, 26*(2), 84–89.

Rempusheski, V. F. (1992). A researcher as resource, mentor, and preceptor. *Applied Nursing Research, 5*(2), 105–107.

Rettig, R. (1991). History, development, and importance to nursing of outcomes research. *Journal of Nursing Quality Assurance, 5*(2), 13–17.

Rew, L., & Barrow, E. M. (1987). Intuition: A neglected hallmark of nursing knowledge. *Advances in Nursing Science, 10*(1), 49–62.

See, E. M. (1977). The ANA and research in nursing. *Nursing Research, 26*(3), 165–171.

Shively, M., Riegel, B., Waterhouse, D., Burns, D., Templin, K., & Thomason, T. (1997). Testing a community level research utilization intervention. *Applied Nursing Research, 10*(3), 121–127.

Shoaf, J., & Oliver, S. (1992). Efficacy of normal saline injection with and without heparin for maintaining intermittent intravenous site. *Applied Nursing Research, 5*(1), 9–12.

Topp, R., & Stevenson, J. S. (1994). The effects of attendance and effort on outcomes among older adults in a long-term exercise program. *Research in Nursing & Health, 17*(1), 15–24.

Vyhlidal, S. K., Moxness, D., Bosak, K. S., Van Meter, F. G., & Bergstrom, N. (1997). Mattress replacement or foam overlay? A prospective study on the incidence of pressure ulcers. *Applied Nursing Research, 10*(3), 111–120.

Werley, H. H., & Fitzpatrick, J. J. (1983). *Annual review of nursing research* (Vol. 1). New York: Springer.

Winslow, E. H., Lane, L. D., & Gaffney, F. A. (1985). Oxygen uptake and cardiovascular responses in control adults and acute myocardial infarction patients during bathing. *Nursing Research, 34*(3), 164–169.

CHAPTER 2

Introduction to the Quantitative Research Process

OBJECTIVES

Completing this chapter should enable you to:

1. *Define quantitative research and discuss its importance in generating knowledge for nursing practice.*
2. *Define terms relevant to the quantitative research process: basic research, applied research, rigor, and control.*
3. *Compare and contrast the use of control in quantitative research.*
4. *Discuss the natural, partially controlled, and highly controlled settings in which quantitative research is conducted.*
5. *Compare and contrast the problem-solving process, nursing process, and research process.*
6. *Describe the steps of the quantitative research process.*
7. *Explain the purposes of a pilot study.*
8. *Identify sources that publish nursing research reports.*
9. *Read research reports.*
10. *Identify the steps of the quantitative research process in a research article.*
11. *Conduct an initial critique of a research report.*
12. *Examine the different types of quantitative research reports: descriptive, correlational, quasi-experimental, and experimental.*

RELEVANT TERMS

Abstract
Applied (practical) research
Assumptions
Basic (pure) research
Control
Correlational research
Data analysis
Data collection
Descriptive research
Design
Experimental research
Framework
Generalization
Interpretation of research outcomes
Limitations
    Methodological limitations
    Theoretical limitations
Literature review
Measurement
Nursing process
Pilot study
Population
Problem-solving process
Process

Quantitative research
Quantitative research process
Quasi-experimental research
Reading research reports
    Analyzing research reports
    Comprehending research reports
    Skimming research reports
Research outcomes
Research problem
Research process
Research purpose
Research report
Rigor
Sample
Sampling
Setting
    Highly controlled setting
    Natural (field) setting
    Partially controlled setting
Theory
Variables
    Conceptual definition
    Operational definition

*W*hat do you think of when you hear the word *research*? Frequently, the word *experiment* comes to mind. One might equate experiments with randomizing subjects into groups, collecting data, and conducting statistical analyses. Frequently, one thinks that an experiment is conducted to "prove" something, such as proving that a drug is an effective treatment for an illness. These ideas are associated with quantitative research. Quantitative research includes specific steps that are detailed in research reports. Reading and critiquing quantitative studies requires learning new terms, understanding the steps of quantitative research, and applying a variety of analytical skills.

This chapter provides you with an introduction to quantitative research and a background for reading a research report. Relevant terms are defined, and the problem-solving and nursing processes are presented to provide a basis for understanding the quantitative research process. The steps of the quantitative research process are introduced, and a descriptive correlational study is presented as an example to promote understanding of the process. The chapter concludes with a discussion of the analytical skills needed for reading research reports and guidelines for conducting an initial critique of these reports. The appendix to this chapter identifies the steps of the research process from a published quasi-experimental study and an experimental study.

What Is Quantitative Research?

Quantitative research is a formal, objective, rigorous, systematic process for generating information about the world. Quantitative research is conducted to describe new situations, events, or concepts in the world, such as describing new illnesses like AIDS or HIV; to examine relationships among concepts or ideas, such as the relationship between wine consumption and cholesterol level; and to determine the effectiveness of treatments on the health of patients and families. The classic experimental designs to test the effectiveness of treatments were originated by Sir Ronald Fisher (1935). He is noted for adding structure to the steps of the research process with such ideas as the hypothesis, research design, and statistical analysis. Fisher's studies provided the groundwork for what is now known as experimental research.

Throughout the years, a number of other quantitative approaches have been developed. Campbell and Stanley (1963) developed quasi-experimental approaches to study the effects of treatments under less controlled conditions. Karl Pearson developed statistical approaches for examining relationships between variables, which increased the conduct of correlational research. The fields of sociology, education, and psychology are noted for their development and expansion of strategies for conducting descriptive research. A broad range of quantitative research approaches is needed to develop knowledge for nursing practice. This section introduces you to the different types of quantitative research and provides definitions of terms relevant to the quantitative research process.

Types of Quantitative Research

Four types of quantitative research are included in this book: (1) descriptive, (2) correlational, (3) quasi-experimental, and (4) experimental. The type of research conducted is influenced by the current knowledge of a research problem. When little knowledge is available, descriptive studies often are conducted. As the knowledge level increases, correlational, quasi-experimental, and experimental studies are conducted.

Descriptive Research

Descriptive research is the exploration and description of phenomena in real-life situations; it provides an accurate account of characteristics of particular individuals, situations, or groups (Kerlinger, 1986). Through descriptive studies, researchers discover new meaning, describe what exists, determine the frequency with which something occurs, and categorize information. The outcomes of descriptive research include the description of concepts, identification of relationships, and development of hypotheses that provide a basis for future quantitative research.

Correlational Research

Correlational research involves the systematic investigation of relationships between or among two or more variables. To do this, the researcher measures the selected variables in a sample and then uses correlational statistics to determine the relationships among the variables. Using correlational analysis, the researcher is able to determine the degree or strength and type (positive or negative) of a relationship. The strength of a relationship varies from -1 (perfect negative correlation) to $+1$ (perfect positive correlation), with 0 indicating no relationship. The positive relationship indicates that the variables vary together, that is, both variables either increase or decrease together. For example, research has shown that the more people smoke, the more lung damage they experience. The negative relationship indicates that the variables vary in opposite directions; thus, as one variable increases, the other will decrease. For example, research has indicated that increased years of smoking is related to a decreased life span. The primary intent of correlational studies is to explain the nature of relationships in the real world, not to determine cause and effect. However, correlational studies are the means for generating hypotheses to guide quasi-experimental and experimental studies that do focus on examining cause-and-effect relationships.

Quasi-experimental Research

The purpose of *quasi-experimental research* is to examine causal relationships or to determine the effect of one variable on another. Quasi-experimental studies involve implementing a treatment and examining the effects of this treatment using selected methods of measurement. Quasi-experimental studies differ from experimental studies by the level of control achieved by the researcher. Quasi-experimental studies usually lack a certain amount of control over the manipulation of the treatment, management of the setting, or selection of the subjects. When studying human behavior, especially in clinical settings, researchers are frequently unable to manipulate or control certain variables or the setting. Thus, nurse researchers conduct more quasi-experimental studies than experimental studies.

Experimental Research

Experimental research is an objective, systematic, controlled investigation for the purpose of predicting and controlling phenomena in nursing practice. In an experimental study, causality between the independent and dependent variables is examined under highly controlled conditions (Kerlinger, 1986). Experimental research is considered the most powerful quantitative method because of the rigorous control of variables. The three main characteristics of experimental studies are (1) controlled manipulation of at least one treatment variable (independent variable), (2) exposure of some of the subjects to the treatment (experimental group) and some of them not (control group), and (3) random selection of subjects for the study. The degree of control achieved in experimental studies varies based on the variables being examined.

Defining Terms Relevant to Quantitative Research

Understanding quantitative research requires an introduction to the terms *basic research, applied research, rigor,* and *control.* In this section, these terms are defined and examples are provided from quantitative studies.

Basic Research

Basic research (or *pure research*) is a scientific investigation that involves the pursuit of "knowledge for knowledge's sake" or for the pleasure of learning and finding truth (Miller, 1991). Basic scientific investigation seeks new knowledge about health phenomena with the hope of establishing general principles. The purpose of basic research is to generate and refine theory; thus, the findings are frequently not directly useful in practice (Wysocki, 1983). Basic nursing research on physiological variables might include laboratory investigations of animals or humans to develop principles about physiological functioning, pathology, or the effects of treatments on physiological and pathological functioning. These studies might focus on increasing our understanding of oxygenation, perfusion, fluid and electrolyte balance, acid-base status, eating and sleeping patterns, and comfort status, as well as pathophysiology of the immune system (Bond & Heitkemper, 1987).

The study by McCarthy, Lo, Nguyen, and Ney (1997) is an example of basic research. This laboratory study was conducted to determine if increasing the protein density of food would positively influence total protein and food intake of tumor-bearing rats. The findings indicated that increasing the protein density of the food consumed resulted in an increase in net protein intake but also in a decrease in food intake of both the healthy and tumor-bearing animals. Thus, the increased protein intake did not affect the nutritional status of the tumor-bearing rats, as indicated by their body weight and serum level of total protein, insulin, or insulin-like growth factor-1. Basic research usually precedes or is the basis for applied research. There is little research to support the hypothesis that increased nutritional intake affects the morbidity and mortality of cancer patients. McCarthy et al.'s (1997) basic study provides a basis for studying the effects of nutritional interventions on appetite and food intake of cancer patients.

Applied Research

Applied research (or *practical research*) is a scientific investigation conducted to generate knowledge that will directly influence or improve clinical practice (Abdellah & Levine, 1979). The purpose of applied research is to solve problems, make decisions, or predict or control outcomes in real-life practice situations. The findings from applied studies can also be invaluable to policymakers as a basis for making changes to address social problems (Miller, 1991). Many of the studies conducted in nursing are applied because researchers have chosen to focus on clinical problems, such as testing the effectiveness of nursing interventions. Applied research is also used to test theory and validate its usefulness in clinical practice. Often the new knowledge discovered through basic research is examined for usefulness in practice by applied research, making these approaches complementary (Wysocki, 1983).

Neuberger et al. (1997) conducted an applied study to determine the effects of exercise on fatigue, aerobic fitness, and disease activity in persons with rheumatoid arthritis (RA). The subjects participated in a 12-week program of low-impact aerobic exercise (treatment or independent variable), and the dependent or outcome variables of fatigue, aerobic fitness, and disease activity level were measured three times during the study. Study findings indicated that the fatigue level decreased for moderate- to high-frequency exercisers and increased for low-frequency exercisers. All subjects participating in the exercise program experienced increased aerobic fitness and increased grip strength, decreased walk time, and decreased pain. These improvements in fatigue level and aerobic fitness occurred without significant changes in the subjects' RA disease, as measured by joint count and sedimentation rate.

Neuberger et al.'s (1997) study addressed the problem in clinical practice of maintaining the mobility, strength, and independence of individuals with RA. The findings from this study can be applied directly to practice. Nurses can use this research information to develop low-impact aerobic exercise programs for persons with RA to decrease their fatigue and increase their aerobic fitness without worsening their arthritis.

Rigor in Quantitative Research

Rigor is the striving for excellence in research and involves discipline, adherence to detail, and strict accuracy. A rigorously conducted quantitative study has precise measurement tools, a representative sample, and a tightly controlled study design. To critique the rigor of a study, one must examine the reasoning and precision used in conducting the study. Logical reasoning, including deductive and inductive reasoning, is essential to the development of quantitative studies. The research process includes specific steps that are developed with meticulous detail and are logically linked. These steps, such as design, measurement, sample, data collection, and statistical analysis, need to be examined for errors and weaknesses.

Another aspect of rigor is precision, which encompasses accuracy, detail, and order. Precision is evident in the concise statement of the research purpose and detailed development of the study design. But the most explicit example of precision is the measurement or quantification of the study variables. For example, a researcher might use a cardiac monitor to measure the heart rate of subjects during an exercise program rather than palpating a radial pulse.

Control in Quantitative Research

Control involves the imposing of rules by the researcher to decrease the possibility of error and thus increase the probability that the study's findings are an accurate reflection of reality. The rules used to achieve control in research are referred to as *design*. Through control, the researcher can reduce the influence of extraneous variables. Extraneous variables exist in all studies and can interfere with obtaining a clear understanding of the relationships among the study variables. For example, if a study focused on the effect of relaxation therapy on perception of incisional pain, the extraneous variables, such as type of surgical incision and time, amount, and type of pain medication administered following surgery, would have to be controlled to prevent their influence on the patient's perception of pain. Some of these extraneous variables might be controlled by selecting only patients with abdominal incisions, who receive only one type of pain medication following surgery. Controlling extraneous variables enables the researcher to identify relationships among the study variables accurately and to examine the effect of one variable on another.

Quantitative research is performed using varying degrees of control, ranging from uncontrolled to highly controlled, depending on the type of study (Table 2-1). Descriptive studies are usually conducted without researcher control because subjects are examined as they exist in their natural setting, such as home, work, or school. Experimental studies are highly controlled and often are conducted on animals in laboratory settings to determine the effectiveness

TABLE 2-1. Control in Quantitative Research

Type of Quantitative Research	Researcher Control	Sampling	Research Setting
Descriptive	Uncontrolled	Nonrandom/ random	Natural setting/partially controlled
Correlational	Uncontrolled/ partially controlled	Nonrandom/ random	Natural setting/partially controlled
Quasi-experimental	Partially controlled/ highly controlled	Nonrandom/ random	Partially controlled
Experimental	Highly controlled	Random	Highly controlled/ laboratory

of a treatment. Researchers use varying levels of control in the selection of subjects (sampling) and identification of research settings (Cook & Campbell, 1979; Miller, 1991).

Sampling. *Sampling* is a process of selecting subjects who are representative of the population being studied. Random sampling usually provides a sample that is representative of a population because each member of the population is selected independently and has an equal chance or probability of being included in the study. In quantitative research, both random and nonrandom samples are used (see Table 2-1). Descriptive studies are often conducted with nonrandom or nonprobability samples, in which the subjects are selected based on convenience. Correlation and quasi-experimental studies may include either nonrandom or random sampling methods, but highly controlled experimental studies have a randomly selected sample. A randomly selected sample is very difficult to obtain in nursing research, so quantitative studies are often conducted with convenience samples. To increase the control and rigor of a study and to decrease the potential for bias, the subjects who are part of a convenience sample are randomly assigned to a treatment or control group.

Research Settings. The *setting* is the location where a study is conducted. There are three common settings for conducting research: natural, partially controlled, and highly controlled (see Table 2-1). A *natural setting,* or *field setting,* is an uncontrolled, real-life situation or environment (Miller, 1991). Conducting a study in a natural setting means that the researcher does not manipulate or change the environment for the study. Descriptive and correlational studies are often conducted in natural settings. For example, Flynn (1997) conducted a correlational study to examine the relationships of learned helplessness, self-esteem, and depression with the health practices of homeless women in a natural setting. The study setting was "six homeless shelters located in urban and suburban areas of New Jersey and Washington, D.C." (p. 73). Those women in the shelter at the time of data collection were provided packets of information to complete and return to the investigator. No attempts were made during the study to manipulate, change, or control the environment of the shelters. Thus, the researcher's intent was to study these homeless women in a natural, real-life environment of a shelter.

A *partially controlled setting* is an environment that is manipulated or modified in some way by the researcher. An increasing number of nursing studies are being conducted in partially controlled settings. Neuberger et al. (1997) conducted a quasi-experimental study to examine the effects of exercise on fatigue, aerobic fitness, and the disease process of persons with RA in a partially controlled setting. The study involved implementing an exercise regimen that was "designed by two physical therapists, an aerobic instructor hired to teach the class, and the principle investigator. The class consisted of four phases: warm-up exercises, strengthening exercises, low-impact aerobic exercises, and cool-down exercises. . . . The exercise class was held in a room in the exercise facility on the medical center campus" (p. 199). The researchers controlled the development of the exercise class treatment and the implementation of the treatment by a specific instructor in a selected room of an exercise facility. However, the researcher did not control other aspects of the environment, such as the interactions of the subjects during the class, the physical activities of the subjects outside of the class, the family support for the exercise program, and the subjects' interactions with other health professionals during the program. The personal characteristics of the subjects, such as their motivation level and physical fitness status, were not controlled. These factors could have influenced the fatigue, aerobic fitness, and disease status of the subjects during the study.

A *highly controlled setting* is an artificially constructed environment developed for the sole purpose of conducting research. Laboratories, research or experimental centers, and test units in hospitals or other health care agencies are highly controlled settings where experimental studies are often conducted. This type of setting reduces the influence of extraneous variables, which enables the researcher to examine accurately the effect of one variable on another. McCarthy et al. (1997) conducted their study on the effect of protein density of food on food intake and nutritional status of tumor-bearing rats in a laboratory setting. The environment of the rats was highly controlled by the researcher, with each rat being "housed individually and maintained on a 12-hr light-dark cycle commencing at 6:00 a.m. Food and water were freely available. The animals were conditioned to the housing for 5 days before the start of the experiment and were treated at all times in a manner consistent with Department of Health, Education, and Welfare *Guidelines for the Care and Use of Laboratory Animals*. . . . The animals were matched according to weight and a total of 30 were randomly selected for tumor implant, leaving 30 healthy animals as controls" (pp. 132–133). The study clearly indicates the use of a highly controlled setting, random selection of subjects for the treatment and control groups, and the controlled implementation of study procedures that are essential in the conduct of experimental research.

Problem Solving and Nursing Processes: Basis for Understanding the Quantitative Research Process

Research is a process and is similar in some ways to other processes. Therefore, the background you acquired early in your nursing education in problem solving and the nursing process is also useful in research. A *process* includes a purpose, a series of actions, and a goal. The purpose provides direction for the implementation of a series of actions to achieve an identified goal. The specific steps of the process can be revised and reimplemented in order to reach the endpoint or goal. The problem-solving process, nursing process, and research process are presented in Table 2-2. Relating the research process to problem solving and the nursing process may be helpful to you in understanding the steps of the quantitative research process.

Comparing Problem Solving with the Nursing Process

The *problem-solving process* involves the systematic identification of a problem, determination of goals related to the problem, identification of possible ap-

TABLE 2-2. Comparison of the Problem-solving Process, Nursing Process, and Research Process

Problem-solving Process	Nursing Process	Research Process
Data Collection	Assessment Data Collection Data interpretation	Knowledge of the world of nursing Clinical experiences Literature review
Problem definition	Nursing diagnosis	Problem and purpose identification
Plan Setting goals Identifying solutions	Plan Setting goals Planned interventions	Methodology plan Design Sample Methods of measurement Data collection Data analysis
Implementation	Implementation	Implementation
Evaluating and revising process	Evaluation and modification	Outcomes, communication of findings, and use of findings in practice

proaches to achieve those goals (planning), implementation of selected approaches, and evaluation of goal achievement. Problem solving is frequently used in daily activities and in nursing practice. For example, you use problem solving when you select your clothing, decide where to live, and turn a patient with a fractured hip.

The *nursing process* is a subset of the problem-solving process. The steps of the nursing process are assessment, diagnosis, plan, implementation, evaluation, and modification (see Table 2-2). Assessment involves the collection and interpretation of data for the development of nursing diagnoses. These diagnoses guide the remaining steps of the nursing process, just as the step of identifying the problem directs the remaining steps of the problem-solving process. The planning step in the nursing process is the same as in the problem-solving process. Both processes involve implementation (putting the plan into action) and evaluation (determining the effectiveness of the process). If the process is ineffective, all steps are reviewed and revised (modified) as necessary. The process is implemented until the problems/diagnoses are resolved and the identified goals are achieved.

Comparing the Nursing Process with the Research Process

The nursing process and the research process have important similarities and differences. The two processes are similar because they both involve abstract, critical thinking and complex reasoning (Miller & Babcock, 1996). Using these processes, you are able to identify new information, discover relationships, and make predictions about phenomena. In both processes information is gathered, observations are made, problems are identified, plans are developed (methodology), and actions are taken (data collection and analysis) (Whitney, 1986). Both processes are reviewed for effectiveness and efficiency; the nursing process is evaluated, and outcomes are determined in the research process (see Table 2-2). Implementing the two processes expands and refines the user's knowledge. With this growth in knowledge and critical thinking, the user is able to implement increasingly complex nursing processes and studies.

The research and nursing processes also have definite differences. Knowledge of the nursing process will not enable you to conduct the research process. The *research process* is more complex than the nursing process, requires an understanding of a unique language, and involves the rigorous application of a variety of research methods (Burns, 1989). The research process also has a broader focus than the nursing process, in which the nurse focuses on a specific patient and family. In the research process, the researcher focuses on groups of patients and their families. In addition, researchers must be knowledgeable about the world of nursing in order to identify problems that require study. This knowledge is obtained from clinical and other personal experiences and by conducting a review of the literature.

The theoretical underpinnings of the research process are much stronger than those of the nursing process. All steps of the research process are logically linked and are also linked to the theoretical foundations of the study (Burns & Grove, 1997). The conduct of research requires greater precision, rigor, and control than the implementation of the nursing process. The outcomes from research are frequently shared with a large number of nurses and other health professionals through presentations and publications. In addition, the outcomes from several studies can be synthesized and used by nurses to create a lasting impact on nursing practice.

Identifying the Steps of the Quantitative Research Process

The *quantitative research process* involves conceptualizing a research project, planning and implementing that project, and communicating the findings. Figure 2-1 identifies the steps of the quantitative research process that are usually included in a research report. This figure indicates the logical flow of the process as one step builds progressively on another. The steps of the quantitative research process are briefly introduced in this chapter and are presented in

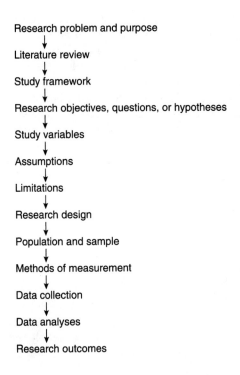

FIGURE 2-1
Steps of the quantitative research process.

detail in Chapters 3 through 10. The descriptive correlational study conducted by Hulme and Grove (1994) on the symptoms of female survivors of child sexual abuse is used as an example to introduce the steps of the quantitative research process.

Research Problem and Purpose

A *research problem* is a situation in need of a solution, alteration, or improvement or a discrepancy between the way things are and the way they ought to be (Adebo, 1974; Diers, 1979). The problem statement in a study usually identifies an area of concern for a particular population that requires investigation. The *research purpose* is generated from the problem and identifies the specific goal or aim of the study. The goal of a study might be to identify, describe, or explain a situation; predict a solution to a situation; or control a situation to produce positive outcomes in practice. The purpose includes the variables, population, and setting for the study. A detailed discussion of the research problem and purpose is presented in Chapter 3. Hulme and Grove (1994) identified the following problem and purpose for their study of female survivors of child sexual abuse.

Research Problem

"The actual prevalence of child sexual abuse is unknown but is thought to be high. Bagley and King (1990) were able to generalize from compiled research that at least 20% of all women in the samples surveyed had been victims of serious sexual abuse involving unwanted or coerced sexual contact up to the age of 17 years. Evidence indicates that the prevalence is greater for women born after 1960 than before (Bagley, 1990).

The impact of child sexual abuse on the lives of the girl victims and the women they become has only lately received the attention it deserves . . . the knowledge generated from research and theory has slowly forced the recognition of the long-term effects of child sexual abuse on both the survivors and society as a whole. . . . Recently, Brown and Garrison (1990) developed the Adult Survivors of Incest (ASI) Questionnaire to identify the patterns of symptoms and the factors contributing to the severity of these symptoms in survivors of childhood sexual abuse. This tool requires additional testing to determine its usefulness in identifying symptoms and contributing factors of adult survivors of incest and other types of child sexual abuse." (pp. 519–520)

continued

Research Purpose

"Thus, the purpose of this study was twofold: (a) to describe the patterns of physical and psychosocial symptoms in female sexual abuse survivors using the ASI Questionnaire, and (b) to examine relationships among the symptoms and identify contributing factors." (p. 520).

Literature Review

Researchers conduct a *literature review* to generate a picture of what is known and not known about a particular problem. Relevant literature or only those sources that are pertinent or highly important in providing the in-depth knowledge needed to study a selected problem is reviewed. The literature review indicates whether adequate knowledge exists to make changes in practice or whether additional research is needed. The process for reviewing the literature is described in Chapter 4. Hulme and Grove's (1994) review of the literature covered relevant theories and studies related to child sexual abuse and its contributing factors and long-term effects.

"Theorists indicated that . . . the act of child sexual abuse can be explained as an abuse of power by a trusted parent figure, usually male, on a dependent child, violating the child's body, mind, and spirit. The family, which normally functions to nurture and protect the child from harm, is viewed as not fulfilling this function, leaving the child to feel further betrayed and powerless. Acceptance of the immediate psychological trauma of child sexual abuse has given impetus for acknowledging the long-term effects.

Studies of both nonclinical and clinical populations have lent support to these theoretical developments. When compared with control groups consisting of women who had not been sexually abused as children, survivors of child sexual abuse consistently have higher incidence of depression and lower self-esteem. Other psychosocial long-term effects encountered include suicidal plans, anxiety, distorted body image, decreased sexual satisfaction, poor general social adjustment, lower positive affect, negative personality characteristics, and feeling different from significant others. . . . The physical long-term effects suggested by research include gastrointestinal problems such as ulcers, spastic colitis, irritable bowel syndrome, and chronic abdominal pain; gynecological disorders; chronic headache; obesity; and increased lifetime surgeries.

Studies of contributing factors that may affect the traumatic impact of child sexual abuse are less in number and less conclusive than those that identify long-term effects. However, poor family functioning, increased age difference between the victim and perpetrator, threat or use of force or violence, multiple abusers, parent or primary caretaker as perpetrator, prolonged or intrusive abuse, and strong emotional bond to the perpetrator with betrayal of trust may all contribute to the increased severity of the long-term effects." (pp. 521–522)

Study Framework

A *framework* is the abstract, theoretical basis for a study that enables the researcher to link the findings to nursing's body of knowledge. In quantitative research, the framework is a testable theory that has been developed in nursing or in another discipline, such as psychology, physiology, or sociology. A *theory* consists of an integrated set of defined concepts and relational statements that present a view of a phenomenon and can be used to describe, explain, predict, or control the phenomenon. The relational statements of the theory, not the theory itself, are tested through research. A study framework can be expressed as a map or a diagram of the relationships that provide the basis for a study or can be presented in narrative format. Chapter 5 provides a background for understanding and critiquing study frameworks. The framework for Hulme and Grove's (1994) study is based on Browne and Finkelhor's (1986) theory of Traumagenic Dynamics in the Impact of Child Sexual Abuse and is expressed in a map.

". . . As shown in Figure 2-2, child sexual abuse is at the center of the adult survivor's existence. Arising from the abuse are four trauma-causing dynamics: traumatic sexualization, betrayal, powerlessness, and stigmatization. These traumagenic dynamics lead to behavioral manifestations and collectively indicate a history of child sexual abuse. The behavioral manifestations were operationalized as physical and psychosocial symptoms for the purposes of this study. Penetrating the core of the adult survivors are the contributing factors, including the characteristics of the child sexual abuse and other factors occurring later in the survivor's life, that affect the severity of behavioral manifestations (Follette, Alexander, & Follette, 1991). The contributing factors examined in this study were age when the abuse began, duration of the abuse, and other victimizations. Other victimizations included past or present physical and emotional abuse, rape, control by others, and prostitution." (pp. 522–523)

continued

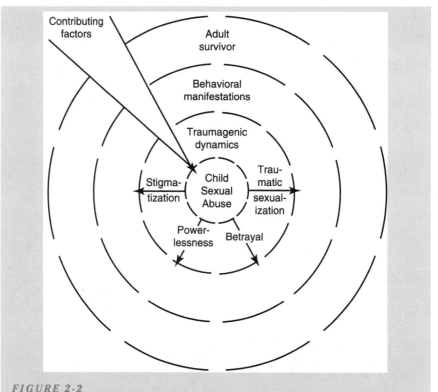

FIGURE 2-2

Long-term effects of child sexual abuse. (From Symptoms of female survivors of sexual abuse. *Issues in Mental Health Nursing, 15*[5], 123. Hulme, P. A., and Grove, S. K. [1994]. Taylor & Francis, Inc., Washington, DC. Reproduced with permission. All rights reserved.)

Research Objectives, Questions, and Hypotheses

Research objectives, questions, or hypotheses are formulated to bridge the gap between the more abstractly stated research problem and purpose and the study design and plan for data collection and analysis. Objectives, questions, and hypotheses are more narrow in focus than the purpose and often specify only one or two research variables, identify the relationship between the variables, and indicate the population to be studied. Some descriptive studies include only a research purpose, while others include a purpose and either objectives or questions to direct the study. Some correlational studies include a purpose and specific questions or hypotheses. Quasi-experimental and experimental studies need to include hypotheses to direct the conduct of the studies and the interpretation of findings. Chapter 3 provides guidelines for critiquing objectives, questions, and hypotheses in research reports. Hulme and Grove (1994) developed the following research questions to direct their study.

1. "What patterns of physical and psychosocial symptoms are present in women 18 to 40 years of age who have experienced child sexual abuse?
2. Are there relationships among the number of physical and psychosocial symptoms, the age when the abuse began, the duration of abuse, and [the] number of other victimizations?" (p. 523).

Study Variables

The research purpose and the objectives, questions, or hypotheses identify the variables to be examined in a study. *Research variables* are concepts at various levels of abstraction that are measured, manipulated, or controlled in a study. The more concrete concepts like temperature, weight, or blood pressure are referred to as *variables* in a study. The more abstract concepts like creativity, empathy, or social support are sometimes referred to as research *concepts*.

The variables or concepts in a study are operationalized by identifying conceptual and operational definitions. A *conceptual definition* provides a variable or concept with theoretical meaning (Fawcett & Downs, 1992) and is derived from a theorist's definition of the concept or is developed through concept analysis. An *operational definition* is developed so that the variable can be measured or manipulated in a study. The knowledge gained from studying the variable will increase understanding of the theoretical concept that the variable represents. A more extensive discussion of variables is provided in Chapter 3. Hulme and Grove (1994) provided conceptual and operational definitions of the study variables, physical and psychosocial symptoms, age when the abuse began, duration of abuse, and victimizations, identified in their purpose and research questions. Only the definitions for physical symptoms and victimizations are presented as examples.

Conceptual Definition. "behavioral manifestations that result directly from the traumagenic dynamics of child sexual abuse." (p. 522)

Operational Definition. ASI Questionnaire was used to measure physical symptoms.

Conceptual Definition. Adult survivor who has experienced multiple forms of abuse, including "past and present physical and emotional abuse, rape, control by others, and prostitution." (p. 523)

continued

Operational Definition. ASI Questionnaire was used to measure victimizations.

Assumptions

Assumptions are statements that are taken for granted or are considered true, even though they have not been scientifically tested. Assumptions are often embedded (unrecognized) in thinking and behavior, and uncovering these assumptions requires introspection. Sources of assumptions are universally accepted truths ("all humans are rational beings"), theories, previous research, and nursing practice (Myers, 1982).

In studies, assumptions are embedded in the philosophical base of the framework, study design, and interpretation of findings. Theories and research instruments are developed based on assumptions that may or may not be recognized by the researcher. These assumptions influence the development and implementation of the research process. The recognition of assumptions by the researcher is a strength, not a weakness. Assumptions influence the logic of the study, and their recognition leads to more rigorous study development. Williams (1980) reviewed published nursing studies and other health care literature to identify 13 commonly embedded assumptions:

1. "People want to assume control of their own health problems.
2. Stress should be avoided.
3. People are aware of the experiences that most affect their life choices.
4. Health is a priority for most people.
5. People in underserved areas feel underserved.
6. Most measurable attitudes are held strongly enough to direct behavior.
7. Health professionals view health care in a different manner than do lay persons.
8. Human biological and chemical factors show less variation than do cultural and social factors.
9. The nursing process is the best way of conceptualizing nursing practice.
10. Statistically significant differences relate to the variable or variables under consideration.
11. People operate on the basis of cognitive information.
12. Increased knowledge about an event lowers anxiety about the event.
13. Receipt of health care at home is preferable to receipt of care in an institution." (p. 48)

Hulme and Grove (1994) did not identify assumptions for their study, but the following assumptions seem to provide a basis for this study: (1) the child victim bears no responsibility for the sexual contact, (2) survivors remember and are willing to report their past child sexual abuse, and (3) behavioral manifestations (physical and psychological symptoms) indicate altered health and functioning.

Limitations

Limitations are restrictions in a study that may decrease the credibility and generalizability of the findings. *Generalization* is the extension of the implications of the research findings from the sample to a larger population. For example, the findings from studying adult female survivors of child sexual abuse might be extended to all females who have been abused. The two types of limitations are theoretical and methodological. *Theoretical limitations* restrict the abstract generalization of the findings and are reflected in the study framework and the conceptual and operational definitions of the variables. Theoretical limitations might include (1) a concept that lacks clarity of definition in the theory used to develop the study framework; (2) the unclear relationships among some concepts in the theorist's work; (3) a study variable lacking a clear link to a concept in the framework; or (4) an objective, question, or hypothesis lacking a clear link to the study framework.

Methodological limitations can limit the credibility of the findings and restrict the population to which the findings can be generalized. Methodological limitations result from such factors as unrepresentative sample, weak designs, single setting, limited control over treatment implementation, instruments with limited reliability and validity, limited control over data collection, and improper use of statistical analyses. Hulme and Grove (1994) identified the following methodological limitation.

Methodological Limitation

". . . [T]his study has limited generalizability due to the relatively small nonprobability sample . . ." (p. 528)

"Additional replications drawing from various social classes and age groups are needed to improve the generalizability of Brown and Garrison's (1990) findings and establish reliability and validity of their tool." (p. 529)

Research Design

Research *design* is a blueprint for the conduct of a study that maximizes control over factors that could interfere with the study's desired outcome. The type of design directs the selection of a population, sampling procedure, methods of

measurement, and a plan for data collection and analysis. The choice of research design depends on the researcher's expertise, the problem and purpose
of the study, and the desire to generalize the findings. Sometimes the design
of a study indicates that a pilot study was conducted. A *pilot study* is frequently
defined as a smaller version of a proposed study conducted to refine the methodology. It is often developed similarly to the proposed study, using similar
subjects, the same setting, the same treatment, and the same data collection
and analysis techniques. Prescott and Soeken (1989), however, believe a pilot
study can be conducted to develop and refine any of the steps in the research
process. The reasons for conducting pilot studies are to:

1. determine whether the proposed study is feasible (e.g., are the subjects
   available, does the researcher have the time and money to do the
   study?);
2. develop or refine a research treatment;
3. develop a protocol for the implementation of a treatment;
4. identify problems with the design;
5. determine whether the sample is representative of the population or
   whether the sampling technique is effective;
6. examine the reliability and validity of the research instruments;
7. develop or refine data collection instruments;
8. refine the data collection and analysis plan;
9. give the researcher experience with the subjects, setting, methodology,
   and methods of measurement; and
10. implement data analysis techniques (Prescott & Soeken, 1989; Van Ort,
    1981).

Designs have been developed to meet unique research needs as they
emerge; thus, a variety of descriptive, correlational, quasi-experimental, and
experimental designs have been generated over time. In descriptive and correlational studies, no treatment is administered, so the purpose of the study design is to improve the precision of measurement. Quasi-experimental and experimental study designs usually involve treatment and control groups, and
focus on achieving high levels of control as well as precision in measurement.
A study's design is usually described in the methodology section of a research
report. In the study by Hulme and Grove (1994), a descriptive correlational
design was used to direct the conduct of the study. A diagram of the design is
presented in Figure 2-3 and indicates the variables described and the relationships examined. The findings generated from correlational research provide a
basis for generating hypotheses for testing in future research.

Population and Sample

The *population* is all elements (individuals, objects, or substances) that meet
certain criteria for inclusion in a study (Kerlinger, 1986). A *sample* is a subset

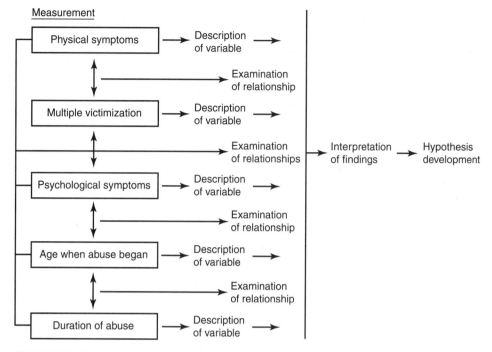

Measurement

FIGURE 2-3

Proposed descriptive correlational design for Hulme and Grove (1994) study of symptoms of female survivors of child sexual abuse. (From Hulme, P. A. & Grove, S. K. [1994]. *Physical and psychosocial symptomatology of female survivors of child sexual abuse, 55.* With permission.)

of the population that is selected for a particular study, and the members of a sample are the subjects. *Sampling* defines the process of selecting a group of people, events, behaviors, or other elements with which to conduct a study. Chapter 8 provides a background for critiquing populations and samples in research reports. The following quote identifies the sampling method, setting, sample size, population, sample criteria, and sample characteristics for the study conducted by Hulme and Grove (1994).

> "The convenience sample [sampling method] was obtained by advertising for subjects at three state universities in the southwest [setting]. Despite the sensitive nature of the study, 22 [sample size] usable interviews were obtained. The sample included women between the ages of 18 and 39 years (X = 28 years, SD = 6.5 years) who were identified as survivors of child sexual abuse [population] [sample criteria]. The majority of these women were white (91%) and students (82%). A little more than half (54%) were single, seven (32%) were divorced, and three (14%) were married. Most (64%) had no children. A small percentage (14%) were on some form of
> *continued*

public assistance and only 14% had been arrested. Although 27% of the subjects had step family members, the parents of 14 subjects (64%) were still married. Half the fathers were working class or self-employed; the rest were professionals. Mothers were either working class or self-employed (50%), homemakers (27%), or professionals (11%). Most subjects (95%) had siblings, and 36% knew or suspected their siblings also had been abused" [sample characteristics]. (pp. 523–524)

Methods of Measurement

Measurement is the process of assigning "numbers to objects (or events or situations) in accord with some rule" (Kaplan, 1964, p. 177). A component of measurement is instrumentation, which is the application of specific rules to the development of a measurement device or instrument. An instrument is selected to examine a specific variable in a study. Data generated with an instrument are at the nominal, ordinal, interval, or ratio level of measurement. The level of measurement, with nominal being the lowest form of measurement and ratio being the highest, determines the type of statistical analysis that can be performed on the data.

Critiquing a method of measurement in a study requires examining its reliability and validity. Reliability is concerned with how consistently the measurement technique measures a variable or concept. Validity is the extent to which the instrument actually reflects or measures what it is supposed to measure. For example, if an instrument was developed to measure chronic pain, the validity is the extent to which the instrument actually measures chronic pain and the reliability is how consistently it measures chronic pain. Chapter 9 introduces the concept of measurement and explains the different types of reliability and validity. Hulme and Grove (1994) used the ASI Questionnaire to measure the study variables.

"The ASI Questionnaire contains 10 sections: demographics; family origin; educational history, occupational history and public assistance; legal history; characteristics of the child sexual abuse (duration, perpetrator, pregnancy, type, and threats); past and present other victimizations; past and present physical symptoms; past and present psychosocial symptoms; and relationship with own children. Each section is followed by a response set that includes space for 'other.' Content validity was established by Brown and Garrison (1990) using an in-depth review of 132 clinical records. . . . For this descriptive correlational study . . . content validity of the tool was examined by asking an open-ended question: 'Is there additional information you would like to share?'" (p. 524)

Data Collection

Data collection is the precise, systematic gathering of information relevant to the research purpose or the specific objectives, questions, or hypotheses of a study. In order to collect data, the researcher must obtain permission from the setting or agency where the study is to be conducted. Consent must also be obtained from the research subjects to indicate their willingness to participate in the study. Frequently, the subjects are asked to sign a consent form, which describes the study, promises the subjects confidentiality, and indicates that the subjects can withdraw from the study at any time. Obtaining permission from an agency to conduct a study and consent from the subjects to participate in the study should be documented in the research report (see Chapter 6).

During data collection, the study variables are measured using a variety of techniques, such as observation, interview, questionnaires, or scales. In an increasing number of studies, nurses are measuring physiological variables with high-technology equipment. The data are collected and recorded systematically on each subject and are organized in a way that facilitates computer entry. Data collection is usually described in the methodology section of a research report under the subheading of "Procedures". Hulme and Grove (1994) identified the following procedure for data collection.

"Although the tool can be self-reporting, it was administered by personal interview to allow for elaboration of 'other' responses. The interviews lasted about one hour and were conducted in a private room provided by The University of Texas at Arlington. Each interview started with a discussion of the study benefits and risks and included signing a consent form. Risks included possible painful memories, anger, and sadness during the interview as well as emotional and physical discomfort after the interview. Sources of public and private counseling were provided to assist subjects with any difficulties experienced related to the study." (pp. 524–525)

Data Analysis

Data analysis is conducted to reduce, organize, and give meaning to the data. Analysis techniques conducted in quantitative research include descriptive and inferential analyses (see Chapter 10) and some sophisticated, advanced analyses. The analysis techniques implemented are determined primarily by the research objectives, questions, or hypotheses and the level of measurement achieved by the research instruments. The data analysis process is described in the results section of the research report and this section is usually organized by the research objectives, questions, or hypotheses. Hulme and Grove (1994) conducted frequencies, percents, means, standard deviations, and Pearson correlations to answer their research questions.

Results

"The first research question focused on patterns of physical and psychosocial symptoms. Six physical symptoms occurred in 50% or more of the subjects: insomnia, sexual dysfunction, overeating, drug abuse, severe headache, and two or more major surgeries. . . . Eleven psychosocial symptoms occurred in 75% or more of the subjects: depression, guilt, low self-esteem, inability to trust others, mood swings, suicidal thoughts, difficulty in relationships, confusion, flashbacks of the abuse, extreme anger, and memory lapse. . . . Self-injurious behavior was reported by eight subjects (33%)." (pp. 527–528)

"The second research question focused on the relationships among the number of physical and psychosocial symptoms and three contributing factors (age abuse began, duration of abuse, and other victimizations). There were five significant correlations among study variables: physical symptoms with other victimizations ($r = .59, p = .002$), physical symptoms with psychosocial symptoms ($r = .56, p = .003$), age abuse began with duration of abuse ($r = -.50, p = .009$), psychosocial symptoms with other victimizations ($r = .40, p = .033$), and duration of abuse with psychosocial symptoms ($r = .40, p = .034$)." (p. 528)

Research Outcomes

The results obtained from data analyses require interpretation to be meaningful. *Interpretation of research outcomes* involves examining the results from data analysis, forming conclusions, considering the implications for nursing, exploring the significance of the findings, generalizing the findings, and suggesting further studies. The research outcomes are presented in the discussion section of a research report. Hulme and Grove (1994) provided the following discussion of their findings, with implications for nursing and suggestions for further study.

Discussion

"While this study may have limited generalizability due to the relatively small nonprobability sample, the findings do support previous research. . . . In addition, the findings support Browne and Finkelhor's (1986) framework that a wide range of behavioral manifestations (physical and psychosocial symptoms) comprise the long-term effects of child sexual abuse." (p. 528)

"Brown and Garrison's (1990) ASI Questionnaire was effective in identifying patterns of physical and psychosocial symptoms in women with a history of child sexual abuse. . . . As data on the behavioral manifestations (physical and psychosocial symptoms) and the effect of each of the contributing factors accumulate, hypotheses need to be formulated to further test Browne and Finkelhor's (1986) framework explaining the long-term effects of child sexual abuse. . . . With additional research, the ASI Questionnaire might be adapted for use in clinical situations. This questionnaire might facilitate identification and delivery of appropriate treatment to female survivors of child sexual abuse in clinical settings." (pp. 529–530)

Reading Research Reports

Understanding the steps of the research process and learning new terms related to those steps will assist you in reading research reports. A *research report* summarizes the major elements of a study and identifies the contributions of that study to nursing knowledge. Research reports are presented at professional meetings and conferences and are published in journals and books. These reports are often overwhelming to nursing students and new graduates. Maybe you have had difficulty locating research articles or understanding the content of these articles. Research reports are usually written to communicate with other researchers, not with clinicians. Thus, the style of the report is often technical and sometimes filled with jargon, which is very confusing to students and practicing nurses. We would like to help you overcome some of these barriers and assist you in understanding the research literature by (1) identifying sources that publish research reports, (2) describing the content of a research report, and (3) providing tips for reading the research literature.

Sources of Research Reports

The most common sources for nursing research reports are professional journals. Research reports are the major focus of the following nursing research journals: *Advances in Nursing Science, Applied Nursing Research, Clinical Nursing Research: An International Journal, Image: Journal of Nursing Scholarship, Nursing Research, Research in Nursing & Health, Scholarly Inquiry for Nursing Practice: An International Journal,* and *Western Journal of Nursing Research.* Two of these journals, *Applied Nursing Research* and *Clinical Nursing Research*, have focused on communicating research findings to practicing nurses. Thus, the journals include less detail on the methodology of the study and the results of the data analysis and more on discussion of the findings and the implications for practice. Many of the nursing clinical specialty journals also place a high

TABLE 2-3. Journals That Focus on Research Articles

Journal Title	Percent of the Journal Focused on Research
Research Journals	
Applied Nursing Research	100
Image: Journal of Nursing Scholarship	70
Nursing Research	80
Research in Nursing & Health	100
Scholarly Inquiry for Nursing Practice	60
Western Journal of Nursing Research	90
Clinical Journals	
American Journal of Alzheimer's Care & Related Disorders and Research	60
Birth	70
Cardiovascular Nursing	60
Computers in Nursing	50
Heart & Lung: Journal of Critical Care	70
Issues in Comprehensive Pediatric Nursing	100
Issues in Mental Health Nursing	67
Journal of Child and Adolescent Psychiatric and Mental Health Nursing	75
Journal of Continuing Education in Nursing	50
Journal of Holistic Nursing	50
Journal of National Black Nurses' Association	75
Journal of Nursing Education	80
Journal of Pediatric Nursing: Nursing Care of Children and Families	50
Journal of Transcultural Nursing	87
Maternal-Child Nursing Journal	75
Nursing Diagnosis	80
Public Health Nursing	75
Rehabilitation Nursing	50
The Diabetes Educator	75

Data from Swanson, E. A., McCloskey, J. C., & Bodensteiner, A. (1991). Publishing opportunities for nurses: A comparison of 92 U.S. journals. *Image: Journal of Nursing Scholarship, 23*(1), 33–38.

priority on publishing research findings. Table 2-3 identifies the clinical journals in which research reports compose 50% or more of the journal content. Currently, 92 nursing journals are published in the United States, and many of them include research articles (Swanson, McCloskey, & Bodensteiner, 1991).

Some research reports, such as those for complex qualitative studies, are lengthy and might be published as books or as chapters in books. Research reports of master's degree students are published as theses, and doctorate students produce dissertations summarizing their research projects. Prior to publication, many research reports are presented at local, national, and international nursing and health care conferences. Often brochures for conferences will indicate whether research reports are part of the program. The findings from many studies are now being communicated through the Internet as journals are being placed online, and selected Web sites include the most current health research (Gibbs, Sullivan-Fowler, & Rowe, 1996). Conducting a review of relevant literature is the focus of Chapter 4.

Content of Research Reports

At this point, you are probably overwhelmed by the appearance of a research report. You might find it easier to read and comprehend these reports if you understand each of the component parts. A research report often includes six parts: (1) abstract, (2) introduction, (3) methods, (4) results, (5) discussion, and (6) reference list. These parts are described in this section, and the study by Neuberger et al. (1997) that examined the effects of exercise on the health status of persons with RA is presented as an example.

Abstract

The report usually begins with an *abstract,* which is a clear, concise summary of a study (Crosby, 1990). Abstracts range from 100 to 250 words and usually include the study purpose, design, setting, sample size, major results, and conclusions. Researchers hope their abstracts will concisely convey the findings from their study and capture your attention so you will read the entire report. Neuberger et al. (1997) developed the following clear, concise abstract that conveys the critical information about their study.

ABSTRACT. "The effects of 12 weeks of low-impact aerobic exercise on fatigue, aerobic fitness, and disease activity were examined in a quasi-experimental time series study of 25 adults with rheumatoid arthritis (RA). Measures were obtained preintervention, midtreatment (after 6 weeks of exercise), end of treatment (after 12 weeks of exercise), and at a 15-week follow-up. ANOVAs (analysis of variances) for repeated measures showed that those subjects who participated more frequently reported decreased fatigue, while those who participated less frequently reported an increase in fatigue. All subjects, on average, showed increased aerobic fitness and increased right and left hand grip strength, decreased pain, and decreased walk time. There were no significant increases in joint count or sedimentation rate. Significant improvement measures at 15-week follow-up also were found. Findings indicate that persons with RA who participate in appropriate exercises may lessen fatigue levels, and experience other positive effects without worsening their arthritis." (p. 195)

TABLE 2-4. Content of a Research Report

Abstract

Introduction
Statement of the problem, with background and significance
Statement of the purpose
Brief literature review
Identification of the framework
Identification of the research objectives, questions, or hypotheses (if applicable)

Methods
Identification of the research design
Description of the treatment of intervention (if applicable)
Description of the sample and setting
Description of the methods of measurement (including reliability and validity)
Discussion of the data collection process

Results
Description of the data analysis procedures
Presentation of results in tables, figures, or narrative organized by the purpose and/
   or objectives, questions, or hypotheses

Discussion
Discussion of major findings
Identification of the limitations
Presentation of conclusions
Implications of the findings for nursing practice
Recommendations for further research

Following the abstract are usually four major content sections of a research report: introduction, methods, results, and discussion. The content covered in each of these sections is outlined in Table 2-4 and is briefly discussed in the following sections.

Introduction

The introduction section of a research report identifies the nature and scope of the problem being investigated and provides a case for the conduct of the study. You should be able to clearly identify the significance of conducting the study to generate knowledge for nursing practice. Neuberger et al.'s (1997) study was significant because it generated knowledge to assist individuals with a chronic illness to promote their health and maintain their independence. The purpose of their study was clearly stated in the first sentence of the abstract.

Depending on the type of research report, the literature review and the framework may be separate sections or part of the introduction. The literature review documents the current knowledge of the problem investigated and includes the sources that were used to develop the study and interpret the findings. For example, Neuberger et al. (1997) summarized literature that focused on the concepts: fatigue, exercise, and RA. A research report also needs to include a framework, but only about half of the published studies identify one (Moody, Wilson, Smyth, Schwartz, Tittle, & Van Cott, 1988). Neuberger et al. (1997) clearly identified their framework as a biobehavioral framework that was "based on concepts of self-regulation and self-monitoring which refer to unconscious as well as conscious mechanisms used by individuals to maintain homeostasis and prevent fatigue. The four concepts of this framework are resources, utilization, activity, and restoration" (p. 197). The framework concepts were clearly defined and interrelated to provide a theoretical basis for the study. A model or map is sometimes developed to clarify the logic within the framework but was not included in this study.

The literature review and framework are presented in such a way as to stress the importance of and to provide support for the study being reported. Often the introduction ends with an identification of the objectives, questions, or hypotheses that were used to direct the study. Neuberger et al. (1997) identified the following hypotheses: "Participation in a low-impact aerobic exercise program (a) will decrease fatigue in outpatients with RA; (b) will increase aerobic fitness levels of subjects; and (c) will not increase measures of disease activity" (p. 197).

Methods

The methods section of a research report describes how the study was conducted and usually includes the study design, sample, setting, methods of measurement, and data collection process. This section of the report needs to be presented in enough detail so that the reader can critique the adequacy of the study methods to produce reliable findings (Tornquist, Funk, Champagne, & Wiese, 1993). Neuberger et al. (1997) identified their design as quasi-experimental time series. They included the subsection "Sample," which described the population, sampling method, sample size, sample characteristics, and setting. Another subsection under "Methods" was "Measurement," which detailed the instruments used to measure the independent variables of fatigue, aerobic fitness, and disease activity. The validity and reliability of the instruments were examined for previous studies and for this study. The subsection "Procedure" detailed the exercise intervention (treatment) and the implementation of the study, including who implemented the treatment, who collected the data, the procedure for collecting data, and the type and frequency of measurements obtained. The effectiveness of the treatment needs to be determined, as well as the feasibility of using the treatment in the real world of clinical practice. The protection of subjects' rights and the informed consent process were also covered in the "Procedure" subsection.

Results

The results section presents what was found by conducting the study and the significance of the findings. This section is best organized by the research purpose or objectives, questions, or hypotheses formulated in the study. The statistical analyses conducted to address the purpose or each objective, question, or hypothesis are identified, and the specific results obtained from the analyses are presented in tables, figures, or narrative of the report (Burns & Grove, 1997). Try not to be confused by the statistical results, and focus more on the summary of the study results and their significance than on the numbers. Neuberger et al. (1997) conducted statistical analyses to address their study hypotheses. The analyses were comprehensive and clearly presented using tables and narrative. Repeated measures analysis of variance (ANOVA) was used to test differences among the three measurement points (6 weeks, 12 weeks, and 15 weeks). Results indicated a significant decrease in fatigue and an increase in aerobic fitness without a worsening of the disease status.

Discussion

The discussion section ties the other sections of the research report together and gives them meaning. This section includes the major findings, limitations of the study, conclusions drawn from the findings, implications of the findings for nursing, and recommendations for further research. Neuberger et al. (1997) discussed their findings in detail, and compared and contrasted them with the findings of previous research. They also linked their findings to their framework with the statement: "The findings suggest that improvements in aerobic fitness, hand grip strength, walk time, and pain levels after the exercise intervention may have contributed to increased energy resources and decreased levels of fatigue" (p. 203). The limitations of the study were small sample size, lack of a separate control group, and lack of completely blinded observers. Following these limitations were directions for further research. Implications of the study findings for practice were addressed with a discussion of the importance of low-impact exercise for individuals with RA.

The conclusions drawn from a research project can be useful in at least three different ways. First, the intervention or treatment tested in a study can be used with patients to improve their care and promote a positive health outcome. Second, reading research reports might change your view of a patient's situation or give you greater insight into the situation. Lastly, studies heighten your awareness of the problems experienced by patients and assist you in assessing and working toward solutions for these problems (Tornquist et al., 1993).

References

Following the discussion section is a reference list that includes all sources cited in the research report. The reference list includes the studies and theories that provide a basis for the conduct of the study. These sources provide an opportunity to read in greater depth on the problem studied. I strongly encourage you to read the Neuberger et al. (1997) article to identify the sections of

a research report and to examine the content in each of these sections. Neuberger et al. detail a rigorously conducted quasi-experimental study that provides excellent knowledge for use in practice.

Tips for Reading Research Reports

When you start reading research reports, you will probably be overwhelmed by the new terms and complex information presented. Hopefully, you will not be discouraged but will see the challenge of examining new knowledge generated through research. You will probably need to read the report slowly two or three times and will need to use the glossary at the end of this textbook to review the definitions of unfamiliar terms. We recommend that you read the abstract first and then the discussion section of the report. This will enable you to determine the relevance of the findings to you personally and to your practice. Initially, focus on research reports that you believe can provide relevant knowledge for your practice.

Reading a research report requires the use of a variety of critical thinking skills, such as skimming, comprehending, and analyzing to facilitate your understanding of the study (Miller & Babcock, 1996). *Skimming* a research report involves quickly reviewing the source to gain a broad overview of the content. You would probably read the title, the author's name, the abstract or introduction, and the discussion section. Knowing the findings of the study provides you with a standard for evaluating the rest of the article (Tornquist et al., 1993). Then you would read the major headings and sometimes one or two sentences under each heading. Lastly, you would examine the summary and/or conclusions from the study. Skimming enables you to make a preliminary judgment about the value of a source and a determination about reading the report in depth.

Comprehending a research report requires that the entire study be read carefully. You need to focus on understanding major concepts and the logical flow of ideas within the study. You might highlight information about the researchers, such as their education, their current positions, and any funding they received for the study. As you read the study, highlight the steps of the research process. You might record notes in the margin so that you can easily identify the problem, purpose, framework, major variables, study design, treatments, sample, measurement methods, data collection process, analysis techniques, results, and study outcomes. You might also record creative ideas or questions you have in the margin of the report.

We encourage you to highlight the parts of the article that you do not understand and ask your instructor or other nurse researchers for clarification. Your greatest difficulty in reading the research report will probably be understanding the statistical analyses. Information in Chapter 10 will help you comprehend the analyses. Basically, you need to identify the particular statistics used, the results from each statistical analysis, and the meaning of the results. Statistical analyses are conducted to address the study purpose or specific

objectives, questions, or hypotheses. Therefore, you need to link each analysis technique to its results and then to the study purpose or objectives, questions, or hypotheses presented in the study.

The final reading skill is *analysis* of a research report, which involves determining the value of the report's content. Break the content of the report into parts, and examine the parts in depth for accuracy, completeness, uniqueness of information, and organization. Note whether the steps of the research process build logically on each other or whether steps are missing or incomplete. Examine the discussion section of the report and determine if the researchers have provided a critical argument for using the study findings in practice. Using the skills of skimming, comprehending, and analyzing in reading research reports will increase your comfort with studies, allow you to become an informed consumer of research, and expand your knowledge for making changes in practice. These skills for reading research reports are critical for conducting a comprehensive research critique. The guidelines for critiquing quantitative and qualitative studies are the focus of Chapter 12.

Conducting an Initial Critique of a Research Report

Being able to read research reports and identify the steps of the research process enable you to conduct an initial critique of a report.

THE FOLLOWING QUESTIONS are important in conducting an initial critique of a quantitative research report.

1. *Was a quantitative or a qualitative study conducted?*
2. *If the research was quantitative, was the study descriptive, correlational, quasi-experimental, or experimental?*
3. *Was the setting for the study natural, partially controlled, or highly controlled?*
4. *Were the steps of the study clearly identified?*
5. *Can you identify the following steps in the research report: problem, purpose, literature review, framework, variables, definitions of variables, design, sample, measurement methods, data collection, data analyses, and outcomes?*
6. *Were any of the steps of the research process missing?*
7. *Were the steps of the study logically linked? Thus, the study problem and purpose need to provide a basis for the literature review and the framework presented. The purpose and framework provide a basis for the objectives, questions, or hypotheses identified. The objectives, questions, or hypotheses provide a basis for the study design, measurement, data collection, and data analyses. The findings from the study need to be linked to the framework and to previous studies cited in the literature review.*

SUMMARY

Quantitative research is the traditional research approach in nursing. Nurses use a broad range of quantitative approaches, including descriptive, correlational, quasi-experimental, and experimental, to develop nursing knowledge. Some of the terms relevant to quantitative research include basic and applied research, rigor, and control. Basic, or pure, research is a scientific investigation that involves the pursuit of "knowledge for knowledge's sake" or for the pleasure of learning and finding truth. Applied, or practical, research is a scientific investigation conducted to generate knowledge that will directly influence or improve clinical practice.

Conducting quantitative research involves rigor, which is the striving for excellence in research. Rigor requires discipline, adherence to detail, and strict accuracy. A rigorous quantitative researcher constantly strives for more precise measurement tools, representative samples, and tightly controlled study designs. Control involves the imposing of rules by the researcher to decrease the possibility of error and thus increase the probability that the study's findings are an accurate reflection of reality. Some of the mechanisms for control within quantitative research include the selection of subjects and the setting. Sampling is a process of selecting subjects who are representative of the population being studied. The three settings for conducting research are natural, partially controlled, and highly controlled.

Research is a process and is similar in some ways to other processes. Therefore, the background you acquired early in your nursing education in problem-solving and the nursing process is also useful in research. A comparison of the problem-solving process, the nursing process, and the research process shows the similarities and differences in these processes and provides a basis for understanding the research process.

The quantitative research process involves conceptualizing a research project, planning and implementing that project, and communicating the findings. The following steps of the quantitative research process are briefly introduced in this chapter and are presented in detail in Chapters 3 through 10.

1. ***Research Problem and Purpose.*** The research problem is a situation in need of a solution, improvement, or alteration. The research purpose is generated from the problem and identifies the specific goal or aim of the study.
2. ***Literature Review.*** The review of relevant literature is conducted to generate a picture of what is known and unknown about a particular topic.
3. ***Study Framework.*** The framework is the theoretical basis for a study that guides the development of the study and enables the researcher to link the findings to nursing's body of knowledge.
4. ***Research Objectives, Questions, or Hypotheses***. Research objectives, questions, or hypotheses are formulated to bridge the gap between the more abstractly stated research problem and purpose and the study design and plan for data collection and analysis.
5. ***Study Variables.*** Variables are concepts at various levels of abstraction that are measured, manipulated, or controlled in a study.
6. ***Assumptions.*** Assumptions are statements that are taken for granted or are considered true even though they have not been scientifically tested.
7. ***Limitations.*** Limitations are restrictions in a study that may decrease the generalizability of the findings.
8. ***Research Design.*** Research design is a blueprint for conducting a study that maxi-

mizes control over factors that could interfere with the study's desired outcome.

9. ***Population and Sample.*** The population is all the elements that meet certain criteria for inclusion in a study. A sample is a subset of the population that is selected for a particular study; the members of a sample are the subjects.

10. ***Methods of Measurement.*** Measurement is the process of assigning numbers to objects, events, or situations in accord with some rule. Methods of measurement are identified to measure each of the variables in a study.

11. ***Data Collection.*** The data collection process involves the precise, systematic gathering of information relevant to the research purpose or the objectives, questions, or hypotheses of a study.

12. ***Data Analyses.*** Data analyses are conducted to reduce, organize, and give meaning to the data.

13. ***Research Outcomes.*** Research outcomes include the conclusions or findings, generalization of findings, implications for nursing, and suggestions for further research.

Understanding of the steps of the research process provides a background for reading research reports. To assist you in reading the research literature, sources of research reports are identified, the content of a research report is described, and the critical skills for reading the report are detailed. The chapter concludes with guidelines for conducting an initial critique of a quantitative study. In the appendix of this chapter are examples of the steps of the research process excerpted from quasi-experimental and experimental published studies.

REFERENCES

Abdellah, F. G., & Levine, E. (1979). *Better patient care through nursing research* (2nd ed.). New York: Macmillan.

Adebo, E. O. (1974). Identifying problems for nursing research. *International Nursing Review, 21*(2), 53–54, 59.

Bagley, C. (1990). Development of a measure of unwanted sexual contact in childhood, for use in community health surveys. *Psychology Reports, 66*(2), 401–402.

Bagley, C. & King, K. K. (1990). *Child sexual abuse. The search for healing.* New York: Travistock/Routledge.

Bond, E. F., & Heitkemper, M. M. (1987). Importance of basic physiologic research in nursing science. *Heart & Lung, 16*(4), 347–349.

Brown, B. E., & Garrison, C. J. (1990). Patterns of symptomatology of adult women incest survivors. *Western Journal of Nursing Research, 12*(5), 587–600.

Browne, A., & Finkelhor, D. (1986). Initial and long-term effects: A review of the research. In D. Finkelhor (Ed.), *A source book on child sexual abuse* (pp. 143–179). Beverly Hills, CA: Sage.

Burns, N. (1989). The research process and the nursing process: Distinctly different. *Nursing Science Quarterly, 2*(4), 157–158.

Burns, N., & Grove, S. K. (1997). *The practice of nursing research: Conduct, critique, and utilization* (3rd ed.). Philadelphia: Saunders.

Campbell, D. T., & Stanley, J. C. (1963). *Experimental and quasi-experimental designs for research.* Chicago: Rand McNally.

Cook, T. D., & Campbell, D. T. (1979). *Quasi-experimentation: Design and analysis issues for field settings.* Chicago: Rand McNally.

Crosby, L. J. (1990). The abstract: An important first impression. *Journal of Neuroscience Nursing, 22*(3), 192–194.

Diers, D. (1979). *Research in nursing practice.* Philadelphia: Lippincott.

Fawcett, J., & Downs, F. S. (1992). *The relationship of theory and research* (2nd ed.). Norwalk, CT: Appleton-Century-Crofts.

Fisher, Sir R. A. (1935). *The designs of experiments.* New York: Hafner.

Flynn, L. (1997). The health practices of homeless women: A causal model. *Nursing Research, 46*(2), 72–77.

Follette, N. M., Alexander, P. C., & Follette, W. C. (1991). Individual predictors of outcome in group treatment for incest survivors. *Journal of Consulting and Clinical Psychology, 59*(1), 150–155.

Gibbs, S. R., Sullivan-Fowler, M., & Rowe, N. W. (1996). *Medical surfari: A guide to exploring the Internet and discovering the top health care resources.* St. Louis: Mosby.

Hastings-Tolsma, M. T., Yucha, C. B., Tompkins, J., Robson, L., & Szeverenyi, N. (1993). Effect of warm and cold applications on the resolution of IV infiltrations. *Research in Nursing & Health, 16*(3), 171–178.

Hulme, P. A., & Grove, S. K. (1994). Symptoms of female survivors of child sexual abuse. *Issues in Mental Health Nursing, 15*(5), 519–532.

Kaplan, A. (1964). *The conduct of inquiry: Methodology for behavioral science.* New York: Chandler.

Kerlinger, F. N. (1986). *Foundations of behavioral research* (2nd ed.). New York: Holt, Rinehart & Winston.

Lewis, G. B. H., & Hecker, J. F. (1991). Radiological examination of failure of intravenous infusions. *British Journal of Surgery, 78*(4), 500–501.

MacCara, M. E. (1983). Extravasation: A hazard of intravenous therapy. *Drug Intelligence and Clinical Pharmacy, 17*(10), 713–717.

McCarthy, D. O., Lo, C., Nguyen, H., & Ney, D. M. (1997). The effect of protein density of food on food intake and nutritional status of tumor-bearing rats. *Research in Nursing & Health, 20*(2), 131–138.

Metheny, N., Eisenberg, P., & McSweeney, M. (1988). Effect of feeding tube properties and three irrigants on clogging rates. *Nursing Research, 37*(3), 165–169.

Millam, D. A. (1988). Managing complications of I.V. therapy. *Nursing 88, 18*(3), 34–42.

Miller, D. C. (1991). *Handbook of research design and social measurement* (5th ed.). Newbury Park, CA: Sage.

Miller, M. A., & Babcock, D. E. (1996). *Critical thinking applied to nursing.* St. Louis: Mosby.

Moody, L. E. , Wilson, M. E., Smyth, K., Schwartz, R., Tittle, M., & Van Cott, M. L. (1988). Analysis of a decade of nursing practice research: 1977–1986. *Nursing Research, 42*(4), 197–203.

Myers, S. T. (1982). The search for assumptions. *Western Journal of Nursing Research, 4*(1), 91–98.

Neuberger, G. B., Press, A. N., Lindsley, H. B., Hinton, R., Cagle, P. E., Carlson, K., Scott, S., Dahl, J., & Kramer, B. (1997). Effects of exercise on fatigue, aerobic fitness, and disease activity measures in persons with rheumatoid arthritis. *Research in Nursing & Health, 20*(3), 195–204.

Prescott, P. A., & Soeken, K. L. (1989). Methodology corner: The potential uses of pilot work. *Nursing Research, 38*(1), 60–62.

Swanson, E. A., McCloskey, J. C., & Bodensteiner, A. (1991). Publishing opportunities for nurses: A comparison of 92 U.S. journals. *Image: Journal of Nursing Scholarship, 23*(1), 33–38.

Tornquist, E. M., Funk, S. G., Champagne, M. T., & Wiese, R. A. (1993). Advice on reading research: Overcoming the barriers. *Applied Nursing Research, 6*(4), 177–183.

Van Ort, S. (1981). Research design: Pilot study. In S. D. Krampitz & N. Pavlovich (Eds.), *Readings for nursing research* (pp. 49–53). St. Louis: Mosby.

Whitney, F. W. (1986). Turning clinical problems into research. *Heart & Lung, 15*(1), 57–59.

Williams, M. A. (1980). Editorial: Assumptions in research. *Research in Nursing and Health, 3*(2), 47–48.

Wysocki, A. B. (1983). Basic versus applied research: Intrinsic and extrinsic considerations. *Western Journal of Nursing Research, 5*(3), 217–224.

Examples of Quantitative Studies

Quasi-experimental Study

Hastings-Tolsma, Yucha, Tompkins, Robson, and Szeverenyi (1993) conducted a quasi-experimental study of the "effect of warm and cold applications on the resolution of IV infiltrations" (p. 171). The steps of this study are outlined following.

Steps of the Research Process

1. **Research Problem.** "It has been estimated that as many as 80% of hospitalized patients receive intravenous (IV) therapy each day (Millam, 1988). IV infiltration, or extravasation, occurs in as many as 23% of all IV infusion failures (MacCara, 1983) and is second only to phlebitis as a cause of IV morbidity (Lewis & Hecker, 1991). The resulting tissue injury depends on the clinical condition of the patient, the nature of the infusate, and the volume infiltrated, and may range from little apparent injury to serious damage. In addition, considerable patient suffering, prolonged hospitalization, and significant costs may be incurred. Despite the frequency and potential severity of injury, little is known about how to treat IV infiltration effectively once it is identified" (Hastings-Tolsma et al., 1993, p. 171).

2. **Research Purpose.** "The purpose of this research was to determine the effect of warm versus cold applications on the pain intensity and the speed of resolution of the extravasation of a variety of commonly used intravenous solutions" (p. 172).

3. **Review of Literature.** The literature review included relevant, current sources that ranged from 1976 to 1991. The journal article was received in April 1992 and was accepted for publication in January 1993. The signs and symptoms of IV infiltration were identified, and the tissue damage that occurs with IV infiltration was described. The effects of the pH and osmolarity of different types of IV solutions on IV infiltration were also discussed. The literature review concluded with a description of the effects of a variety of treatments, including warm and cold applications, on the resolution of IV infiltrations. Hastings-Tolsma et al. (1993) concluded that "examination of warm and cold application with less toxic infiltrates has not been studied carefully under controlled conditions" (p. 172).

4. **Framework.** Hastings-Tolsma and colleagues did not identify a framework for their study. They did identify relevant concepts (IV therapy, nature of infusate, vessel damage, extravasation, tissue damage, treatment, and reso-

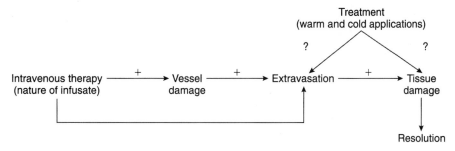

FIGURE 2A-1

Proposed framework map for Hastings-Tolsma, Yucha, Tompkins, Robson, and Szeverenyi's (1993) study of the effect of warm and cold applications on the resolution of intravenous infiltrations.

lution) and discuss the relationships among these concepts in their literature review. A possible map for their study framework is presented in Figure 2A-1. The map indicates that the more IV therapy patients receive, the more likely they are to experience vessel damage that leads to extravasation or IV infiltration. The nature of the IV infusate (solution) also affects the severity of the vessel damage and extravasation. Extravasation leads to tissue damage, and the greater the extravasation, the greater the tissue damage. The treatment with warm and cold applications has an unknown effect on the extravasation and tissue damage. If the extravasation and tissue damage are decreased by either the cold or the warm treatment, then the patient experiences resolution of the extravasation.

5. ***Research Questions.*** "(a) What are the differences in tissue response as measured by pain, erythema and induration, and interstitial fluid volume between warm versus cold applications to infiltrated IV sites? (b) What is the effect of warm versus cold applications in the resolution of infiltrated solutions of varying osmolarity when pH is held constant?" (Hastings-Tolsma et al., 1993, pp. 172–173).

6. ***Variables.*** The independent variables were temperature applications (warm and cold) and osmolarity of the IV solution. The dependent variables were pain, erythema, induration, and interstitial fluid volume.

Temperature Applications

Conceptual Definition. Topical warm and cold applications to the sites of extravasation to promote the reabsorption of infusate and resolution of the infiltration.

Operational Definition. Warm (43°C) or cold (0°C) topical applications using a thermostated pad to the sites of IV infiltration.

Osmolarity of the IV Solution

Conceptual Definition. The osmolar concentration expressed as osmoles per liter of solution.

Operational Definition. IV solutions of ½ saline (154 mOsm), normal saline (308 mOsm), or 3% saline (1027 mOsm).

Pain

Conceptual Definition. Sensation of discomfort caused by tissue damage and the inflammatory response.

Operational Definition. Pain was measured with the Analogue Chromatic Continuous Scale (ACCS), a self-report, unidimensional visual analogue scale for quantifying pain intensity.

Erythema

Conceptual Definition. Redness at the IV infiltration site due to an inflammatory response.

Operational Definition. Indelible ink was used to mark the borders of erythema. Then a centimeter ruler was used to measure the widest perpendicular widths, and the two widths were multiplied to estimate surface area of erythema.

Induration

Conceptual Definition. The swelling at the IV infiltration site created by the IV solution, tissue damage, and inflammatory response.

Operational Definition. Indelible ink was used to mark the borders of induration. Then a centimeter ruler was used to measure the widest perpendicular widths, and the two widths were multiplied to estimate the surface area of induration.

Interstitial Fluid Volume

Conceptual Definition. The amount of fluid that leaks from the damaged blood vessel into the surrounding tissues.

Operational Definition. Magnetic resonance imaging (MRI) was used to quantify the amount of infiltrate remaining at the IV site.

7. **Design.** The design most closely resembles an interrupted time series, with each subject receiving both treatments of warm and cold applications.
8. **Sample.** "The sample was composed of 18 healthy adult volunteers. All participants were nonpregnant and taking no medications. . . . Of the 18 participants studied, 78% were female ($n = 14$) and 22% were male ($n = 4$), and they ranged in age from 20 to 45 years with a mean age of 35 years (SD = 7). All subjects were Caucasian. The research was approved by the

Health Science Center Institutional Review Board for the Protection of Human Subjects. After the study was explained to interested individuals, written informed consent was obtained from volunteers. All individuals were offered financial compensation for their participation" (Hastings-Tolsma et al., 1993, p. 173).

9. ***Procedures.*** "All measurements were taken in the Health Science Center's Department of Radiology NMR Laboratory. After obtaining written informed consent, participants were taken to the MR imaging suite where infiltrations and subsequent measurements were made. . . . Total data collection time was approximately 3½ hours. One of three solutions was infiltrated into the cephalic vein of the forearm: ½ saline (154 mOsm), normal saline (308 mOsm), or 3% saline (1027 mOsm). These solutions were selected because of the varying osmolarity range, as well as relatively common clinical use. Solutions were infiltrated sequentially so that each participant was given a different solution in the order of recruitment into the study. Randomization was used to determine right or left arm, as well as which application, warm or cold, would be used" (p. 174).

10. ***Results.*** "Warm and cold treatments to the infiltrated IV sites using three solutions revealed significant differences in tissue response as measured by the interstitial fluid volume . . . For all three solutions, the volume remaining was always less with warm than with cold application, F (1, 15) = 46.69, $p < .001$. There was no difference in pain with warm or cold applications. . . . Surface area measurement failed to demonstrate the presence of erythema with any of the solutions. . . . Surface induration reflected a significant decrease over time, F (2, 16) = 14.38, $p = .001$, although accurate measurement of the infiltrate was nearly impossible after the first or second imaging period as the borders were so poorly defined. . . . There was no significant effect of warmth or cold on surface area" (p. 175).

11. ***Discussion.*** This section includes the study conclusions, recommendations for further research, and implications of the findings for nursing practice. "These findings demonstrate that the application of warmth to sites of IV infiltration produces faster resolution of the extravasation than does cold, as monitored over one hour. . . . It is interesting to note that cold appeared to have a more immediate dramatic effect on the increase in interstitial edema than warmth when applied to the hyperosmolar infiltrate. Presumably this is due to osmosis of fluid from the plasma and surrounding tissues into the area of infiltration. . . .

Other factors that might influence accurate assessment and treatment of infiltrations need to be examined. These should include the use of larger amounts of extravasate and other more varied and caustic solutions, as well as other treatments such as elevation, differing IV site placement, differing gauge needles, and the study of patients of varying ages and clinical conditions. . . ." (p. 176).

"The nurse generally has responsibility for IV therapy and criteria for accurate assessment and appropriate intervention clearly are needed. Find-

ings from this research support the use of warm application to sites of infiltration of noncaustic solutions of varying osmolarity, but raise questions
about the adequacy of currently used indicators of IV infiltrations. Continued scientific scrutiny should contribute to the development of standards
useful in the assessment and treatment of IV extravasation" (p. 177).

Experimental Study

The planning and implementation of experimental studies are highly controlled
by the researcher, and these studies often are conducted on animals in a laboratory setting. For example, Metheny et al. (1988) conducted an experimental
study of the effects of feeding-tube properties and irrigants on the incidence
of tube clogging. The treatments and the tube properties and irrigants were
highly controlled in a laboratory setting, and the tubes were randomly selected
for this study. The steps of the study are outlined following.

Steps of the Research Process

1. **Research Problem.** "Luminal obstruction of feeding tubes is one of the most
    common mechanical complications associated with enteral feedings. . . .
    Inability to clear a clogged tube necessitates its removal and replacement
    with a new tube. Not only does this add to the patient's discomfort and
    risk of trauma, but it interrupts the administration of nutrients and results
    in increased cost" (Metheny et al., 1988, p. 165).
2. **Research Purpose.** "The purpose of this laboratory study was to examine
    the effect of selected feeding tube properties (material and diameter) on
    the incidence of tube clogging and the efficacy of three irrigants (cranberry
    juice, water, and Coca-Cola) in preventing tube clogging" (p. 165).
3. **Review of Literature.** The literature review included studies that examined
    the effects of feeding tube properties on flow rate and the effects of irrigants
    on tube patency. Previous research had indicated that the flow rate was
    greater for polyurethane tubes than for silicone tubes. "There are no direct
    references for the effect of the tube diameter on clogging rates. . . ." (Meth-
    eny et al., 1988, p. 165). Different studies indicated that water, Coca-Cola,
    and cranberry juice were effective irrigants for feeding tubes.
4. **Framework.** Metheny and associates did not identify a framework, but the
    concepts of tube properties, irrigants, flow rate, and luminal obstruction
    were identified in the literature review. The relationships among these con-
    cepts are presented in Figure 2A-2. Certain tube properties and irrigants
    were proposed to affect the flow rate through the feeding tube, but the
    effect is unknown, as indicated by the question marks. An increase in flow
    rate would result in the delivery of substances, and a decrease in flow
    rate could result in luminal obstruction or clogging of the tube.
5. **Variables.** The independent variables were physical tube properties (mate-

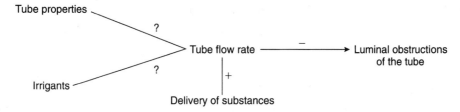

FIGURE 2A-2
Proposed framework map for Metheny, Eisenberg, and McSweeny's (1988) study of the effects of feeding tube properties and irrigants of tube clogging rates.

rial and diameter) and irrigants (cranberry juice, water, and Coca-Cola), and the dependent variable was tube clogging.

Physical Tube Properties

Conceptual Definition. The physical elements or properties (material and diameter) of the tube that influence flow rate.

Operational Definition. Polyurethane and silicone tubes of the following diameters were used: 12 Fr., 10 Fr., and 8 Fr.

Irrigant

Conceptual Definition. The substance used to flush the internal surface of the tube.

Operational Definition. Three irrigants were used: cranberry juice, water, and Coca-Cola.

Tube Clogging

Conceptual Definition. Mechanical complication of the tube that results in decreased flow rate through the tube and ultimate obstruction of the lumen of the tube.

Operational Definition. Clogging was defined by flow rates. "Flow rates were considered free flowing if the volume was greater than 0.7 ml/minute, slowed if less than 0.7 ml/minute but greater than 0.4 ml/minute, almost stopped if less than 0.4 ml/minute but greater than zero, and completely stopped if zero ml/minute. When tubes became irreversibly clogged, they were removed from the study and not replaced" (Metheny et al., 1988, pp. 166–167).

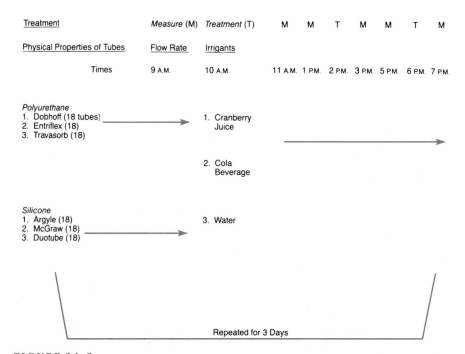

Treatment	Measure (M)	Treatment (T)	M	M	T	M	M	T	M
Physical Properties of Tubes	Flow Rate	Irrigants							
Times	9 A.M.	10 A.M.	11 A.M.	1 P.M.	2 P.M.	3 P.M.	5 P.M.	6 P.M.	7 P.M.

Polyurethane
1. Dobhoff (18 tubes)
2. Entriflex (18)
3. Travasorb (18)

1. Cranberry Juice

2. Cola Beverage

Silicone
1. Argyle (18)
2. McGraw (18)
3. Duotube (18)

3. Water

Repeated for 3 Days

FIGURE 2A-3
Repeated measures design for Metheny, Eisenberg, and McSweeny's (1988) study of the effect of feeding tube properties and irrigants on clogging rates.

6. **Design.** An experimental design of repeated measures was used in this study (Fig. 2A-3). The diagram indicates the manipulation of two treatments, physical tube properties (material and diameter) and irrigants (cranberry juice, water, and Coca-Cola). The treatment of tube properties (T_1) was held constant throughout the data collection process. The treatment (T_2) of the irrigants was implemented three times a day for 3 days, and the flow rates through the different tubes were measured (M) every 2 hours for 3 days.

7. **Sample.** "One hundred and eight feeding tubes were studied over 3 consecutive 12-hour days. There were 54 polyurethane and 54 silicone tubes equally divided among external diameters of 8 Fr, 10 Fr, and 12 Fr" (Metheny et al., 1988, p. 166). The number and type of tubes used in the study are identified in Figure 2A-3.

8. **Data Collection.** "Each tube was connected to a gravity flow feeding bag containing 200 ml of isotonic enteral formula. . . . To facilitate collection of data, six 'stations' were set up. At each station, there were three sets of tubes (a set was defined as one of each of the six types of tubes). . . . One set of tubes at each station was irrigated with cranberry juice, one with Coca-Cola, and one with tap water. . . . Actual amounts of formula delivered

per tube were monitored at 2-hour intervals (9:00 A.M., 11:00 A.M., 1:00 P.M., 3:00 P.M., 5:00 P.M., and 7:00 P.M.) for three days" (Metheny et al., 1988, p. 166) (Fig. 2A-3).

9. ***Results.*** "On each of the 3 days, both the univariate and multivariate ANO-VAs revealed significant, $p < .05$, effects of tube material, of cranberry juice contrasted with Coca-Cola and water as irrigants, and of time. Polyurethane was consistently superior to silicone as a tube material, and cranberry juice was consistently inferior to both Coca-Cola and water as an irrigant" (p. 167).

10. ***Discussion.*** "Among the tube properties examined the only significant finding was the superiority of polyurethane over silicone in promoting flow of enteral formula. . . . Contrary to some reports in the literature, cranberry juice is not an effective irrigant to prevent tube clogging. . . . Although it was hypothesized that Coca-Cola would be a more effective irrigant than water because of its carbonation and relatively low pH, this was not supported. . . . Thus, considering all of the above factors, it is logical to use polyurethane tubes of 10 Fr or 12 Fr diameters. Awareness of the effect of feeding tube properties on flow rate and ability to check placement gives the nurse more influence with the purchasing department when it is time to order feeding tubes. Selection of a tube least likely to clog during use is cost-effective, even though it may be somewhat more expensive than another tube of lesser quality" (p. 168).

Research Problems, Purposes, and Hypotheses

Completing this chapter should enable you to:

1. Define the concepts research topic, problem, and purpose.
2. Differentiate the research problem from the purpose.
3. Identify research topics, problems, and purposes in published quantitative, qualitative, and outcomes studies.
4. Examine the significance of research problems and purposes in published studies.
5. Critique the feasibility of a study problem and purpose by examining the researcher's expertise; money commitment; availability of subjects, facilities, and equipment; and the study's ethical considerations.
6. Examine the use of objectives, questions, and hypotheses in published studies.
7. Differentiate among the types of hypotheses (simple versus complex, nondirectional versus directional, associative versus causal, and statistical versus research).
8. Critique the quality of objectives, questions, and hypotheses presented in published studies.
9. Describe the different types of variables.
10. Differentiate between conceptual and operational definitions of variables.
11. Critique the conceptual and operational definitions of variables in published studies.
12. Use critical thinking in determining the significance and clarity of the problem, purpose, and definitions of variables in published studies.

Conceptual definition
Hypothesis
    Associative hypothesis
    Causal hypothesis
    Complex hypothesis
    Directional hypothesis ·
    Nondirectional hypothesis
    Null (statistical) hypothesis
    Research hypothesis
    Simple hypothesis
    Testable hypothesis
Operational definition
Research objective
Research problem

Research purpose
Research question
Research topic
Sample characteristics
Variables
    Confounding variable
    Demographic variables
    Dependent variable
    Environmental variable
    Extraneous variables
    Independent (treatment or
        experimental) variable
    Research variable or concept

*W*e are constantly asking questions to gain a better understanding of ourselves and the world around us. This human ability to wonder and ask creative questions is the first step in the research process. By asking questions, nurse researchers are able to identify significant research topics and problems that require study. A *research topic* is a concept or broad issue that is important to nursing, such as pain management, health promotion, or chronic illness. Each topic contains numerous potential research problems. For example, chronic pain is a research topic that includes potential problems such as these: What is chronic pain? How can chronic pain be assessed? What is it like to live with chronic pain? What are effective interventions for managing chronic pain? The problem or area of concern provides the basis for developing the research purpose. The purpose or goal of a study is closely linked to the objectives, questions, or hypotheses that guide the conduct of the study. Objectives, questions, or hypotheses are included in a study to bridge the gap between the more abstractly stated problem and purpose and the detailed design and plan for data collection and analysis. Objectives, questions, and hypotheses include the variables, the relationships among the variables, and often the population to be studied. Variables are concepts at various levels of abstraction that are measured, manipulated, or controlled in a study.

This chapter includes content that will assist you in differentiating a problem from a purpose and critiquing the problems and purposes in published quantitative, qualitative, and outcomes studies. Objectives, questions, and hypotheses are also discussed, and the different types of study variables are introduced. The chapter concludes with critical thinking exercises that guide the critique of the objectives, questions, hypotheses, and variables in published studies.

What Are a Research Problem and Purpose?

A *research problem* is a situation in need of solution, improvement, or alteration (Adebo, 1974) or "a discrepancy between the way things are and the way they ought to be" (Diers, 1979, p. 12). In a published study, the research problem identifies an area of concern for a particular population and outlines the need for additional study. Not all published studies include a clearly expressed problem, but the problem can usually be identified in the first or second paragraph of the article. The research problem from Palmer, Myers, and Fedenko's (1997) study of "Urinary continence changes after hip-fracture repair" is presented as an example.

> "A hip fracture is a significant event, adversely affecting an older adult's functional and psychosocial well-being. Despite an increasingly shorter hospital length of stay and rapid postoperative ambulation, surgical repair of a hip fracture signifies a sudden and perhaps prolonged period of altered mobility. There is a well-known relation-

ship between mobility status and urinary continence in older adults (Diokno, Brock, Herzog, & Bromberg, 1990; Jirovec, 1991; Ouslander, Palmer, Rovner, & German, 1994). Although the urinary tract may be normal, lack of access to the toilet for bladder emptying may lead to a transient state of incontinence until access is achieved, or if access and assistance are denied, to a permanent or chronic condition.

Cognitive impairment is also associated with urinary incontinence (Skelly & Flint, 1995). One population study found incontinence in more than 6% of the adults with some degree of cognitive impairment. . . ." (pp. 8–9)

"Urinary incontinence and urinary tract infections are genitourinary complications that may be present after hip fracture (Gordon, 1989). **However, the prevalence, incidence, and risk factors of incontinence and bacteriuria after hip fracture in older adults have not been investigated**." (p. 9)

The first two paragraphs of this study provide the background for and significance of the problem statement that is highlighted in boldface. The background for this problem includes previous studies conducted on the research topic of urinary incontinence and the associated risk factors of altered mobility and cognitive impairment. The problem is significant because of the incidence and seriousness of hip fractures in the elderly and the possible complication of incontinence. In addition, this problem is significant to nurses who are responsible for the postoperative care of patients with hip-fracture repairs. The highlighted problem statement identifies the area of concern as "the prevalence, incidence, and risk factors of incontinence and bacteriuria" and the study population as older adults experiencing hip-fracture repair. These researchers clearly expressed their study problem and documented that little is known about changes in continence status after hip-fracture repair and the need for additional research.

The *research purpose* is a clear, concise statement of the specific aim or intent of a study. The aim of a study might be to identify, describe, or explain a situation or predict a solution to a problem. The purpose also includes the variables, the population, and often the setting for the study. A clearly stated research purpose can capture the essence of a study in a single sentence and is essential to direct the remaining steps of the research process (Creswell, 1994). In a published study, the purpose statement is often presented after the problem or the literature review. In addition, the purpose is often reflected in the title of the study and is the first line of the study abstract. Palmer et al. (1997) presented the purpose of their study in the title of their research article,

"Urinary continence changes after hip-fracture repair." In addition, the purpose was stated after the study problem: "The purpose of this study was to determine the prevalence, incidence, and [risk factors] of the postoperative complication urinary incontinence [in the older adult following hip-fracture repair]" (p. 10).

The aim of this study is **descriptive** of the prevalence, incidence, and risk factors of urinary incontinence. The study variables are urinary incontinence and risk factors of incontinence, the population is older adults with hip-fracture repair, and the setting is the hospital. The purpose statement would have been more complete if the variable of risk factors, which included cognitive impairment and mobility status, had not been omitted and the population had been identified.

Identifying the Problem and Purpose in Quantitative, Qualitative, and Outcomes Studies

Quantitative, qualitative, and outcomes research approaches enable nurses to investigate a variety of research problems and purposes. Examples of research topics, problems, and purposes for different types of quantitative studies (descriptive, correlational, quasi-experimental, and experimental) are presented in Table 3-1. Not all published studies include a clearly expressed problem and purpose, and these must be extracted from the article. The research purpose usually reflects the type of study that was conducted. The purpose of descriptive research is to describe concepts or variables, identify possible relationships, and describe differences among groups. Edel, Houston, Kennedy, and LaRocco (1998) described the number and types of microbes found on artificial, polished, and natural nails following a 5-minute surgical scrub. These authors found that artificial nails harbored a significantly higher number of bacteria than polished or natural nails and that polished nails harbored a significantly higher number of bacteria than natural nails. Thus, this study provides clear direction for practice in that natural nails are safer in preventing the transmission of bacteria.

The purpose of correlational research is to examine the strength (low, moderate, or high) and type (positive or negative) of relationships among study variables. Bournaki (1997) conducted a correlational study to examine the relationships of selected variables to the pain-related responses to venipuncture in school-age children (see Table 3-1). This researcher found significant correlations between pain intensity, pain quality, behavioral responses, and heart rate, which support the multidimensionality of children's pain. These findings support the need to assess children's pain in practice and to identify factors that may aggravate their pain.

Quasi-experimental and experimental studies are conducted to determine the effect of a treatment or independent variable on designated dependent or outcome variables. Meek (1993) studied the effects of slow-stroke back massage on the relaxation of hospice patients and found this treatment extremely effective in promoting the comfort of the terminally ill. Thus, slow-stroke back massage is a research-based nursing intervention that you could use in your practice to promote the comfort and relaxation of your patients. If little is known about a topic, the researcher usually starts with a descriptive study and progresses to the other types of studies. By examining the problems and purposes in Table 3-1, you can note the differences and similarities among the types of quantitative research.

The problems formulated for qualitative research identify areas of concern that require investigation to gain new insights, expand understanding, or improve comprehension of the whole. The purpose of a qualitative study indicates the focus of the study, which might be a concept such as pain, an event such as loss of a child, or a facet of a culture such as the healing practices of the American Indian. In addition, the purpose often identifies the qualitative approach used and the basic assumptions for this approach (Creswell, 1994). Examples of research topics, problems, and purposes for some of the types of qualitative research conducted in nursing are presented in Table 3-2.

Phenomenological research is conducted to promote an understanding of human experiences from an individual researcher's perspective, like patients' lived experience of comfort (Morse, Bofforff, & Hutchinson, 1995). In grounded theory research, the problem identifies the area of concern and the purpose indicates the focus of the theory to be developed from the research. For example, Logan and Jenny (1997) investigated patients' work during mechanical ventilation and weaning to develop a theory of ventilator weaning. You could use this theory to facilitate the weaning of patients from ventilators. In ethnographic research, the problem and purpose identify the culture and the specific attributes of the culture that are to be examined and described. The problem and purpose in historical research focus on a specific individual, a characteristic of society, an event, or a situation in the past and identify the time period in the past that was examined by the study. For example, Wilderquist (1992) examined the life of Florence Nightingale to gain an understanding of her beliefs and spirituality and the link to spiritual issues surrounding nursing today.

Outcomes research is conducted to examine the end results of care. Table 3-3 includes the topics, problem, and purpose from an outcomes study by Rudy, Daly, Douglas, Montenegro, Song, and Dyer (1995). This study was conducted to determine the patient outcomes for the chronically critically ill in the special care unit (SCU) versus the intensive care unit (ICU). Common outcomes of cost, patient satisfaction, length of stay, complications, and readmissions were examined to determine the impact of care from these two units on the patients and the health care system. The findings from this 4-year study demonstrated that nurse case managers in an SCU setting can produce patient outcomes equal to or better than those obtained in the traditional ICU environment for long-term, critically ill patients. In addition, the SCU group showed significant cost savings compared to the ICU group.

Text continued on page 74

TABLE 3-1. Quantitative Research: Topics, Problems, and Purposes		
Type of Research	*Research Topic*	*Research Problem and Purpose*
Descriptive Research	Aseptic technique (scrubbing for operating room), microbial flora, hygiene of fingernails	*Title of Study:* "Impact of a 5-minute scrub on the microbial flora found on artificial, polished, or natural fingernails of operating room personnel" (Edel, Houston, Kennedy, & LaRocco, 1998).
		Problem: "For many years, maintaining short and polish-free fingernails has been part of the Recommended Standards of Practice for scrubbing and gowning of operating room (OR) personnel. . . . However, in recent years as artificial nails have become more popular, some physicians, OR nurses, and other health care providers have challenged these guidelines, claiming that nails with frequent care provided by nail technicians are healthier than unmanicured natural nails. . . . A limited number of studies have been conducted to determine the relationship of artificial nails to bacterial colonization. . . . Only one study has examined bacterial colonization associated with polished nails" (Edel et al., 1998, pp. 54–55).
		Purpose: "The purpose of this study was to determine whether differences exist in the presence and type of microbes found on the nails and nail beds of OR personnel with natural, polished, or artificial nails before and after a 5-minute surgical scrub" (Edel et al., 1998, p. 55). Comparative descriptive study examining the number and type of microbes on three types of nails (three-group descriptive comparison).
Correlational Research	Pain-related responses, venipuncture	*Title of Study:* "Correlates of pain-related responses to venipunctures in school-age children" (Bournaki, 1997).
		Problem: "Venipunctures are described as painful procedures by hospitalized children (Van Cleve, Johnson, & Pothier, 1996; Wong & Baker, 1988) and the most difficult to deal with by adolescent oncology survivors. . . . However, not all children respond similarly to venipunctures. . . . Factors that account for variability in children's responses to venipunctures have not been fully identified" (Bournaki, 1997, p. 147).
		Purpose: "The purpose of this study, therefore, was to examine the relationship of a set of correlates, including age, gender, past painful experiences, temperament, general and medical fears, and child-rearing practices, on school-age children's subjective, behavioral, and heart rate responses to

TABLE 3-1. *Continued*		
Type of Research	*Research Topic*	*Research Problem and Purpose*
		a venipuncture'' (Bournaki, 1997, p. 147). Predictive correlational study in which selected variables were correlated and used to predict children's responses to venipuncture.
Quasi-experimental Research	Nonpharmacologic intervention of slow stroke back massage, relaxation	*Title of Study:* ''Effects of slow stroke back massage on relaxation in hospice clients'' (Meek, 1993).
		Problem: ''Alleviation of symptoms and pain control to increase comfort are the primary goals of palliative nursing care. . . . Therefore, it is essential to investigate nursing interventions such as relaxation techniques which may add to the comfort of terminally ill people'' (Meek, 1993, p. 17).
		Purpose: ''The purpose of this study was to examine the effects of a nonpharmacologic intervention, slow stroke back massage (SSBM), on systolic and diastolic blood pressure, heart rate, and skin temperature as indicators of relaxation in hospice clients'' (Meek, 1993, p. 9).
Experimental Research	Sleep deprivation, wound healing	*Title of Study:* ''Effects of 72 hours of sleep deprivation on wound healing in the rat'' (Landis & Whitney, 1997).
		Problem: ''Sleep is thought to be essential for recovery from injury, and lost or disturbed sleep is believed to hinder postinjury wound healing (tissue repair). Disrupted and lost sleep are common experiences in the immediate postoperative period . . . and patients often express concern about losing sleep after surgery. . . . The consequences of lost sleep are of particular concern to nurses and other clinicians who provide or guide care for patients after acute surgical or accidental injury and are in a position to facilitate or educate patients about sleep. Questions regarding the possible effects of sleep loss on tissue repair and mechanisms by which sleep loss might negatively affect wound healing have been raised (Lee & Stotts, 1990), but no investigators have systematically evaluated the impact of sleep loss on tissue repair at cellular and subcellular levels'' (Landis & Whitney, 1997, p. 259).
		Purpose: ''The purpose of this study was to determine the effects of 72 hours of sleep loss on cellular markers of the proliferative and early collagen biosynthesis phases of wound healing'' (Landis & Whitney, 1997, p. 261).

TABLE 3-2. Qualitative Research: Topics, Problems, and Purposes		
Type of Research	*Research Topic*	*Research Problem and Purpose*
Phenomenological Research	Comfort, illness, injury, lived experience	*Title of Study:* "The paradox of comfort" (Morse, Bottorff, & Hutchinson, 1995).
		Problem: "What is comfort? In nursing, the term appears frequently in clinical texts, where 'making the patient comfortable' is a nursing goal. . . . Interestingly, although relatively little attention has been paid to the concept of comfort, nurses are often judged by their ability to make their patients comfortable . . . comfort remains an illusive goal for nursing, and we know little about how it is experienced by patients" (Morse et al., 1995, p. 14).
		Purpose: "In this study, the phenomenological method as described by van Manen (1990) was used to explore and reflect on patients' experiences of illness or injury. The aim of this study was to uncover and gain a deeper understanding of the meaning of comfort as an everyday experience" (Morse et al., 1995, p. 15).
Grounded Theory Research	Mechanical ventilation, weaning, patient's experience	*Title of Study:* "Qualitative analysis of patients' work during mechanical ventilation and weaning" (Logan & Jenny, 1997).
		Problem: "Mechanical ventilation and weaning present significant challenges for clinicians. A substantial minority of patients who receive mechanical ventilation support have considerable weaning difficulties and account for a disproportionate amount of health care costs. . . . Predictors of weaning success have been studied extensively, primarily from physiologic and technologic perspectives. Less attention has been paid to patients' subjective experience of mechanical ventilation and weaning, even though psychologic factors have been proposed as important determinants of outcomes in some patients, particularly for those requiring prolonged ventilator support" (Logan & Jenny, 1997, p. 140).
		Purpose: "The purpose of this study was to examine patients' subjective experiences of mechanical ventilation and weaning to validate and extend previous work. The study also contributes another perspective to an evolving theory of ventilator weaning" (Logan & Jenny, 1997, p. 141).

TABLE 3-2. *Continued*		
Type of Research	*Research Topic*	*Research Problem and Purpose*
Ethnography Research	Inner-city ghettos, survival, elders, drug activity	*Title of Study:* "Center as haven: Findings of an urban ethnography" (Kauffman, 1995).
		Problem: "In underserved, inner-city ghettos known for drug-related violence and crime, active participation in community life is dangerous and even life-threatening. This is especially true for elders burdened with the infirmities of aging and lacking the means to provide for alternatives to social isolation. Few researchers have ventured into inner-city communities known for troublesome and dangerous public spaces. . . . Therefore, little is known about the social lives of people in these communities, in particular, vulnerable older people who are frequently victims of illegal drug activity" (Kauffman, 1995, p. 231).
		Purpose: "This urban ethnography was conducted over a period of three years in a predominantly African American inner-city ghetto. The main question to be answered was: How do elders survive in the midst of 'drug warfare' in an inner-city community known for its dangerous streets and public spaces?" (Kauffman, 1995, p. 231).
Historical	Spirituality, beliefs, morals, religion	*Title of Study:* "The spirituality of Florence Nightingale" (Widerquist, 1992).
		Problem: "Rigid morals characterize the nineteenth century in the minds of most twentieth-century people. . . . While Nightingale's moral beliefs are well documented, less is known about why she held them. Moral and spiritual are not necessarily the same. . . . To simply define Florence Nightingale's beliefs, however does not describe her spirituality—the force that motivated her life" (Widerquist, 1992, p. 49).
		Purpose: "An examination of Nightingale's life—what influenced her beliefs, how she arrived at them, and what she did about them—offers a deeper understanding of her spirituality and a greater awareness of the spiritual issues surrounding nursing" (Widerquist, 1992, p. 49).

TABLE 3-3. Outcomes Research: Topics, Problem, and Purpose		
Type of Research	*Research Topic*	*Research Problem and Purpose*
Outcomes Research	Patient outcomes, special care unit, intensive care unit, chronically critically ill	*Title of Study:* "Patient outcomes for the chronically critically ill: Special care unit versus intensive care unit" (Rudy, Daly, Douglas, Montenegro, Song, & Dyer, 1995, p. 324).
		Problem: "The original purpose of intensive care units (ICUs) was to locate groups of patients together who had similar needs for specialized monitoring and care so that highly trained health care personnel would be available to meet these specialized needs. As the success of ICUs has grown and expanded, the assumption that a typical ICU patient will require only a short length of stay in the unit during the most acute phase of an illness has given way to the recognition that stays of more than one month are not uncommon. . . . These long-stay ICU patients represent a challenge to the current system, not only because of costs, but also because of concern for patient outcomes. . . . While ample evidence confirms that this subpopulation of ICU patients represents a drain on hospital resources, few studies have attempted to evaluate the effects of a care delivery system outside the ICU setting on patient outcomes, costs, and nurse outcomes" (Rudy et al., 1995, p. 324).
		Purpose: "The purpose of this study was to compare the effects of a low-technology environment of care and a nurse case management care delivery system (specific care unit, SCU) with the traditional high-technology environment (ICU) and primary nursing care delivery system on the patient outcomes of length of stay, mortality, readmission, complications, satisfaction, and cost" (Rudy et al., 1995, p. 324).

Determining the Significance of a Study Problem and Purpose

A research problem is significant in nursing when it has the potential to generate or refine relevant knowledge for practice. In critiquing the significance of the problem and purpose in a published study, you need to determine whether the knowledge generated in the study (1) impacts nursing practice, (2) builds on previous research, (3) promotes theory testing or development, and/or (4) addresses current concerns or priorities in nursing (Moody, Vera, Blanks, & Visscher, 1989).

Impacts Nursing Practice

The practice of nursing needs to be based on empirical knowledge or knowledge that is generated through research. Thus, studies that address clinical concerns and generate findings to improve nursing practice are considered significant. Several research problems and purposes have focused on the effects of nursing interventions or on ways to improve these interventions. For example, researchers have examined the effects of (1) pelvic muscle exercises on stress urinary incontinence (Sampselle & DeLancey, 1992); (2) pulmonary rehabilitation program on self-efficacy, perception of dyspnea, and physical endurance (Scherer & Schmieder, 1997); and (3) warm and cold applications on the resolution of intravenous infiltrations (Hastings-Tolsma, Yucha, Tompkins, Robson, & Szeverenyi, 1993). These studies generated knowledge that can be used to improve the care provided to patients and their families.

Builds on Previous Research

A significant study problem and purpose are based on previous research. In a research article, the introduction and literature review sections include relevant studies that provide a basis for a study. Often a summary of the current literature indicates what is known and not known in the area being studied. The gaps in the current knowledge base provide support for and document the significance of the study's purpose. For example, Palmer et al. (1997) provided documentation from several sources that mobility status and cognitive impairment influence the incidence of urinary incontinence. Thus, this study was based on previous research. In addition, they indicated what was not known, which was the prevalence, incidence, and risk factors of urinary incontinence in older adults with hip fractures. What was not known regarding the topic of urinary incontinence became the focus of the Palmer et al. (1997) study. The intent was to generate knowledge about the risk factors of urinary incontinence in the elderly to improve their care postoperatively following hip fracture repair.

Promotes Theory Testing or Development

Significant problems and purposes are supported by theory. A study might focus on either testing or developing theory (Chinn & Kramer, 1991). For example, Jemmott and Jemmott (1991) tested the theory of reasoned action (Ajzen & Fishbein, 1980) in their study of condom use among black women. They tested the following proposition or relational statement from the theory: "A behavioral intention is seen as determined by the attitude toward the specific behavior and the subjective norm regarding that behavior" (p. 228). They then linked the proposition to their study by stating: "Thus, a woman's intention to use condoms is a function of her attitude—positive or negative—toward using condoms and her perception of what significant others think she should do"

(p. 229). Based on this theoretical proposition, Jemmott and Jemmott developed the following hypotheses:

> "First, women who express more favorable attitudes toward condoms will report stronger intentions to use condoms than will women who express less favorable attitudes. Second, women who perceive subjective norms more supportive of condom use will report stronger intentions to use condoms than will their counterparts who perceive subjective norms less supportive of condom use."
> (pp. 229–230)

By conducting this study, Jemmott and Jemmott tested the theory of reasoned action (Ajzen & Fishbein, 1980) to determine its usefulness in describing people's attitudes and behavior about condom use. The study findings supported the hypotheses that attitudes and perceived subjective norms influence black women's use of condoms. Thus, the proposition from the theory was supported.

Addresses Nursing Research Priorities

Since 1975, expert researchers, specialty groups, and the National Institute for Nursing Research (NINR) have identified research priorities. Lindeman (1975) developed an initial list of research priorities for clinical practice, which identified such priorities as nursing interventions related to stress, care of the aged, pain management, and patient education. The American Association of Critical-Care Nurses (AACN) determined initial research priorities in the early 1980s (Lewandowski & Kositsky, 1983) and revised these priorities for the 1990s (Lindquist et al., 1993). The top clinical research priorities for critical-care nursing in the 1990s included:

> 1. "Techniques to optimize pulmonary functioning and prevent pulmonary complications.
> 2. Weaning of mechanically ventilated patients.
> 3. Effect of nursing activities/interventions on hemodynamic parameters.
> 4. Techniques for real-time monitoring of tissue perfusion and oxygenation.
> 5. Nutritional support modalities and patient outcomes.
> 6. Interventions to prevent infection.
> 7. Pain assessment and pain management techniques." (p. 115)

In 1994, Bayley, Richmond, Noroian, and Allen conducted a study to identify research priorities for trauma nursing. The four top priority questions included: "(1) What are the most effective nursing interventions in the prevention of pulmonary and circulatory complications in trauma patients? (2) What are the most effective methods for preventing aspiration in the trauma patient during the postoperative phase? (3) What psychological and lifestyle changes result from traumatic injury? and (4) What is the effect of early mobilization on the incidence of complications and length of stay in trauma patients?" (Bayley et al., 1994, p. 213).

The American Association of Occupational Health Nurses (AAOHN) identified research priorities for occupational health nursing. The top two priorities were "(1) the effectiveness of primary health care delivery at the worksite, and (2) effectiveness of health promotion nursing intervention strategies" (Rogers, 1989, p. 497).

In 1991, the Oncology Nursing Society (ONS) published the research priorities for the 1990s by surveying 310 ONS members (Mooney, Ferrell, Nail, Benedict, & Haberman, 1991). The top 10 research topics identified were quality of life, symptom management, outcome measures, pain control and management, cancer survivorship, prevention and early detection, research utilization, cancer rehabilitation, cost containment, and economic influences.

As more health care is provided in the home, Albrecht (1992) recognized the importance of developing a list of the research priorities for home health nursing. These priorities were generated by surveying 50 experts in the field of home health, and the top 10 research priorities identified were (1) outcomes of care, (2) cost of home care, (3) policy analysis and reimbursement, (4) client classification systems, (5) uniform data set, (6) predictors of care/managed care, (7) coordination of care/managed care, (8) productivity, (9) documentation, and (10) use of health care services.

The American Organization of Nurse Executives (AONE) identified research priorities for nurses in executive practice. The priority research strategies identified include (1) examining the impact of redesign on patient care outcomes, (2) determining the role of nursing leadership in the current health care system, (3) managing cultural/workforce diversity, (4) examining the impact of information systems technology, and (5) implementing models for widespread dissemination and effective utilization of research information in practice (Beyers, 1997). Nurse executives support of the use of research findings in practice is critical to the implementation of quality nursing care. Hopefully, this indicates that you will receive support as you attempt to use research findings in your practice.

A major initiative of the NINR is the development of a National Nursing Research Agenda that will involve identifying nursing research priorities, outlining a plan for implementing priority studies, and obtaining resources to support these priority projects. Initially, seven broad priority areas (research topics) for nursing research were identified in 1989: "(1) low birth weight: mothers and infants; (2) HIV infection: prevention and care; (3) long-term care for older adults; (4) symptom management; (5) information systems; (6) health promotion; and (7) technology dependency across the life span" (Bloch, 1990, p. 4). These topics were then analyzed by a Priority Expert Panel (PEP), and research priorities were selected to guide a portion of the NINR's funding through 1999. The funding priority for 1996 was research focused on the effectiveness of nursing interventions in HIV/AIDS, especially for individuals of different cultures and women. Cognitive impairment was the research funding priority for 1997, with a focus on research to develop and test biobehavioral and environmental approaches to manage cognitive impairment. Living with chronic illness was the funding priority for 1998, with a focus on research to test interventions that might increase individuals' resources in dealing with their chronic illnesses. In 1999, the research funding priorities are biobehavioral factors related to immunocompetence, with research focused on identifying biobehavioral factors and testing interventions to promote immunocompetence (NINR, 1993). NINR is also exploring opportunities in genetic research including basic genetic studies and applied studies to translate basic scientific findings into interventions to manage current clinical problems (Sigmon, Grady, & Amende, 1997).

Another federal agency that is having a major impact on setting research priorities for funding is the Agency for Health Care Policy and Research (AHCPR). This agency funds health services research that examines patient outcomes and the effectiveness of clinical practice (Rettig, 1990). The goals of outcomes research are to (1) avoid adverse effects of care, (2) improve the patient's physiological status, (3) reduce the patient's signs and symptoms, (4) improve the patient's functional status and well-being, (5) achieve patient satisfaction, (6) minimize the cost of care, and (7) maximize revenues (Davies, Doyle, Lansky, Rutt, Stevic, & Doyle, 1994). Outcomes research is not a new methodology in nursing but has received limited attention over the last 25 years. Heater, Becker, and Olson (1988) conducted a meta-analysis of the studies from 1977 to 1984 that were focused on nursing interventions and patient outcomes. Eighty-four studies were analyzed, and the findings indicated that "patients who receive research-based nursing interventions can expect 28% better outcomes than 72% of the patients who receive standard care" (Heater et al., 1988, p. 303).

Expert researchers, professional organizations, and federal agencies have identified research priorities to direct the future conduct of health care research. When critiquing a study, you need to determine whether the problem and purpose are based on previous research, theory, and current research priorities. You also need to question whether the findings will have an impact on nursing practice. These elements document the significance of the study in developing and refining nursing knowledge.

Examining the Feasibility of a Problem and Purpose

In critiquing a study, you need to determine whether the problem and purpose were feasible for the researcher to study. The feasibility of a research problem and purpose is determined by examining the researchers' expertise; money commitment; availability of subjects, facilities, and equipment; and the study's ethical considerations (Kahn, 1994; Rogers, 1987). The feasibility of the Palmer et al. (1997) study of urinary continence changes after hip-fracture repair is critiqued and presented as an example.

Researcher Expertise

The research problem and purpose studied need to be within the area of expertise of the researchers. Research articles usually identify the education of the researchers and their current positions. This information indicates their research expertise and their area of clinical specialization.

THE FOLLOWING QUESTIONS might be used to assess the researchers' expertise in a research report:

1. *Were the researchers adequately prepared to conduct the study? Nurses with a doctorate degree, who have a strong background in conducting research, often collaborate with master's-prepared nurses, who have strong clinical expertise, to conduct studies.*
2. *Do the researchers have the clinical experience and/or expertise to conduct the study?*
3. *Do the researchers cite other studies they have conducted in this area?*
4. *Do the researchers acknowledge the assistance of others in the conduct of the study?*

The purpose of the Palmer et al. (1997) study was to determine the prevalence, incidence, and risk factors of the postoperative complication urinary incontinence in the older adult following hip-fracture repair. Palmer has a doctorate degree and is a faculty member and researcher at the University of Maryland School of Nursing. Myers also has a doctorate and is a senior staff fellow at the Laboratory of Behavioral Sciences at the National Institute on Aging. Both Palmer and Myers have a history of conducting research on urinary incontinence in the elderly, and their previous studies are cited in the study's reference list. Fedenko is a nurse practitioner in medical oncology at the Greenbaum Cancer Center. These authors' credentials indicate strong research and clinical expertise for conducting this study. In addition, Palmer et al. (1997) expressed thanks to individuals who assisted them with data collection, management, and analysis, as well as manuscript preparation, which indicates collaboration with others to facilitate the conduct of a quality research project.

Money Commitment

The problem and purpose studied are influenced by the amount of money available to the researcher. The cost of a research project can range from a few dollars for a student's small study to hundreds of thousands of dollars for complex projects. Did the researchers have the resources to complete a quality study? Sources of funding for a study are usually identified in the article. For example, the study might have been funded by a federal research grant or by a professional organization such as Sigma Theta Tau or the American Nurses Association. The researchers might have received financial assistance from companies that provided the equipment they needed.

Receiving funding for a study indicates a quality study that has been reviewed by peers. Palmer et al. (1997) did not indicate that their study was funded but did state that the study was part of a larger research project that might have been funded. The focus of the study was limited, and the study could have been accomplished without external funding. The research center at the University of Maryland School of Nursing probably provided support for data entry and analysis.

Availability of Subjects, Facilities, and Equipment

Researchers need to have adequate subjects, facilities, and equipment to implement their study. Most published studies indicate the sample size and setting(s) in the methods section of the research report. The following questions might be used to assess the adequacy of the sample and setting: Was the sample size adequate to address the research purpose? Was the facility appropriate and adequate for the research problem and purpose? Was an adequate sample size obtained from the designated setting? Did the study require a highly specialized laboratory or was a natural setting appropriate?

Most nursing studies are conducted in natural settings, such as a hospital unit, clinic, or client's home. Many of these facilities are easy to access. Palmer et al. (1997) obtained an adequate sample of 100 medical records for patients 55 years and older admitted for a fractured hip to the orthopedic units of a university-affiliated hospital and a community metropolitan hospital. The hospital personnel were supportive of the study and facilitated the record reviews. The sample size seems adequate to address the research purpose of this descriptive study.

Review the data collection section of the research article to determine if adequate equipment was available. Did the equipment function accurately during the study? Nursing studies frequently require a limited amount of equipment such as a tape or video recorder for interviews or physiological instruments such as an electrocardiogram (ECG) or thermometer. The Palmer et al. (1997) study required no equipment, and the record review was conducted with a standardized form to obtain the essential information from the patients' medical records.

Ethical Considerations

The purpose selected for investigation must be ethical, which means that the subjects' rights and the rights of others in the setting are protected (Burns & Grove, 1997). The following questions might be used to assess the ethical nature of a study: Does the study purpose appear to infringe upon the rights of the subjects? There are usually some risks in every study, but the value of the knowledge generated should outweigh the risks. Was it ethical to conduct this study based on the risks and benefits? Chapter 6 includes the steps for determining the benefit-risk ratio of a study.

In the Palmer et al. (1997) study, the benefits of determining the prevalence, incidence, and risk factors for urinary incontinence following hip-fracture repair of the elder outweigh any potential risks. Determining the risk factors for incontinence can provide the basis for implementing interventions to prevent this problem postoperatively. The investigators conducted record reviews and presented their results in such a manner that subjects could not be identified individually. The methods used in this study are thought to have minimal to no risks for the subjects. Thus, the study would probably be considered exempt from review by the hospital's Institutional Review Board (IRB) (Department of Health and Human Services, 1991).

Critiquing Problems and Purposes in Published Studies

THE PROBLEM and purpose should be clearly and concisely expressed in a published study. In addition, the significance and feasibility of the problem and purpose should be examined.

1. *Is the problem clearly and concisely expressed early in the study?*
2. *Is the problem sufficiently delimited in scope without being trivial?*
3. *Is the purpose clearly expressed?*
4. *Does the purpose narrow and clarify the focus and aim of the study?*
5. *Does the purpose identify the variables, population, and setting for the study?*
6. *Are the problem and purpose significant in generating nursing knowledge? Is the study based on previous research, theory, and/or current research priorities? Will the findings have an impact on nursing practice?*
7. *Was it feasible for the researchers to study the problem and purpose identified? Did the researchers have the expertise to conduct the study? Did they have adequate money, subjects, setting, and equipment to conduct the study? Was the purpose of the study ethical?*

Examining Research Objectives, Questions, and Hypotheses in Research Reports

Research objectives, questions, and hypotheses evolve from the problem, purpose, and study framework and direct the remaining steps of the research process. In a published study, the objectives, questions, or hypotheses are usually presented after the literature review section and right before the methods section. The content in this section is provided to assist you in identifying and critiquing objectives, questions, and hypotheses in published studies.

Research Objectives

A *research objective* is a clear, concise, declarative statement that is expressed in the present tense. For clarity, an objective usually focuses on one or two variables and indicates whether they are to be identified or described. Sometimes the purpose of objectives is to identify relationships among variables or to determine differences between two groups regarding selected variables. Sometimes the purpose statement is divided into two or three objectives. A descriptive study by Brown (1997) demonstrates the logical flow from research problem and purpose to research objectives.

Research Problem

"In the United States, cardiovascular disorders cause more deaths among adults than all other diseases combined. Approximately one third of all deaths in the United States are caused by ischemic heart disease, and of these, one half result from an acute myocardial infarction (AMI). . . . Today, there is a new population at risk for the development of cardiovascular disease, the cocaine user. . . . The use of cocaine as a recreational drug by young adults has increased markedly since the early 1980s and has resulted in a significant increase in hospital emergency room admissions, mortality, and morbidity. . . . Traditionally, only case studies, animal studies, and small samples of patients with AMI attributed to cocaine use have been reported. Little is known about chest pain syndromes after cocaine use, the patient's clinical symptomatology in the emergency department, or the risk factor profile of the cocaine user." (p. 136)

Research Purpose

"The purpose of this study was to examine the incidence of chest pain and cocaine use in 18–40 year olds who were seen in a public inner city emergency department." (p. 136)

Research Objectives

The objectives of this study were expressed in a detailed purpose statement indicating that the study was conducted "(1) to describe the incidence of cocaine use in 18–40 year old persons seen in a hospital emergency department with complaints of chest pain, and (2) to determine if there is a relationship among demographics, physiological, diagnostic, and patient history data associated with chest pain and cocaine use" (p. 136).

The cardiac problems with cocaine use identified by Brown (1997) are a significant health care concern that is increasing in prevalence in today's society. The purpose of the study identifies the goal or aim of the research and includes the study variables (cocaine use and risk profile of the cocaine user), population, and setting. The purpose of the first objective is to describe the incidence of cocaine use (variable) in 18- to 40-year-old persons with complaints of chest pain (populations) seen in hospital emergency departments (setting). The second objective focuses on the examination of relationships among selected variables that comprise the risk factor profile of a cocaine user (demographics, physiological, diagnostic, and patient history data) and the incidence of chest pain with cocaine use. The problem provides a basis for the purpose, and the objectives evolve from the purpose and clearly indicate the focus of the study.

Research Questions

A *research question* is a concise interrogative statement that is worded in the present tense and includes one or more variables (or concepts). The foci of research questions are description of the variable(s), examination of relationships among variables, and determination of differences between two or more groups regarding selected variable(s). Bostrom, Mechanic, Lazar, Michelson, Grant, and Nomura (1996) conducted a descriptive correlational study to examine the nursing practices, costs, and outcomes of preventing skin breakdown. The problem, purpose, and research questions used to guide this study are presented following.

Research Problem

"Operating efficiently within the constraints of shrinking financial parameters is a major concern of nursing administrators. Nurses are challenged to determine not only which nursing interventions are effective but also the cost impact of the various interventions. One nursing intervention that holds great potential for possible refinement of protocol and resultant cost reduction is prevention and management of skin breakdown. The cost of treatments for maintaining skin integrity ranges from $20 for a barrier dressing to several thousand dollars for a specialty bed. . . . A variety of intervention studies aimed at prevention of pressure sores have been conducted with patients identified at risk for altered skin integrity. . . . Cost analyses related to the use of these various interventions have not been published." (pp. 184–185)

Research Purpose

"The specific purpose of the investigation was to assess the relationships between the development of pressure ulcers during acute

continued

hospitalization and (a) skin breakdown risk and (b) types and costs of prevention strategies used by nurses." (p. 184)

Research Questions

The following questions were addressed in this study:

1. "What is the relationship between the Braden risk-factors scores for skin breakdown and actual skin breakdown in acute settings?
2. What is the relationship between the Braden risk-factors scores for skin breakdown and the strategies chosen for prevention of skin breakdown?
3. What is the relationship of both Braden risk-factors scores and strategies chosen for prevention of skin breakdown to actual skin breakdown?
4. What are the costs of skin breakdown prevention strategies?" (p. 185)

Skin breakdown is a significant health care problem that requires cost-effective nursing interventions to prevent. The research purpose clearly identifies the aim of the study: to assess the relationships between the development of pressure ulcers and skin breakdown risk and the types and costs of prevention strategies (variables) used on patients (population) during acute hospitalization (setting). The first, second, and third research questions focus on examining relationships (associations) among the study variables (Braden risk-factors scores for skin breakdown, incidence of skin breakdown, and prevention strategies). The fourth research question focuses on describing the costs of skin breakdown prevention strategies. The research questions reflect the problem and purpose and clearly indicate the focus of the study. These questions were presented just before the methods section of the article and were used to direct the implementation of the study procedures and the analysis of study data.

Hypotheses

A *hypothesis* is a formal statement of the expected relationship(s) between two or more variables in a specified population. The hypothesis translates the research problem and purpose into a clear explanation or prediction of the expected results or outcomes of the study. A clearly stated hypothesis includes the variables to be manipulated or measured, identifies the population to be examined, and indicates the proposed outcomes for the study. Hypotheses also influence the study design, sampling technique, data collection and analysis methods, and interpretation of findings. In this section, types of hypotheses are described and a testable hypothesis is discussed.

Types of Hypotheses

Different types of relationships and numbers of variables are identified in hypotheses. A study might have one, three, five, or more hypotheses, depending on its complexity. The type of hypothesis developed is based on the purpose of the study. Hypotheses can be described using four categories: (1) associative versus causal, (2) simple versus complex, (3) nondirectional versus directional and (4) null versus research.

Associative versus Causal Hypotheses. The relationships identified in hypotheses are associative or causal. An *associative hypothesis* proposes relationships among variables that occur or exist together in the real world, and when one variable changes, the other changes (Reynolds, 1971). Associative hypotheses are usually expressed using the following formats:

1. Variable X is related to variables Y and Z in a specified population. (Predicts relationships among variables but does not indicate the types of relationships.)
2. Variable X increases as variable Y increases in a specified population. (Predicts a positive relationship.)
3. Variable X decreases as variable Y decreases in a specified population. (Predicts a positive relationship.)
4. Variable X increases as variable Y decreases in a specified population. (Predicts a negative relationship.)

Associative hypotheses identify relationships among variables in a study but do not indicate cause and effect between variables or that one variable causes another variable to change. Lanza, Kayne, Pattison, Hicks, and Islam (1996) studied the relationship of behavioral cues to assaultive behavior and formulated the following problem, purpose, and associative hypotheses.

Research Problem

"Violence is now the Center for Disease Control's (CDC's) top priority (Rosenberg, 1993). Assault by patients on other patients and staff is reaching epidemic proportions both within hospital units and outpatient areas. The high rate of assault is a significant problem across types of institutions. . . . The assault rate increase in hospitals, reflecting the rising violence in society, has become a major public health problem. . . . Better understanding of the problem of assaultive behavior will enable clinicians to make more accurate assessments and design more effective interventions to reduce assault incidence." (pp. 6–7)

continued

Research Purpose

"The purpose of this study was to characterize patients who assaulted one or more times during the period of observation and to compare them to patients who had not assaulted. Factors compared were behavioral assessments and sociodemographic variables." (p. 8)

Hypotheses

1. "Patients who assault during the period of observation will differ from patients who do not in being more likely to have a history of violence and being more likely to have a history of alcohol abuse;
2. . . . patients who assault will exhibit more visibility cues (hostile verbalizations, increased motor activity, suspiciousness) than will nonassaultive patients;
3. . . . patients who assault and exhibit high-visibility cues (hostile verbalization, increased motor activity, suspiciousness) will score lower on the Withdrawal-Retardation Subscale. . . ." (p. 10)

The problem indicates the area of concern, that is, violence in health care settings, and the need for further study to manage this problem. The purpose is based on the problem and clearly identifies the goal of the study. The purpose also identifies the study variables (assaults, behavioral assessment, and sociodemographic variables) and population (patients) and indicates the setting (hospital). Hypotheses 1 and 2 state positive associations, which means that as variable X increases, there is an increase in variable Y. Hypothesis 1 predicts that an increase in assaults (X) is associated with an increase in history of violence (Y) and alcohol abuse (Z). Hypothesis 2 predicts that an increase in assaults (X) is related to an increase in visibility cues (Y). Hypothesis 3 includes two different types of relationships: increased assaults (X) is associated with increased high-visibility cues (Y) (positive relationship), and increased assaults (X) is associated with lower Withdrawal-Retardation Subscale scores (Z) (negative relationship). These hypotheses clearly identify the study variables and population and indicate the study outcomes. The results from the study only partially supported the hypotheses. Assaultive behavior was linked to a history of violence but not to alcohol dependence. Threatening language and increased motor activity were important signs of assault, but suspiciousness was not. There was no difference between the assaultive and nonassaultive patients on the Withdrawal-Retardation Subscale (Lanza et al., 1996).

A *causal hypothesis* proposes a cause-and-effect interaction between two or more variables, which are referred to as independent and dependent variables. The independent variable (treatment or experimental variable) is manipulated by the researcher to cause an effect on the dependent variable. The dependent variable (outcome or criterion variable) is measured to examine the effect created by the independent variable. A format for stating a causal hypothesis is: The subjects in the experimental group who are exposed to the independent variable demonstrate greater change, as measured by the dependent variable, than do the subjects in the control group who are not exposed to the independent variable. Coyne and Hoskins (1997) conducted a study "to determine the effects of directed verbal prompts and positive reinforcement on the level of eating independence (LEI) of elderly nursing home patients with dementia" (p. 275). The independent variables are the treatments of verbal prompts and positive reinforcement, and the dependent variable is LEI. The population is clearly identified as nursing home patients with dementia, and the setting is a nursing home. Coyne and Hoskins (1997) formulated the following causal hypothesis to direct their study: "subjects in the experimental group would exhibit higher independence and frequency scores when eating solid foods and liquids than the control group at posttest T2 (short-term effects) and T3 (long-term effects)" (p. 278). The experimental group received the treatment of verbal prompts to encourage eating and positive reinforcement when completing eating tasks that the control group did not receive. These treatments were proposed to cause a change in the dependent variable of increasing the level of eating independence in demented nursing home patients. The findings from this study supported the hypothesis, indicating that the treatments were effective in increasing eating behaviors in patients with dementia.

Simple versus Complex Hypotheses. A *simple hypothesis* states the relationship (associative or causal) between two variables. A *complex hypothesis* predicts the relationship (associative or causal) among three or more variables. In complex, causal hypotheses, relationships are predicted between two (or more) independent variables and/or two (or more) dependent variables. For example, Deiriggi (1990) conducted a quasi-experimental study "to test the effects of nonoscillating waterbed flotation on indicators of energy expenditure in preterm infants: motor activity, heart rate, and behavioral state" (p. 140). Table 3-4 includes the study's hypotheses, which are labeled "simple" or "complex" based on the number of independent and dependent variables in each hypothesis. These hypotheses might have been more reflective of the population studied rather than of the sample if they had been expressed in the present tense ("is") rather than the future tense ("will be"). This idea is expanded in the section on testable hypotheses in this chapter.

Nondirectional versus Directional Hypotheses. A *nondirectional hypothesis* states that a relationship exists but does not predict the nature of the relationship. If the direction of the relationship being studied is not clear in clinical practice or in the theoretical or empirical literature, the researcher has no clear indication of the nature of the relationship. Under these circumstances, nondirec-

TABLE 3-4. Simple and Complex Hypotheses		
	Independent Variables	*Dependent Variables*
Simple Hypotheses		
Motor activity over all states as well as within a given state will be (is) reduced during the on-waterbed period.	Waterbed flotation	Motor activity
Heart rate will be (is) reduced during the on-waterbed period.	Waterbed flotation	Heart rate
There will be (is) a greater percentage of time spent in sleep states versus awake states during the on-waterbed period.	Waterbed flotation	Sleep versus awake state
There will be (are) fewer sleep-to-wake transitions during the on-waterbed period. (Deiriggi, 1990, p. 141)	Waterbed flotation	Sleep-to-wake transitions
Complex Hypothesis		
The duration of sleep state epochs will be (is) greater during the on-waterbed period. The duration of waking activity and fuss state epochs will be (is) greater during the off-waterbed period (expressed as one hypothesis). (Deiriggi, 1990, p. 141)	Waterbed flotation	Sleep state epochs Waking activity Fuss state epochs

tional hypotheses are developed, such as those developed by Jirovec and Kasno (1990) to direct their study.

> 1. "Elderly nursing home residents' self-appraisals of their self-care abilities are related to the basic conditioning factors of sex, sociocultural orientation, health, and family influences.
> 2. Elderly nursing home residents' self-appraisals of their self-care abilities are related to their perceptions of the nursing home environment." (p. 304)

The first hypothesis is complex (five variables), associative, and nondirectional. The second hypothesis is simple (two variables), associative, and nondirectional. Both hypotheses state that a relationship exists but do not indicate the direction of the relationship. The hypotheses also clearly identify the study variables (self-appraisals of self-care abilities, basic conditioning factors, and perceptions of nursing home environment), population (elderly), and setting (nursing home) and indicate the expected outcomes of the study.

A *directional hypothesis* states the nature (positive or negative) of the interaction between two or more variables. Directional hypotheses are developed from theoretical statements (propositions), findings of previous studies, and clinical experience. As the knowledge on which a study is based increases, the researcher is able to make a prediction about the direction of a relationship between the variables being studied. For example, Baker, Garvin, Kennedy, and Polivka (1993) developed a directional hypothesis to study the effect of environmental sound and communication on coronary care unit patients' heart rate (HR) and blood pressure (BP). They developed their study hypothesis based on previous research and theory, as indicated by the following quotation:

> "Overall, the findings of previous studies suggest that ambient and social stressors in coronary care are associated with cardiovascular (CV) changes in patients. However, it is not known if different CV effects occur with background sounds than with communication. Since stress is viewed as a person-environment relationship (Lazarus, Delongis, Folkman, & Gruen, 1985), the goal of this study was to examine factors in the natural environment that are associated with the stress response. The assumption was made that naturally occurring sounds, such as conversation and equipment, have personal meaning to subjects. The patient appraises the meaning through cognitive processes which in turn can produce autonomic CV arousal. Data suggest that persons with CV disease are more reactive to mental stress than persons without CV disease (Contrada & Krantz, 1988). It was **hypothesized** [emphasis added] that there would be an increase in patients' HR and BP during the high ambient stressors (environmental sounds) and social stressors (room and hall conversation) as compared to low ambient (background) sounds." (p. 416)

The use of terms such as *less, more, increase, decrease, greater, higher,* and *lower* in a hypothesis indicate the direction of the relationship. In Baker et al.'s (1993) hypothesis, environmental sounds and room and hall conversation are positively related to patient HR and BP. Thus, as the environmental sounds and room and hall conversation increase, the patient's HR and BP increase.

A causal hypothesis predicts the effect of an independent variable on a dependent variable, specifying the direction of the relationship. Thus, all causal hypotheses are directional. As discussed earlier, Coyne and Hoskins (1997) formulated a causal hypothesis to direct their study and provided an experimental group with the treatments of verbal prompts to encourage eating and positive reinforcement when completing eating tasks (independent variables) to *increase* the level of eating independence (dependent variable) in demented nursing home patients. Thus, this causal hypothesis is directional, since the treatment is proposed to increase the LEI, and complex, since more than two variables are identified.

Null versus Research Hypotheses. The *null hypothesis* (H_0), also referred to as a *statistical hypothesis,* is used for statistical testing and for interpreting statistical outcomes. Even if the null hypothesis is not stated, it is implied, because it is the converse of the research hypothesis (Kerlinger, 1986). Some researchers state the null hypothesis because it is more easily interpreted based on the results of statistical analyses. The null hypothesis is also used when the researcher believes there is no relationship between two variables and when there is inadequate theoretical or empirical information to state a research hypothesis.

A null hypothesis can be simple or complex and associative or causal. An example of a simple, associative, null hypothesis is "There is no relationship between the number of experiences performing a developmental assessment skill and learning of the skill" (Koniak, 1985, p. 85). Fahs and Kinney (1991) developed the following causal, null hypothesis to direct their study: "There is no difference in the occurrence of bruise at injection site with low-dose heparin therapy when administered in three different subcutaneous sites [abdomen, thigh, and arm]" (p. 204). There was no statistically significant difference in bruising at 60 and 72 hours postinjection for the three sites. Thus, this null hypothesis was supported and provides direction for giving heparin in clinical practice.

A *research hypothesis* is the alternative hypothesis (H_1 or H_A) to the null hypothesis and states that there is a relationship between two or more variables. All the hypotheses stated in previous sections of this chapter were research hypotheses. Research hypotheses can be simple or complex, nondirectional or directional, and associative or causal. Jadack, Hyde, and Keller (1995) formulated both research and null hypotheses to "examine gender differences in knowledge about HIV, the reported incidence of risky sexual behavior, and comfort with safer sexual practices among young adults" (p. 313). Each of the hypotheses is listed following, with a description indicating the type of hypothesis.

1. "There will be (is) no difference between men and women in knowledge about HIV transmission routes (sexual, needle sharing, casual)" (Jadack et al., 1995, p. 315). The type of hypothesis is null, associative, simple, and nondirectional, with two variables of gender and knowledge about HIV transmission routes.
2. "[T]here will be (is) no difference between men and women in

knowledge about the effectiveness of measures to prevent sexual transmission of HIV" (Jadack et al., 1995, p. 315). The type of hypothesis is null, simple, associative, and nondirectional, with two variables of gender and knowledge about effectiveness of measures to prevent sexual transmission of HIV.

3. "[M]en and women will differ with respect to reported frequency and type of behaviors that could lead to the transmission of HIV" (Jadack et al., 1995, p. 315). This hypothesis is research, associative, complex, and nondirectional. The variables are gender, frequency of behaviors, and types of behaviors. This hypothesis is nondirectional because there is no indication of how men and women will differ and associative because a relationship is stated with no indication of cause and effect.

4. "[M]en and women will differ with respect to reported level of comfort and safer sexual practices" (Jadack et al., 1995, p. 315). This hypothesis is research, complex, associative, and nondirectional. The variables are gender, level of comfort, and safer sexual practices. The hypothesis is nondirectional, with no indication of how men and women will differ, and associative because the relationship does not indicate cause and effect between variables.

Testable Hypothesis

A testable hypothesis is clearly stated, predicting a relationship between two or more variables. Hypotheses are clearer without the phrase "There is no *significant* difference" because the level of significance is only a statistical technique applied to sample data (Armstrong, 1981). In addition, hypotheses should not identify methodological points such as techniques of sampling, measurement, and data analysis (Kerlinger, 1986). Therefore, phrases such as "*measured by,*" "in a *random sample* of," and "*using ANOVA*" are inappropriate since they limit the hypotheses to the measurement methods, sample, or analysis techniques identified for one study. In addition, hypotheses need to reflect the variables and population outlined in the research purpose and should be expressed in the present tense, not the future tense. Expressing the hypotheses in the present tense does not limit them to the study being conducted and enables them to be used in additional research.

The value of a hypothesis is ultimately derived from whether it is testable in the real world. A *testable hypothesis* is one that contains variables that are measurable or able to be manipulated. Thus, the independent variable must be clearly defined so that it can be implemented precisely and consistently as a treatment in the study. The dependent variable must be precisely defined to indicate how it will be accurately measured.

A testable hypothesis also needs to predict a relationship that can be "supported" or "not supported" based on data collection and analysis. If the hypothesis states an associative relationship, correlational analyses are conducted on the data to determine the existence, type, and strength of the relationship between the variables studied. The hypothesis that states a causal relationship is evaluated using inferential statistics, such as the *t*-test and ANOVA. It is the null hypothesis (stated or implied) that is tested. The intent of the data analyses is to determine whether the independent variable produced a significant effect on the dependent variable.

Critiquing Research Objectives, Questions, and Hypotheses in Published Studies

The research objectives, questions, and hypotheses need to be clearly focused and concisely expressed in studies. Objectives or questions can be used in descriptive and correlational studies, but questions are more common. Some correlational studies focus on predicting relationships and might include hypotheses. Quasi-experimental and experimental studies need to be directed by hypotheses.

THE FOLLOWING QUESTIONS might help you critique the objectives, questions, and hypotheses in a study.

1. *Are the objectives, questions, or hypotheses formally stated in the study? If they were not stated, were they needed to direct the conduct of the study? If the study is quasi-experimental or experimental, hypotheses are needed to direct the study.*
2. *Are the objectives, questions, or hypotheses clearly focused and concisely expressed in the study? Do they clearly identify the variables and population to be studied?*
3. *Are the study objectives, questions, or hypotheses based on the purpose? They should not contain new concepts and populations that were not identified in the problem or purpose.*
4. *Are the variables and relationships among the variables identified in the objectives, questions, or hypotheses linked to the study framework?*
5. *Does each hypothesis predict a relationship between the variables?*
6. *Are the hypotheses associative or causal, simple or complex, directional or nondirectional, and/or research or null?*
7. *Are the hypotheses testable in this study? Thus, are they clearly stated in the present tense, with measurable dependent variables and appropriate independent variables that can be consistently implemented during the study?*

Understanding Study Variables

The research purpose and objectives, questions, and hypotheses include the variables or concepts to be examined in a study. *Variables* are qualities, properties, or characteristics of persons, things, or situations that change or vary. Variables are also concepts at different levels of abstraction that are concisely defined to promote their measurement or manipulation within a study (Chinn & Kramer, 1991). In this section, different types of variables are described, and conceptual and operational definitions of variables are discussed.

Types of Variables

Variables have been classified into a variety of types to explain their use in research. Some variables are manipulated; others are controlled. Some variables are identified but not measured; others are measured with refined measurement devices. The types of variables presented in this section include independent, dependent, research, extraneous, and demographic.

Independent and Dependent Variables

The relationship between independent and dependent variables is the basis for formulating hypotheses for correlational, quasi-experimental, and experimental studies. An *independent variable* is a stimulus or activity that is manipulated or varied by the researcher to create an effect on the dependent variable. The independent variable is also called a *treatment* or *experimental variable*. A *dependent variable* is the response, behavior, or outcome that the researcher wants to predict or explain. Changes in the dependent variable are presumed to be caused by the independent variable.

The null hypothesis tested by Lim-Levy (1982) was: "Oxygen inhalation by nasal cannula of up to 6 LPM [liters per minute] does not affect oral temperature" (p. 150). The independent variable is oxygen inhalation by nasal cannula, and the oxygen was administered at three levels: 2, 4, and 6 LPM. The dependent variable was oral temperature measured by an electronic thermometer. This null hypothesis was supported in the study, indicating that oxygen inhalation by nasal cannula does not affect oral temperature. These findings provide clear direction for you when you are taking the temperature of patients on nasal oxygen.

Research Variables or Concepts

Qualitative studies and some quantitative (descriptive and correlational) studies involve the investigation of research variables or concepts. *Research variables or concepts* are the qualities, properties, or characteristics identified in the research purpose and objectives or questions that are observed or measured in a study. Research variables or concepts are used when the intent of the study is to observe or measure variables as they exist in a natural setting without the implementation of a treatment. Thus, no independent variables are manipulated, and no cause-and-effect relationships are examined. Logan and Jenny (1997) conducted a qualitative study to describe patients' recollections of their experiences during mechanical ventilation and weaning and to extend an evolving nursing theory of weaning. The authors used grounded theory techniques to investigate the following concepts: (1) experiences with mechanical ventilation and (2) experiences during weaning.

Extraneous Variables

Extraneous variables exist in all studies and can affect the measurement of study variables and the relationships among these variables. Extraneous variables are of primary concern in quantitative studies because they can interfere with obtaining a clear understanding of the relational or causal dynamics within these studies. These variables are classified as recognized or unrecognized and controlled or uncontrolled. Some extraneous variables are not recognized until the study is in progress or is completed, but their presence influences the study outcome.

Researchers attempt to recognize and control as many extraneous variables as possible in quasi-experimental and experimental studies, and specific designs have been developed to control the influence of these variables. Lim-Levy (1982) controlled some of the extraneous variables in her study of the effect of oxygen inhalation by nasal cannula on oral temperature. The subjects who were mouth-breathing or hyperventilating or who had an oral inflammatory process were excluded because these characteristics might have influenced the oral temperature.

The extraneous variables that are not recognized until the study is in process, or are recognized before the study is initiated but cannot be controlled, are referred to as *confounding variables*. Sometimes extraneous variables can be measured during the study and controlled statistically during analysis. However, if these extraneous variables cannot be controlled or measured, this hinders the interpretation of findings. As control decreases in quasi-experimental and experimental studies, the potential influence of confounding variables increases.

Environmental variables are a type of extraneous variable composing the setting in which the study is conducted. Examples of these variables include climate, family, health care system, and governmental organizations. If a researcher is studying humans in an uncontrolled or natural setting, it is impossible and undesirable to control all the extraneous variables. In qualitative and some quantitative (descriptive and correlational) studies, little or no attempt is made to control extraneous variables. The intent is to study subjects in their natural environment without controlling or altering that setting. The environmental variables in quasi-experimental and experimental research can be controlled by using a laboratory setting or a specially constructed research unit in a hospital. Environmental control is an extremely important part of conducting an experimental study.

Demographic Variables

Demographic variables are characteristics or attributes of subjects that are collected to describe the sample. Some common demographic variables are age, education, gender, ethnic origin (race), marital status, income, job classification, and medical diagnosis(es). When a study is completed, the demographic data are analyzed to provide a picture of the sample and are called *sample characteristics*. A study's sample characteristics can be presented in table format or narrative. As discussed earlier in this chapter, Brown (1997) studied the incidence of chest pain and cocaine use in 18- to 40-year-old persons in a sample of 386 subjects. The demographic variables examined in this study included age, gender, race, marital status, education, employment, and insurance status. Table 3-5 presents the demographic profile of the subjects in Brown's (1997) study; this profile is also referred to as the sample characteristics for the study.

Sample characteristics can also be presented in narrative format in the research report. For example, Logan and Jenny (1997), in their study of patients' work during mechanical ventilation and weaning, described their sample of 20 subjects as follows:

> ". . . 11 were women and 9 were men. Their ages ranged from 19 to 83 years (mean 57.5 years). Twelve participants were married. Eleven patients had a variety of medical diagnoses, and nine had had surgical procedures. Severity of illness as measured by the Acute Physiological and Chronic Health Evaluation (APACHE III) scale ranged from 5 to 44 (mean 20.8) at the time of admission. Patients receive mechanical ventilator support from 5 to 214 days (mean 31.5, median 14.5 days). . . . Length of time for weaning ranged from 1 to 45 days (mean 15.1, median 6.24 days)." (p. 141)

Conceptual and Operational Definitions of Variables

A variable is operationalized in a study by the development of conceptual and operational definitions. A *conceptual definition* provides the theoretical meaning of a variable (Fawcett & Downs, 1992) and is often derived from a theorist's definition of a related concept. In a published study, the framework includes concepts and their definitions, and the variables are selected to represent the concepts. Thus, the variables are conceptually defined, indicating the link with the concepts in the framework. An *operational definition* is derived from a set of procedures or progressive acts that a researcher performs to receive sensory impressions (such as sound, visual, or tactile impressions) that indicate the existence or degree of existence of a variable (Reynolds, 1971). Operational definitions need to be independent of time and setting so that variables can be investigated at different times and in different settings using the same operational definitions. An operational definition is developed so that a variable can be measured or manipulated in a concrete situation, and the knowledge gained from studying the variable will increase the understanding of the theoretical concept that this variable represents.

	n	Percent
TABLE 3-5. Demographic Profile of Subjects (*N* = 386)		
Age		
18–24	78	20.2
25–32	136	35.2
33–40	172	44.6
Total	386	100.0
Sex		
Male	235	60.9
Female	151	39.1
Total	386	100.0
Race		
African American	322	83.4
Caucasian	62	16.1
Other	2	0.5
Total	386	100.0
Marital status		
Single	308	79.8
Married	74	19.2
Other	1	0.2
Not recorded	3	0.8
Total	386	100.0
Education		
Less than high school	35	9.1
High school diploma	43	11.1
Some college	9	2.3
College degree	3	0.8
Not recorded	296	76.7
Total	386	100.0
Employment		
Not employed	143	37.0
Employed	45	11.7
Not recorded	198	51.3
Total	386	100.0
Insurance		
Uninsured	190	49.2
Insured	8	2.1
Not recorded	188	48.7
Total	386	100.0

Source: Brown, S. C. (1997). Chest pain and cocaine use in 18 to 40 year-old persons: A retrospective study. *Applied Nursing Research, 10*(3), 137, with permission.

Corff, Seideman, Venkataraman, Lutes, and Yates (1995) conducted a study to determine the "effectiveness of facilitated tucking, a nonpharmacologic nursing intervention, as a comfort measure in modulating preterm neonates' physiologic and behavioral responses to minor pain" (p. 143). The hypothesis for this prospective study was that "preterm neonates would have less variation in heart rate, oxygen saturation, and sleep state (shorter crying and sleep disruption time and less fluctuation in sleep states) in response to

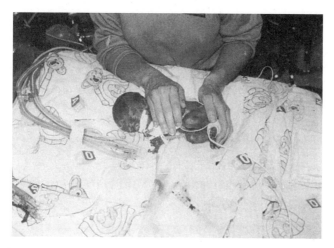

FIGURE 3-1
Facilitated tucking of a premature infant. (From Corff, K. E., Seideman, R., Venkataraman, P. S., Lutes, L., & Yates, B. [1995]. Facilitated tucking: A nonpharmacologic comfort measure for pain in preterm neonates. *Journal of Obstetric, Gynecologic and Neonatal Nursing, 24*[2], 144, with permission.)

the painful stimulus of a heelstick with facilitated tucking than without" (Corff et al., 1995, p. 144). The variables from this study are identified and defined conceptually and operationally in the next section.

Independent Variable—Facilitated Tucking

Conceptual Definition. A nonpharmacologic comfort measure that involves the motoric containment of an infant's arms and legs.

Operational Definition. The infant's arms and legs are contained in "a flexed, midline position close to the infant's trunk with the infant in a side-lying or supine position" (p. 14) (see Figure 3-1).

Dependent Variables—Heart Rate and Oxygen Saturation

Conceptual Definition. Physiologic responses that are influenced by painful stimuli.

Operational Definition. Heart rate and oxygen saturation per pulse oximetry "were recorded visually and were graphed using a System VI Air Shields Infant Monitor With Data Logger" (p. 145).

continued

Dependent Variable—Sleep State

Conceptual Definition. Behavioral responses of crying, sleep disruption time, and fluctuation in sleep state that are influenced by painful stimuli.

Operational Definition. "Sleep states were recorded by one of two observers who reached 90% reliability in reading sleep states, as defined in the Neonatal Individualized Developmental Care and Assessment Program. Sleep states are defined as state 1 = deep sleep; state 2 = light sleep; state 3 = drowsiness; state 4 = awake, alert; state 5 = aroused, fussy; and state 6 = crying. . . . Sleep states were recorded during a 12-minute baseline period, the heelstick period, and a 15-minute post-stick period for both control and experimental trials" (p. 145).

The variables in quasi-experimental and experimental research are narrow and specific in focus and can be quantified (converted to numbers) or manipulated using specified steps. In addition, the variables are objectively defined to decrease researcher bias, as indicated in the previous example. The research variables or concepts in descriptive and correlational studies are usually more abstract and broadly defined than are the variables in quasi-experimental studies. For example, O'Brien (1993) conducted a descriptive correlational study to examine the relationships among self-esteem, social support, and coping behavior in adults with multiple sclerosis. O'Brien identified the following definitions for coping behavior.

Research Variable—Coping Behavior

Conceptual Definition. Coping behaviors are actions "directed toward managing internal or environmental demands, or both, that tax or exceed a person's resources (Lazarus & Folkman, 1984). Coping responses serve two functions: (1) they are efforts to deal directly with the source of stress, such as altering a situation (problem-focused); and (b) they are efforts directed at dealing with the emotional reaction (emotional-focused)" (p. 54).

Operational Definition. "[T]he Ways of Coping Checklist (WCC), a 68-item scale that lists a broad range of behavioral and cognitive coping strategies, was used to measure coping behaviors. . . . The WCC contains eight subscales: one problem-focused scale, six emotion-focused scales, and one problem- and emotion-focused scale" (p. 56).

O'Brien's conceptual definition of coping behavior is based on Lazarus and Folkman's (1984) theory. The operational definition of coping behaviors is reflective of the conceptual definition because the WCC measures the problem- and emotion-focused elements of coping behavior.

Critiquing Study Variables in Published Studies

VARIABLES need to be identified clearly and defined conceptually and operationally in a published study. The following questions might help you critique the variables in a study.

1. *Are the independent, dependent, or research variables identified?*
2. *Are the variables that are manipulated or measure in the study consistent with the variables identified in the purpose or the objectives, questions, or hypotheses?*
3. *Are the variables reflective of the concepts identified in the study framework?*
4. *Are the variables clearly defined conceptually and operationally based on theory and previous research?*
5. *Is the conceptual definition of the variable consistent with the operational definition?*
6. *Were the essential attributes or demographic variables examined and summarized?*
7. *Were the extraneous variables identified and controlled as necessary in the study?*
8. *Are there uncontrolled extraneous variables that may have influenced the findings? Is the potential impact of these variables on the findings discussed?*

SUMMARY

This chapter provides an introduction to the research problem and purpose and the objectives, questions, and hypotheses that are used to direct studies. The problem is a situation in need of solution, improvement, or alteration or a discrepancy between the way things are and the way they ought to be. The research purpose is a concise, clear statement of the specific goal or aim of the study. The goal of a study might be to identify, describe, explain, or predict a solution to a situation in clinical practice.

The problem and purpose of a study need to have professional significance and potential or actual significance for society. In critiquing the significance of the problem and purpose in a published study, you need to determine if the knowledge generated by the study impacts nursing practice, builds on previous research, promotes theory development, and/or addresses current concerns or priorities in nursing. The feasibility of studying an identified problem and purpose is also examined in a research critique. Study feasibility is evaluated by examining the researchers' expertise; money commitments; availability of subjects, facilities, and equipment; and the study's ethical considerations. Guidelines are provided to direct the critique of problems and purposes in quantitative, qualitative, and outcomes research reports.

Research objectives, questions, or hypotheses are formulated to bridge the gap between the more abstractly stated research problem and purpose and the detailed design and plan for data collection and analysis. Research objectives are clear, concise, declarative statements that are expressed in the present tense. Research questions are concise, interrogative statements that are worded in the present tense and include one or more variables. Objectives and questions focus on description of variables, examination of relationships among variables, and determination of differences between two or more groups regarding selected variables.

A hypothesis is the formal statement of the expected relationship(s) between two or more variables in a specified population. The hypothesis translates the research problem and purpose into a clear explanation or prediction of the expected results or outcomes of the study. Hypotheses can be described using four categories: (1) associative versus causal, (2) simple versus complex, (3) nondirectional versus directional, and (4) null versus research. Testable hypotheses contain variables that are measurable or manipulable, and these hypotheses are evaluated using statistical analyses. Guidelines are provided for use in critiquing objectives, questions, and hypotheses in published studies.

The research purpose and objectives, questions, and hypotheses identify the variables to be examined in a study. Variables are qualities, properties, or characteristics of persons, things, or situations that change or vary. The types of variables discussed in this chapter include independent, dependent, research, extraneous, and demographic. An independent variable is a stimulus or activity that is manipulated or varied by the researcher to create an effect on the dependent variable. A dependent variable is the response, behavior, or outcome that the researcher wants to predict or explain. Research variables or concepts are the qualities, properties, or characteristics that are observed or measured in a study. Research variables are often examined in descriptive and correlational quantitative studies, and research concepts or variables might be examined in qualitative studies. Extraneous variables exist in all studies and can affect the measurement of study variables and the relationships among these variables. Environmental variables are a type of extraneous variable that make up the setting in which the study is conducted. Demographic variables are characteristics or attributes of the subjects that are collected and analyzed to describe the study sample.

A variable is operationalized in a study by developing conceptual and operational definitions. A conceptual definition provides the theoretical meaning of a variable and is derived from a theorist's definition of a related concept. The conceptual definition provides a basis for formulating an operational definition. An operational definition is derived from a set of procedures or progressive acts that a researcher performs to receive sensory impressions that indicate the existence or degree of existence of a variable. Operational definitions indicate how a treatment or independent variable will be implemented and how the dependent variable will be measured. Operational definitions need to be independent of time and setting so that variables can be investigated at different times and in different settings using the same definitions. The chapter concludes with guidelines to direct the critique of study variables in research reports.

REFERENCES

Adebo, E. O. (1974). Identifying problems for nursing research. *International Nursing Review, 21*(2), 53–54, 59.

Ajzen, I., & Fishbein, M. (1980). *Understanding attitudes and predicting social behavior.* Englewood Cliffs, NJ: Prentice-Hall.

Albrecht, M. (1992). Research priorities for home health nursing. *Nursing & Health Care, 13*(10), 538–541.

Armstrong, R. L. (1981). Hypothesis formulation. In S. D. Krampitz & N. Pavlovich (Eds.), *Readings for nursing research* (pp. 29–39). St. Louis: Mosby.

Baker, C. F., Garvin, B. J., Kennedy, C. W., & Polivka, B. J. (1993). The effect of environmental sound and communication on CCU patients' heart rate and blood pressure. *Research in Nursing & Health, 16*(6), 415–421.

Bayley, E. W., Richmond, T., Noroian, E. L., & Allen, L. R. (1994). A delphi study on research priorities for trauma nursing. *American Journal of Critical Care, 3*(3), 208–216.

Beyers, M. (1997). The American Organization of Nurse Executives (AONE) research column. Research priorities of the American Organization of Nurse Executives. *Applied Nursing Research, 10*(1), 52–53.

Bloch, D. (1990). Strategies for setting and implementing the National Center for Nursing Research priorities. *Applied Nursing Research, 3*(1), 2–6.

Bostrom, J., Mechanic, J., Lazar, N., Michelson, S., Grant, L., & Nomura, L. (1996). Preventing skin breakdown: Nursing practices, costs, and outcomes. *Applied Nursing Research, 9*(4), 184–188.

Bournaki, M. C. (1997). Correlates of pain-related responses to venipunctures in school-age children. *Nursing Research, 46*(3), 147–154.

Brown, S. C. (1997). Chest pain and cocaine use in 18 to 40 year-old persons: A retrospective study. *Applied Nursing Research, 10*(3), 136–142.

Burns, N., & Grove, S. K. (1997). *The practice of nursing research: Conduct, critique, and utilization* (3rd ed.). Philadelphia: Saunders.

Chinn, P. L., & Kramer, M. K. (1991). *Theory and nursing: A systematic approach* (3rd ed.). St. Louis: Mosby.

Contrada, R. J., & Krantz, D. S. (1988). Stress, reactivity, and type A behavior: Current status and future directions. *Annals of Behavioral Medicine, 10*(2), 64–70.

Corff, K. E., Seideman, R., Venkataraman, P. S., Lutes, L., & Yates, B. (1995). Facilitated tucking: A nonpharmacologic comfort measure for pain in preterm neonates. *Journal of Obstetric, Gynecologic & Neonatal Nursing, 24*(2), 143–147.

Coyne, M. L., & Hoskins, L. (1997). Improving eating behaviors in dementia using behavioral strategies. *Clinical Nursing Research, 6*(3), 275–290.

Creswell, J. W. (1994). *Research design: Qualitative and quantitative approaches*. Thousand Oaks, CA: Sage.

Davies, A. R., Doyle, M. A. T., Lansky, D., Rutt, W., Stevic, M. O., & Doyle, J. B. (1994). Outcomes assessment in clinical settings: A consensus statement on principles and best practices in project management. *The Joint Commission Journal on Quality Improvement, 20*(1), 6–16.

Deiriggi, P. M. (1990). Effects of waterbed flotation on indicators of energy expenditure in preterm infants. *Nursing Research, 39*(3), 140–146.

Department of Health and Human Services (DHHS). (June 18, 1991). Protection of human subjects. *Code of Federal Regulations*, Title 45 Public Welfare, Part 46.

Diers, D. (1979). *Research in nursing practice*. Philadelphia: Lippincott.

Diokno, A., Brock, B., Herzog, R., & Bromberg, J. (1990). Medical correlates of urinary incontinence in the elderly. *Urology 36*(2), 129–138.

Edel, E., Houston, S., Kennedy, V., & LaRocco, M. (1998). Impact of a 5-minute scrub on the microbial flora found on artificial, polished, or natural fingernails of operating room personnel. *Nursing Research, 47*(1), 54–59.

Fahs, P. S. S., & Kinney, M. R. (1991). The abdomen, thigh, and arm as sites for subcutaneous sodium heparin injections. *Nursing Research, 40*(4), 204–207.

Fawcett, J., & Downs, F. S., (1992). *The relationship of theory and research* (2nd ed.). Norwalk, CT: Appleton-Century-Crofts.

Gordon, M. (1989). Restoring functional independence in the older hip fracture patient. *Geriatrics, 44*(12), 48–59.

Hastings-Tolsma, M. T., Yucha, C. B., Tompkins, J., Robson, L., & Szeverenyi, N. (1993). Effect of warm and cold applications on the resolution of IV infiltrations. *Research in Nursing & Health, 16*(3), 171–178.

Heater, B. S., Becker, A. M., & Olson, R. K. (1988). Nursing interventions and patient outcomes: A meta-analysis of studies. *Nursing Research, 37*(5), 303–307.

Jadack, R. A., Hyde, J. S., & Keller, M. L. (1995). Gender and knowledge about HIV, risky sexual behaviors, and safer sex practices. *Research in Nursing & Health, 18*(4), 313–324.

Jemmott, L. S., & Jemmott, J. B., III (1991). Applying the theory of reasoned action to AIDS risk behavior: Condom use among black women. *Nursing Research, 40*(4), 228–234.

Jirovec, M. M. (1991). The impact of daily exercise on the mobility, balance, and urine control of cognitively impaired nursing home residents. *International Journal of Nursing Studies, 28*(2), 145–151.

Jirovec, M. M., & Kasno, J. (1990). Self-care agency as a function of patient-environmental factors among nursing home residents. *Research in Nursing & Health, 13*(5), 303–309.

Kahn, C. R. (1994). Picking a research problem: The critical decision. *The New England Journal of Medicine, 330*(21), 1530–1533.

Kauffman, K. S. (1995). Center as haven: Findings of an urban ethnography. *Nursing Research, 44*(4), 231–236.

Kerlinger, F. N. (1986). *Foundations of behavioral research* (3rd ed.). New York: Holt, Rinehart & Winston.

Koniak, D. (1985). Autotutorial and lecture-demonstration instruction: A comparative analysis of the effects upon students' learning of a developmental assessment skill. *Western Journal of Nursing Research, 7*(1), 80–100.

Landis, C. A., & Whitney, J. D. (1997). Effects of 72 hours of sleep deprivation on wound healing in the rat. *Research in Nursing & Health, 20*(3), 259–267.

Lanza, M. L., Kayne, H. L., Pattison, I., Hicks, C., & Islam, S. (1996). The relationship of behavioral cues to assaultive behaviors. *Clinical Nursing Research, 5*(1), 6–27.

Lazarus, R. S., Delongis, A., Folkman, S., & Gruen, R. (1985). Stress and adaptational outcomes: The problem of confounded measures. *American Psychologist, 40*(7), 770–779.

Lazarus, R. S., & Folkman, S. (1984). *Stress, appraisal, and coping*. New York: Springer.

Lee, K. A., & Stotts, N. A. (1990). Support of the growth hormone-somatomedin system to facilitate healing. *Heart & Lung, 19*(2), 157–164.

Lewandowski, A., & Kositsky, A. M. (1983). Research priorities for critical care nursing: A study by the American Association of Critical Care Nurses. *Heart & Lung, 12*(1), 35–44.

Lim-Levy, F. (1982). The effect of oxygen inhalation on oral temperature. *Nursing Research, 31*(3), 150–152.

Lindeman, C. A. (1975). Delphi survey of priorities in clinical nursing research. *Nursing Research, 24*(6), 434–441.

Lindquist, R., Banasik, J., Barnsteiner, J., Beecroft, P. C., Prevost, S., Riegel, B., Sechrist, K., Strzelecki, C., & Titler, M. (1993). Determining AACN's research priorities for the 90s. *American Journal of Critical Care, 2*(2), 110–117.

Logan, J., & Jenny, J. (1997). Qualitative analysis of patients' work during mechanical ventilation and weaning. *Heart & Lung, 26*(2), 140–147.

Meek, S. S. (1993). Effects of slow stroke back massage on relaxation in hospice clients. *Image: Journal of Nursing Scholarship, 25*(1), 17–21.

Moody, L., Vera, H., Blanks, C., & Visscher, M. (1989). Developing questions of substance for nursing science. *Western Journal of Nursing Research, 11*(4), 393–404.

Mooney, K. H., Ferrell, B. R., Nail, L. M., Benedict, S. C., & Haberman, M. R. (1991). 1991 Oncology Nursing Society research priorities survey. *Oncology Nursing Forum, 18*(8), 1381–1388.

Morse, J. M., Bottorff, J. L., & Hutchinson, S. (1995). The paradox of comfort. *Nursing Research, 44*(1), 14–19.

National Institute of Nursing Research (NINR) (September 23, 1993). *National nursing research agenda: Setting nursing research priorities*. Bethesda, MD: National Institutes of Health.

O'Brien, M. T. (1993). Multiple sclerosis: The relationship among self-esteem, social support, and coping behavior. *Applied Nursing Research, 6*(2), 54–63.

Ouslander, J., Palmer, M., Rovner, B., & German, P. (1994). Urinary incontinence in nursing homes: Incidence, remission, and associated factors. *Journal of the American Geriatrics Society, 41*(10), 1083–1089.

Palmer, M. H., Myers, A. H., & Fedenko, K. M. (1997). Urinary continence changes after hip-fracture repair. *Clinical Nursing Research, 6*(1), 8–24.

Rettig, R. (1990). History, development, and importance to nursing of outcomes research. *Journal of Nursing Quality Assurance, 5*(2), 13–17.

Reynolds, P. D. (1971). *A primer in theory construction.* Indianapolis: Bobbs-Merrill.

Rogers, B. (1987). Research corner: Is the research project feasible? *American Association of Occupational Health Nurses Journal, 35*(7), 327–328.

Rogers, B. (1989). Establishing research priorities in occupational health nursing. *American Association of Occupational Health Nurses Journal, 37*(12), 493–500.

Rosenberg, M. (November 15, 1993). *Understanding violence—A public health perspective*. Paper presented at the American Academy for Nursing Conference, Violence: Nursing Debates the Issues. Washington, DC.

Rudy, E. B., Daly, B. J., Douglas, S., Montenegro, H. D., Song, R., & Dyer, M. A. (1995). Patient outcomes for the chronically critically ill: Special care unit versus intensive care unit. *Nursing Research, 44*(6), 324–330.

Sampselle, C. M., & DeLancey, J. O. L. (1992). The urine stream interruption test and pelvic muscle function. *Nursing Research, 41*(2), 73–77.

Scherer, Y. K., & Schmieder, L. E. (1997). The effect of a pulmonary rehabilitation program on self-efficacy, perception of dyspnea, and physical endurance. *Heart & Lung, 26*(1), 15–22.

Sigmon, H. D., Grady, P. A., & Amende, L. M. (1997). The National Institute of Nursing Research explores opportunities in genetics research. *Nursing Outlook, 45*(5), 215–219.

Skelly, J., & Flint, A. (1995). Urinary incontinence associated with dementia. *Journal of the American Geriatrics Society, 43*(3), 286–294.

Van Cleve, L., Johnson, L., & Pothier, P. (1996). Pain responses of hospitalized infants and children to venipuncture and intravenous cannulation. *Journal of Pediatric Nursing, 11*(3), 161–168.

van Manen, M. (1990). *Researching lived experience. Human science for an action sensitive pedagogy.* London, Ontario: Althouse Press.

Widerquist, J. G. (1992). The spirituality of Florence Nightingale. *Nursing Research, 41*(1), 49–55.

Wong, D. L., & Baker, C. M. (1988). Pain in children: Comparison of assessment scales. *Pediatric Nursing, 14*(1), 9–17.

Review of Literature

Completing this chapter should enable you to:

1. *Describe the sources and content of a literature review in a research report.*
2. *Differentiate between theoretical and empirical sources.*
3. *Discuss the purposes for reviewing the literature in quantitative and qualitative studies.*
4. *Critique the literature review section of a published study.*
5. *Discuss the process for identifying and locating research sources.*
6. *Conduct a computerized and manual search of the literature.*
7. *Use the Internet to search for relevant electronic publications.*
8. *Discuss the importance of replication in generating a body of knowledge for use in practice.*
9. *Use a variety of sources in developing a literature review.*
10. *Summarize the research literature in an area of interest for use in nursing practice.*

Academic library
Catalog
Computer search
Dissertation
Empirical literature
Index
Integrative review of research
Interlibrary loan department
Internet
Landmark studies
Library resources
Library sources
Manual search
Monograph
Paraphrase

Periodicals
Primary source
Public library
Replication studies
   Approximate replication
   Concurrent replication
   Exact replication
   Systematic extension replication
Review of literature
Secondary source
Special library
Synthesis of sources
Theoretical literature
Thesis
World Wide Web (WWW)

*T*he *review of literature* in a research report is a summary of current knowledge about a particular practice problem and includes what is known and not known about the problem. The literature is reviewed to summarize knowledge for use in practice or to provide a basis for conducting a study. This chapter provides essential information to assist you in critiquing the literature review sections of quantitative and qualitative studies. In addition, the steps for conducting a review of the literature are detailed: (1) using the library, (2) identifying sources, and (3) locating sources. The amount of research information available continues to escalate, with the production of approximately 6,000 new scientific articles a day. At this rate, scientific knowledge will double about every 5 years (Naisbitt & Aburdene, 1990). In nursing, the number of journals has increased by more than 575% since 1961, and the Internet has made available a multitude of these research reports. Thus, the literature review process is much more enlightening today than in the past, and computerized databases have greatly facilitated the process of searching the literature. The focus in this chapter is on conducting a literature review to summarize knowledge for use in nursing practice. A literature review on the prediction and prevention of pressure ulcers is presented as an example of research knowledge that is ready for use in practice.

Understanding the Literature Review in Research Reports

In published studies, researchers present literature reviews to provide the reader with a background for the problem studied. The review of literature section includes a description of the current knowledge of a practice problem, the gaps in this knowledge base, and the contribution of the present study to the development of knowledge in this area. The scope of a literature review should be broad enough to allow the reader to become familiar with the research problem and narrow enough to include predominantly relevant sources. To increase your understanding of the literature reviews presented in published studies, the following areas are addressed: (1) the sources included in a literature review and (2) the purposes of the literature review in quantitative and qualitative studies.

Sources Included in a Literature Review

Predominantly two types of sources are cited in the review of literature for research, both theoretical and empirical. Other types of published information such as descriptions of clinical situations, educational literature, and position papers are reviewed but are rarely cited because of their subjectivity (Pinch, 1995). Theoretical and empirical sources can be primary or secondary in origin, but usually primary sources are cited in a literature review. This section describes the theoretical and empirical literature cited in published studies and the use of primary versus secondary sources in literature reviews.

Theoretical and Empirical Literature

Theoretical literature includes concept analyses, models, theories, and conceptual frameworks that support a selected research problem and purpose. Theoretical sources can be found in periodicals and monographs. *Periodicals* are published over time, such as journals, and are numbered sequentially for the years published. *Monographs* are usually written once, such as books, booklets of conference proceedings, or pamphlets, and may be updated with a new edition. Periodicals and monographs are available in a variety of media, such as print, online, or CD-ROMs. In a published study, theoretical and conceptual sources are described and summarized to reflect the current understanding of the research problem and to provide a basis for the study framework.

Empirical literature includes relevant studies that are published in journals or books, as well as unpublished studies, such as master's theses and doctoral dissertations. A *thesis* is a research project completed by a master's student as part of the requirements for a master's degree. A *dissertation* is an extensive, usually original research project that is completed by a doctoral student as part of the requirements for a doctoral degree. The empirical literature reviewed depends on the study problem and the type of research conducted. Research problems that were frequently investigated in the past or are currently being investigated have more extensive empirical literature than new or unique problems. Descriptive studies are usually conducted in new areas of research, so the number of studies available for review is limited compared to those for a quasi-experimental or experimental study.

Primary and Secondary Sources

The published literature includes primary and secondary sources. A *primary source* is written by the person who originated or is responsible for generating the ideas published. In empirical publications, a primary source is written by the person(s) who conducted the research. A primary theoretical source is written by the theorist who developed the theory or conceptual content. A *secondary source* summarizes or quotes content from primary sources. Thus, authors of secondary sources paraphrase the works of researchers and theorists. The problem with secondary sources is that the author has interpreted the works of someone else, and this interpretation is influenced by that author's perception and bias. Sometimes errors and misinterpretations have been promulgated by authors using secondary sources rather than primary sources. Predominantly primary sources are cited in research reports. Secondary sources are used only if primary sources cannot be located or if the secondary source provides creative ideas or a unique organization of information not found in a primary source.

Purpose of the Literature Review in Quantitative Research

The review of literature in quantitative research is conducted to direct the development and implementation of a study. The major literature review is conducted at the beginning of the research process, and a limited review is conducted during the generation of the research report to identify new studies. The purpose of the literature review is similar for the different types of quantitative studies (descriptive, correlational, quasi-experimental, and experimental). Relevant sources are cited throughout a quantitative research report in the introduction, methods, results, and discussion sections. In the introduction section, the background and significance of the research problem are summarized from relevant sources. The review of literature section includes both theoretical and empirical sources that document the current knowledge of the problem studied. The framework section is developed from the theoretical literature and sometimes from empirical literature, depending on the focus of the study. The methods section of the research report describes the design, sample, measurement methods, treatment, and data collection process that are based on previous research. In the results section, the analysis of the data is conducted with knowledge of the results of previous studies. The discussion section of the research report provides conclusions that are a synthesis of the findings from previous research and those from the present study.

Purpose of the Literature Review in Qualitative Research

In qualitative research, the purpose and timing of the literature review vary based on the type of study to be conducted (Table 4-1). Phenomenologists believe the literature should be reviewed after data collection and analysis so that the information in the literature will not influence the researcher's objectivity (Munhall & Oiler, 1993). For example, if a researcher decided to describe the phenomenon of dying, the review of literature would include Kubler-Ross's (1969) five stages of grieving. Knowing the details of these stages could influence the way the researcher views the phenomenon during data collection and analysis. However, after data analyses, the information from the literature is compared with findings from the present study to determine similarities and differences. Then the findings are combined to reflect the current knowledge of the phenomenon.

In grounded theory research, a minimal review of relevant studies is done at the beginning of the research process. This review is only a means of making

TABLE 4-1. Purposes of the Literature Review in Qualitative Research

Type of Qualitative Research	*Purpose of the Literature Review*
Phenomenological research	Compare and combine findings from the study with the literature to determine current knowledge of a phenomenon
Grounded theory research	Use the literature to explain, support, and extend the theory generated in the study
Ethnographic research	Review the literature to provide a background for conducting the study, as in quantitative research
Historical research	Literature is reviewed to develop research questions and is a source of data in the study

the researcher aware of what studies have been conducted, but the information from these studies is not used to direct data collection or theory development from those data. Mainly, the literature is used by the researcher to explain, support, and extend the theory generated in the study (Munhall & Oiler, 1993).

The review of literature in ethnographic research is similar to that in quantitative research. The literature is reviewed early in the research process to provide a general understanding of the variables to be examined in a selected culture. The literature is usually theoretical because few studies have typically been conducted in the area of interest. From these sources, a framework is developed for examining complex human situations in the selected culture (Munhall & Oiler, 1993). The literature review also provides a background for conducting the study and interpreting the findings.

In historical research, an initial literature review is conducted to select a research topic and to develop research questions. Then the investigator develops an inventory of sources, locates these sources, and examines them; thus, the literature is a major source of data in historical research. Since historical research requires an extensive review of literature that is sometimes difficult to locate, the researcher can spend months and even years locating and examining sources. The information gained from the literature is analyzed and organized into a report to explain how an identified phenomenon has evolved over a particular time period (Munhall & Oiler, 1993).

Critiquing the Literature Review in a Published Study

The literature review section of a research report needs to be identified and critiqued for quality. The review of literature might be a clearly identified section in the report or part of the introduction. A quality literature review logically builds a case for the study being reported. Thus, reading the literature review should provide you with a basic understanding of the study problem and evidence that the study conducted was appropriate based on the current knowledge of this problem. This section provides guidelines for critiquing the literature review in a published study and an example literature review critique.

Guidelines for Conducting a Critique of the Literature Review

Critiquing the literature review of a published study involves examining the quality of the content and sources presented. The content of the literature review includes what is known and not known about the study problem and identifies the focus of the present study. Thus, the review needs to provide a basis for the study purpose and is often organized by the variables in the purpose. The sources cited need to be relevant and current for the problem and purpose of the study. To determine if sources cited in a research report are relevant, you would need to locate the sources or abstracts of the sources and review them. This is very time-consuming and is usually not done when critiquing an article. However, you can review the reference list and determine the focus of the sources, the number of empirical and theoretical sources cited, and where the sources were published. Some of the research and clinical nursing journals that include quality studies and theoretical literature are identified in Chapter 2. Reading a variety of professional journals will strengthen your ability to judge the relevance and quality of sources.

The literature review needs to include current sources from the last 5–10 years prior to publication of the report. Sources cited need to be comprehensive as well as current, and that depends on whether the problem studied has existed for years or is relatively new. Some problems have been studied for decades, and the literature review often includes landmark studies that were conducted years ago. *Landmark studies* are significant research projects that generate knowledge that influences a discipline and sometimes society. These studies are frequently replicated or are the basis for the generation of additional studies. For example, Williams (1972) studied factors that contribute to skin breakdown, and these findings provided the basis for numerous studies on the prevention and treatment of pressure ulcers. Many of these studies have been summarized to provide guidelines for the prediction and prevention of pressure ulcers in clinical practice (Harrison, Wells, Fisher, & Prince, 1996; Panel for the Prediction and Prevention of Pressure Ulcers in Adults, 1992).

CRITIQUING the literature review section of a published study is often difficult because you are less familiar with the topic than are the authors of the article. In addition, the literature review sections frequently seem too concise to present the current knowledge on selected topics because the review is often reduced to comply with space limitations for publication. The following questions might help you determine the quality of a literature review in a study.

1. Are relevant studies identified and described?
2. Are relevant theories identified and described?
3. Are primary sources cited in the review?
4. Are the references current?
5. Are relevant landmark studies described?
6. Are the sources paraphrased to promote the flow of the content presented?
7. Is the literature review clearly organized and logically developed?
8. Is the current knowledge about the research problem described?
9. Does the literature review clearly provide a basis for the study conducted?

Example Critique of a Study's Literature Review

The review of literature section from Vyhlidal, Moxness, Bosak, Van Meter, and Bergstrom's (1997) study of the effects of selected mattress surfaces on the incidence of pressure ulcers is presented as an example. "The purpose of the study was to compare the incidence of pressure ulcers in 40 newly admitted at-risk (Braden Scale score <18) skilled-nursing-facility residents, randomly assigned to Iris 3000 (Bio Clinic of Sunrise Medical Corp, Ontario, CA) foam mattress overlays ($n = 20$) or a MAXIFLOAT (BG Industries, North-ridge, CA) foam mattress replacements ($n = 20$)" (p. 111). The literature review is presented on pages 112–113 of the research article, and the references are on page 120.

Background or Literature Review

"Landis (1930) found that the average arteriolar capillary pressure among healthy subjects was 32 mm Hg. Based largely on the Landis findings, practitioners and developers of support surfaces contend that unrelieved pressure greater than 32 mm Hg creates tissue ischemia which can lead to pressure ulcer development (Hedrick-Thompson, Halloran, Strader, & McSweeney, 1993; Jester & Weaver, 1990; Krouskop, Williams, Krebs, Herszkowicz, & Garber, 1985; Panel for Prediction and Prevention of Pressure Ulcers, 1992). Furthermore, high pressures of short duration and low pressures of long duration are known to be capable of producing pressure ulcers (Husain, 1953; Kosiak, 1959). Manufacturers of support surfaces use the 32 mm Hg capillary closing pressure as a benchmark to evaluate product pressure reduction capabilities. Support surfaces that reduce pressure between skin overlying bony prominences and support surfaces (interface pressure) below 32 mm Hg should hypothetically reduce the risk of pressure ulcer development.

Product studies have examined interface pressure using healthy subjects rather than subjects at-risk for developing ulcers (Hedrick-Thompson et al., 1993; Jester & Weaver, 1990). The Jester and Weaver study compared families of products with low-risk or normal volunteers lying on the support surfaces for unknown periods of time. MAXIFLOAT replacement foam mattresses had lower interface pressure readings among four product groups (overlays, air mattresses, foam mattresses, and other mattresses), but these pressures were not as low as air-fluidized or low air-loss specialty beds. A study of 4-in. convoluted foam mattress overlays reported the overlays to have significantly lower pressure readings than the standard bed (Krouskop et al., 1985). Hedrick-Thompson et al. (1993) also found 4-in. foam overlays to have lower pressure readings than the standard bed but higher pressures than air mattress overlays and air-loss beds.

A more informative way of evaluating product efficacy is to examine a patient-centered outcome, whether or not patients develop pressure ulcers. However, few investigators have evaluated product efficacy in terms of this outcome. No studies could be found testing the efficacy of the MAXIFLOAT or Iris 3000 foam support surfaces. A few studies were found on other brands of 4-in. foam overlays. Subjects in these studies were usually hospitalized or skilled nursing facility residents. One study reported no statistical difference in skin outcome between 4-in. foam overlays and alternating air pressure mattresses (Whitney, Fellows, & Larson, 1984). In contrast, Stoneberg, Pitcock, and Myton (1986) noted a higher number and greater severity of pressure ulcers with 4-in. foam overlays than with alternating pressure pads. Kemp et al. (1993) found [that] solid 4-in. foam overlays produced statistically fewer ulcers than the convoluted foam overlays when taking into account Braden Scale mobility subscale scores.

Research involving MAXIFLOAT foam mattresses is limited to explaining interface pressures. No research specifically examined the Iris 3000 foam overlay, but conflicting findings on pressure reduction and pressure ulcer incidence were reported with other 4-in. foam overlay products. This study compares these two foam products based on pressure ulcer incidence in an at-risk population. Results will provide clinicians with meaningful data to aid in the selection of a cost-effective beneficial product." (Vyhlidal et al., 1997, pp. 112–113)

The literature review, though brief, includes quality content and relevant sources that provide a basis for the conduct of this study. The review of literature is well organized and focuses on the study variables (pressure ulcer, Iris 3000 foam mattress overlays, and MAXIFLOAT foam mattress replacements). The first two paragraphs describe what is known about the research problem, and the third paragraph focuses on what is not known. The last paragraph briefly summarizes the major points of the literature review and addresses the importance of the current study in contributing to the development of knowledge for practice.

The researchers cited quality, relevant primary sources from excellent medical and nursing research journals, such as the *Journal of the American Medical Association, Journal of ET Nursing, Ostomy/Wound Management, Research in Nursing & Health, Archives of Physical Medicine and Rehabilitation, Journal of Rehabilitation Research and Development, Heart,* and *Journal of Gerontological Nursing.* The clinical practice guideline for the prediction and prevention of pressure ulcers is an excellent source that was developed by health professionals (physicians and nurses), politicians, and consumers who are experts in the field of pressure ulcer prevention, assessment, and treatment (Panel for Prediction and Prevention of Pressure Ulcers in Adults, 1992). The sources are current and comprehensive, ranging from 1930 to 1995. The research by Landis (1930) is a landmark study that documented the pressure at which pressure ulcers develop. Most of the sources were published in the late 1980s and 1990s.

Vyhlidal et al.'s (1997) study did produce useful findings for practice. They found that the MAXIFLOAT foam mattress replacements were significantly more effective in preventing pressure ulcers than the Iris 3000 foam mattress overlay, even when the subjects on the MAXIFLOAT were heavier and used the mattress more days than the subjects on the Iris 3000. "MAXIFLOAT proved to be more effective in preventing pressure ulcers in an at-risk skilled-care population and was cost-effective" (p. 111). This knowledge is valuable in making decisions about the bed surfaces for elderly patients at risk for pressure ulcers.

Reviewing the Research Literature for Use in Practice

A background in reading research reports and critiquing the literature review sections of published studies will assist you in conducting a review of the literature in an area of interest. This section focuses on reviewing relevant literature to generate a picture of what is known and not known about a problem and to determine whether the knowledge is ready for use in practice. Think of a problem that you have experienced in clinical practice. For example, maybe you have noted that many hospitalized patients are elderly, and far too many of them develop pressure ulcers during their hospital stay. Reviewing the research literature might provide you with possible solutions for this practice problem. The steps for reviewing the literature include (1) using the library, (2) identifying relevant research sources, and (3) locating these sources.

Using the Library

This section provides you with information about libraries and some tips on using them. There are three major categories of libraries: public, academic, and special (Strauch, Linton, & Cohen, 1989). The *public library* serves the needs of the community in which it is located and usually contains few research reports. The *academic library* is located within an institution of higher learning and contains numerous research reports in journals and books. Most academic libraries have an *interlibrary loan department*, which can be useful when you cannot find a particular research report. This department can frequently locate and obtain books, booklets, conference proceedings, and articles from other libraries in 1 or 2 weeks.

The *special library* contains a collection of materials on a specific topic or specialty area, such as nursing or medicine. Large hospitals, health care centers, and health research centers have special libraries that contain sources relevant to health care providers and researchers. For example, the most comprehensive collection of national and international nursing literature is available at the Center for Nursing Scholarship in Indianapolis, Indiana. Specialty libraries, such as those in hospitals, often have a librarian who will assist nurses in conducting a literature search.

When using a library for the first time, you might ask the library personnel for an orientation. Most libraries offer tours and handouts to help you locate the resources and sources available in the facility. Essential *library resources* include the library personnel, interlibrary loan department, circulation department, reference department, computer search department, and photocopy services. The library personnel in the reference department are familiar with the library's collections and operations and can provide assistance in using the computers, indexes, abstracts, and other equipment and reference materials in the library. Common *library sources* for research reports include journals, books, conference proceedings, master's theses, and doctoral dissertations (Strauch et al., 1989).

Identifying Relevant Research Sources

Once you have identified a problem in clinical practice, you can search the literature for studies related to this problem. To identify relevant sources, conduct a brief manual search of the literature and then a computer search. A *manual search* involves examining reference sources, such as catalog lists and indexes, by hand to identify relevant sources for an area of interest. Most manual searches are brief, and are conducted to clarify and narrow the research topic and provide direction for a computer search. Through the advancement of technology, *computer searches* can be conducted to scan the citations in different databases and identify sources relevant to a research topic. If you have difficulty finding sources related to a specific topic, identify some synonymous terms using thesauruses, such as the *International Nursing Index's Nursing Thesaurus*. Frequently, word processing programs and dictionaries are helpful in identifying synonymous terms. These terms can be used to conduct a brief manual search of the catalog and indexes to identify key terms, current studies, and researchers in an area.

Searching the Catalog and Indexes

The *catalog* identifies what is available in the library. These listings are usually available on an on-line computer. The catalog listings include books, conference proceedings, audiovisuals, professional organizations' publications, theses, and dissertations. Some individuals overlook the value of books because they believe the content is too old. However, books can be excellent sources for qualitative studies and often include extensive bibliographies that might direct you to additional relevant studies. Conference proceedings usually contain current studies, but the information is frequently limited to an abstract or a brief paper. The researcher could be contacted for more information by phone, E-mail, or fax. Theses and dissertations frequently provide a complete review of the literature for a specific research problem and an extensive bibliography.

An *index* provides assistance in identifying journal articles and other publications relevant to a topic of interest. Indexes are organized into two major sections, subject and author. The research topic, synonymous terms, and subheadings identified are used to guide the search through the subject section of the index. The subject section includes headings and subheadings, and under these headings, several publications (predominantly articles) are listed. Many of these publications are listed under more than one subject heading and subheading for easy access by the searcher. For example, a nursing study of the measurement of chronic pain in the elderly might be listed under the subject headings of pain, elderly, and nursing research and under the subheadings of chronic pain and pain assessment.

If you are familiar with the names of key researchers for a specific topic, you can search the author section of the index to identify recent publications by these individuals. The author section is organized alphabetically by the first author's name; no more than three authors are listed. The second and third authors' names appear as cross references to the full citation under the first author's name. The author's name is followed by the same bibliographic content that is included in the subject section. Two major indexes used in nursing are *Cumulative Index to Nursing & Allied Health Literature* and *Index Medicus*.

Cumulative Index to Nursing & Allied Health Literature (CINAHL) (formerly *Cumulative Index to Nursing Literature*). This index is usually consulted first by nurses, students, and educators because it is published frequently, references a large number of relevant nursing sources, and is the original index for nursing literature. *CINAHL* was first published in 1956 and references more than 400 nursing journals, along with publications of the American Nurses' Association (ANA) and the National League for Nursing (NLN). The index also provides access to allied health and health-related journals and includes numerous pertinent citations from the biomedical journals listed in *Index Medicus*. CINAHL also has an on-line version and a CD-ROM version (Nicoll & Ouellette, 1997).

Index Medicus (IM). IM is the oldest health-related index and was first published in 1879. This index cites articles from approximately 3,500 domestic and foreign journals. IM is published monthly and issues a bound annual volume of cumulated listings. This index covers all aspects of biomedicine and includes allied health fields, such as nursing, the biological and physical sciences, veterinary medicine, and the humanities. IM also includes listings of books related to biomedicine and publications from selected proceedings. This index is available on-line through MEDLARS (MEDical Literature Analysis and Retrieval System) (Mills, Romano, & Heller, 1996).

Conducting a Computer Search of Relevant Databases

After a brief manual search of the literature, you have clear direction for conducting a computer search. A computer search will generate a list of references with complete bibliographic information; for many of the references, abstracts are also available on request. On-line abstracts allow you to determine quickly if a study is relevant to the review you are conducting. Computer searches have the advantages of being comprehensive, affordable, accessible, and easy to conduct (Hebda, Czar, & Mascara, 1998; Nicoll, 1993).

You can search the literature on your own or request the librarian to conduct the search. Most academic libraries have the facilities for you to conduct your own on-line computer search, whereby you can access the catalog listings of the library, and relevant databases with lists of references. Many libraries have on-line access to the catalogs of other libraries in the local area or within the state. Thus, when you are searching the literature for a topic, you have access to all the materials in your library and the surrounding libraries. In most libraries, you can direct the computer to print a copy of the sources selected for review.

You can also use a microcomputer at home or work to conduct searches of library holdings and databases. You might contact your university library to determine what you would need to conduct on-line searches with your microcomputer. In addition to your microcomputer, you need a modem, a telephone line, and a communication software package. The library personnel will provide you with information on how to access the university's on-line system, how to search the library collections, and how to sign off of the system. You also need a number to call if you have any problems or questions while using the system. Most universities now provide students with an account that makes it possible to access the Internet. The *Internet* is a worldwide network that connects computers together. This technology was initiated by the government to encourage researchers at different academic sites to share their findings. The *World Wide Web* (*WWW*) is an information service for access to the Internet resources by content rather than file names (Hebda et al., 1998).

When you are searching databases, you need to organize your search. You can search by subject, journal, or author. The terms you use to search determine the quality of the sources identified. Poor selection of terms can result in identifying an overwhelming number or an inadequate number of sources. You need to spend some time doing a brief manual search of the indexes or reviewing a few significant studies to identify relevant terms and key researchers in an area. For example, if you want information on prevention of pressure ulcers in the elderly, you might search under the topics of pressure ulcer, pressure sore, or decubitus ulcer. You also might want to search selective journals, such as *Applied Nursing Research, Decubitus, Journal of Gerontological Nursing, Nursing Research,* or *Research in Nursing & Health* for relevant sources. If you know authors who publish regularly on the topic of pressure ulcers, you might search under their names for current research articles. Some of the authors who have published on prevention of pressure ulcers include Braden and Bergstrom (1987) and Norton (1989).

Several databases are pertinent to nursing. Conducting a computer search involves identifying which databases to search to generate the references for a selected research problem. The most common databases used by nurse researchers are briefly introduced below (Hebda et al., 1998; Mills et al., 1996; Nicoll & Ouellette, 1997).

CINAHL Information System. This database is the on-line version of the *Cumulative Index to Nursing and Allied Health Literature (CINAHL).* It includes more than 800 journals and 215,000 records. The materials are indexed using *CINAHL's* annually updated thesaurus, which is adapted from the U.S. National Library of Medicine's Medical Subject Headings (MeSH). No abstracts are included. The database was initiated in 1983 and is updated every 2 months. CINAHL's direct on-line service is available but does require the payment of a membership fee (Nicoll & Ouellette, 1997). The online address for CINAHL is http://cinahl.com/.

MEDLARS (MEDical Literature Analysis and Retrieval System). MEDLARS is the computerized system of databases offered by the National Library of Medicine (NLM). This system includes more than 40 databases that are commonly used by nurses, such as MEDLINE (MEDical Literature Analysis and Retrieval System onLINE), AVLINE (AudioVisual catalog onLINE), BIOETHICSLINE, and CANCERLIT (CANR).

MEDLINE. MEDLINE includes about 6 million articles from approximately 3,500 biomedical journals. This database also contains a separate file called "Special List Nursing" that includes citations from approximately 260 nursing journals that are in the *International Nursing Index.* A MEDLINE search generates the following information: author, title, abstract (since 1975 for some citations), language, and indexing terms. This database covers the period from 1966 to the present and is updated semimonthly.

AVLINE (AudioVisual catalog onLINE). This database includes more than 11,000 audiovisual packages covering a broad range of health-related subjects, such as nurse-patient relationships, nursing care, nursing audit, and legal aspects of nursing. The supplier of AVLINE is the National Library of Medicine, and it is updated every month. An AVLINE search produces the following information: title, media type, authorship, physical description, indexing terms, run time, audience level, review rating and date, reviewer, learning method, abstract, continuing education credit note, price, and source for purchase or loan.

BIOETHICSLINE. This database covers citations that deal with ethical questions arising in health care or biomedical research, such as human experimentation, patients' rights, death and dying, and resource allocation. The suppliers of BIOETHICSLINE are the National Library of Medicine and the Kennedy Institute of Ethics. This database includes citations from 1973 to the present and is updated three times a year. The information obtained from this database includes author, title, source, indexing terms, language, and type of publication.

CANCERLIT (CANR). This database contains more than 685,000 citations from over 3,000 journals, books, conference proceedings, theses, and reports. The suppliers of CANCERLIT are the National Library of Medicine and the Cancer Institute. This database covers all aspects of cancer from 1963 to the present and is updated monthly. The information obtained from this database includes author, author's affiliation, title, abstract, language, type of publication, and indexing terms.

Combined Health Information Database (CHID). This database contains more than 44,000 citations and abstracts of information for health professionals, patients, and the general public. Just a few of the topics covered are Alzheimer's disease, AIDS information and education, cholesterol education, and high blood pressure. CHID was initiated in 1973 and is updated four times a year.

CATLINE (CATalog onLINE). This database contains about 500,000 references for books and serials cataloged at the National Library of Medicine. The information obtained includes author, title, source, language, indexing terms, and other data such as edition, series, title, and notes. CATLINE originated in 1965 and is currently updated weekly.

Locating Sources

You are now ready to locate the sources identified by the manual and computer searches. Locating sources involves the following steps: (1) organizing the list of identified sources, (2) searching the Internet and the library for those sources, and (3) systematically recording references.

Organizing the List of Sources

The list of identified sources can be organized in several ways to facilitate locating them through the Internet or within a library. Journal sources might be organized by journal name and year. You can methodically locate all sources within a specific journal and then proceed to the next one. Sources included in the library catalog (such as books, organizational publications, and conference proceedings) can be organized by author or subject. This organization will not only make it easier to find these sources but will also assist you in eliminating any duplicated references.

Searching the Internet and Library for Sources

Some research articles can be obtained using full text retrieval from the Internet (Hebda et al., 1998). For example, Sigma Theta Tau International has just begun to publish *The Online Journal of Knowledge Synthesis for Nursing*. With a computer and a modem, access is possible through a network such as the Internet or CompuServe, or by a modem dial access through the Online Computer Library Center (OCLC) (Barnsteiner, 1994). Using this system, journal articles can be delivered across commercial telecommunications lines to a personal computer. Subscriptions for the on-line journal can be obtained through Sigma Theta Tau International. Many universities have purchased this system for use by faculty and students. Obtaining journal articles electronically is still quite expensive, and many students prefer to locate sources in their university libraries.

Those sources not available by full text retrieval must be obtained from local libraries or through the interlibrary loan department. Your search for sources in the library can be facilitated by talking with library personnel to determine the classification system; the availability of resources and publications; and the location of journals, books, dictionaries, indexes, and abstracts. When locating books, the library call number should be recorded in case you need to find the source a second time. Persistence is required to find library sources, so do not mark a source off the list simply because it was not located on the first search.

You need to identify the sources that were located in the available library(ies), the sources that are available in the library but were not found, and the sources that are unavailable. If certain sources cannot be found in the local library, you should attempt to locate them through the interlibrary loan department. Locating a source might also require contacting the author when a journal article is incomplete or when requesting reprints of a study or other relevant information. Reviewing the literature is an additive process in which identifying and locating sources leads to further identification and location of sources until the relevant sources are identified.

Systematically Recording References

The bibliographical information on a source should be recorded in a systematic manner, according to the format that will be used in the reference list. Many journals and academic institutions use the American Psychological Association (APA) (1994) format. The reference lists in this textbook are presented in a modified APA format. A complete bibliographic citation (according to APA) should be recorded for all articles at the time they are copied. If the article is obtained from interlibrary loan, the complete citation is stapled to the article and should be kept or copied onto the article. Computerized lists of sources usually contain complete citations for references and should be filed for future use. With the use of your personal computer, you can also easily search a computerized database and obtain complete reference citations.

When citing sources in a paper or recording sources in a reference list, be sure to cross-check them two or three times to prevent errors. Damrosch and Damrosch (1996) have identified some of the common APA mistakes that have been made and provide guidelines to avoid them. The sources cited in the reference list need to follow the correct format for print and on-line full text versions.

Print Version

Plawecki, H. M. (1996). Improving a manuscript's chances for acceptance. *Journal of Holistic Nursing, 14,* 3–5.

On-line Full Text Version

Plawecki, H. M. (1996). Improving a manuscript's chances for acceptance. *Journal of Holistic Nursing, 14,* 3–5. Available: Ovid File: Periodical Abstracts Research II Item: 02993150.

Summarizing the Research Literature for Use in Practice

The review of the literature generates a variety of relevant studies that require synthesis for use in practice. Initially, you need to read and critique the studies to determine those that are most relevant. The studies are selected for inclusion in a literature review based on their quality and their relationship to a selected practice problem. Summarizing the research literature involves the synthesis of the study findings and the mechanics of writing the review.

Synthesizing Findings from Relevant Studies

Synthesis is the basis for developing the literature review for a utilization project. Through *synthesis of sources,* you are able to cluster and interrelate ideas from several studies to identify the current knowledge of a topic. Synthesis involves clarifying the meaning obtained from each research report and then paraphrasing it. *Paraphrasing* involves expressing an author's ideas clearly and concisely in your own words. Last, the meanings obtained from all sources are combined, or *clustered,* to determine the current knowledge of a topic.

A comprehensive, scholarly synthesis of the literature is evident in published, integrative reviews of research. An *integrative review of research* is conducted to identify, analyze, and synthesize the results from independent studies to determine the current knowledge (what is known and not known) in a particular area (Ganong, 1987; Smith & Stullenbarger, 1991). The studies in an integrative review have the same focus and sometimes are replications of previous landmark studies (Cooper, 1984). *Replication studies* involve reproducing or repeating another study to determine whether similar findings will be obtained (Taunton, 1989). Replication is essential for knowledge development since it (1) establishes the credibility of the findings, (2) extends the generalizability of the findings over a range of instances and contexts, (3) provides support for theory development, and (4) decreases the acceptance of erroneous results (Beck, 1994). Thus, replication studies are essential to generate knowledge that can be used in practice.

Four different types of replication studies have been conducted to generate scientific knowledge for nursing: (1) exact, (2) approximate, (3) concurrent, and (4) systematic extension (Beck, 1994; Haller & Reynolds, 1986). An *exact,* or identical, *replication* involves duplicating the initial researcher's study to confirm the original findings. All conditions of the original study must be maintained; thus, "there must be the same observer, the same subjects, the same procedure, the same measures, the same locale, and the same time" (Haller & Reynolds, 1986, p. 250). Exact replications might be thought of as ideal to confirm original study findings but are frequently not attainable. An *approximate,* or operational, *replication* involves repeating the original study under similar conditions, following the original methods as closely as possible (Beck, 1994; Haller & Reynolds, 1986). The intent is to determine whether the findings from the original study hold up despite minor changes in the research conditions. If the findings generated through replication are consistent with the original study findings, these findings are more credible and have the potential to be used in practice.

A *concurrent,* or internal, *replication* involves the collection of data for the original study and their replication simultaneously to provide a check of the reliability of the original study (Beck, 1994). The confirmation, through replication, of the original study findings is part of the original study's design. For example, a research team might collect data simultaneously at two different hospitals and compare and contrast the findings. Consistency in the findings increases the credibility and generalizability of the findings. A *systematic extension,* or constructive, *replication* is done under distinctly new conditions. The researchers conducting the replication do not follow the design or methods of the original researchers; rather, "the second investigative team begins with a similar problem statement but formulates new means to verify the first investigator's findings" (Haller & Reynolds, 1986, p. 250). The aim of this type of replication is to extend the findings of the original study and test the limits of generalizability.

Beck (1994) conducted a computerized and manual review of the nursing literature from 1983 through 1992 and found only 49 replication studies. Possibly, the number of replication studies is limited because replication is viewed by some as less scholarly or less important than original research. However, the lack of replication studies severely limits the development of a scientific knowledge base for nursing (Beck, 1994; Martin, 1995). Thus, replication of studies is an important priority for nursing because it will greatly influence the generation of nursing knowledge that can be synthesized for use in practice (Burns & Grove, 1997).

The increased number of studies in nursing and the focus on replication over the last 10 years have generated a body of literature that requires synthesis. Expert researchers and clinicians have developed publications that summarize nursing knowledge on a variety of topics. In 1983 the first volume of the *Annual Review of Nursing Research* was published by Werley and Fitzpatrick. The integrative reviews of research included in these annual publications cover relevant topics about nursing practice, nursing care delivery, nursing education, and the nursing profession. Integrative reviews have also been published in a variety of clinical and research journals.

Integrative reviews of research can be used to identify relevant studies and facilitate the process of reading, critiquing, and synthesizing research reports for use in practice. For example, three integrated reviews of research have been written on pressure ulcer prevention (Carlson & King, 1990; Cooper, 1987; Panel for the Prediction and Prevention of Pressure Ulcers in Adults, 1992).

If the research literature on a topic has not been synthesized and published, you will need to develop your own summary of current knowledge. Initially, you need to read and critique the studies identified through your search of the literature. Often studies will need to be read several times to determine their quality and their relevance to the review of literature you are developing. You then need to select the studies that are of the highest quality and compare their purposes, methods, results, and findings. You might develop a table that includes essential information from each study so that you can make comparisons (Table 4-2) (Martin, 1997). You also might want to identify the common findings noted among the different studies and compare and contrast the out-

TABLE 4-2. Table for Synthesizing Studies to Generate a Review of Literature

Author & Year	Purpose	Sample	Measurement	Treatment	Results	Findings
Allman (1991)						
Bergstrom, Braden, Laguzza, & Holman (1987)						
Berlowitz & Wilking (1989)						
Braden & Bergstrom (1987)						
Harrison, Wells, Fisher, & Prince (1996)						
Norton (1989)						
Norton, McLaren, & Exton-Smith (1975)						
Okamoto, Lamers, & Shurtleff (1983)						

TABLE 4-3. Table to Compare and Contrast Study Findings on the Prediction and Prevention of Pressure Ulcers

Author & Year	Finding 1	Finding 2	Finding 3
Allman (1991)			
Bergstrom, Braden, Laguzza, & Holman (1987)			
Berlowitz & Wilking (1989)			
Braden & Bergstrom (1987)			
Harrison, Wells, Fisher, & Prince (1996)			
Norton (1989)			
Norton, McLaren, & Exton-Smith (1975)			
Okamoto, Lamers, & Shurtleff (1983)			

comes of these studies. Table 4-3 was developed as an example, using the studies conducted on the prediction and prevention of pressure ulcers in adults. These exercises will assist you in determining the essential content to be included in a literature review.

Organizing and Writing the Review of Literature

A literature review should document the current knowledge of a selected topic and indicate the findings that are ready for use in practice. Often a detailed outline is developed to guide the writing of a literature review. The review of literature begins with an introduction, includes a presentation of relevant studies, and concludes with a summary of current knowledge (Burns & Grove, 1997). The headings and essential content of a literature review are briefly described following.

1. *Introduction.* The introduction indicates the focus or purpose of the review; describes the organization of sources; and indicates the basis for ordering the sources—for example, from least to most important or from least to most current. This section should be brief and interesting enough to capture the attention of the reader. The introduction may be rewritten several times based on the development of other sections of the literature review.
2. *Empirical Literature.* Empirical literature includes quality studies that are relevant for a selected utilization project. For each study, the purpose, sample size, design, and specific findings should be presented, with a scholarly but brief critique of the study's strengths and weaknesses. Work for conciseness and clarity, and include only the most relevant studies. The content from these sources is best paraphrased or summarized in your own words. If you use a direct quotation, try to keep it short to promote the flow of ideas. Long quotations are often unnecessary and interfere with the reader's train of thought.

   Ethical issues must be considered in presenting research sources (Gunter, 1981). The content from studies must be presented honestly and not distorted to support a selected utilization project. The weaknesses of a study need to be addressed, but it is not necessary to be highly critical of a researcher's work. The criticism should focus on the content, be relevant in some way to the proposed project, and be stated as possible or plausible explanations, so that it is neutral and scholarly rather than negative and blaming. Also, be sure to document accurately the researchers' works that you cite in the literature review.

3. *Summary.* The summary includes a concise presentation of the research knowledge about a selected topic, including what is known and not known. The Panel for the Prediction and Prevention of Pressure Ulcers in Adults (1992) has summarized the research literature related to the prevention of pressure ulcers in adults. The following quotation presents key information from their summary of risk assessment tools and risk factors.

Risk Assessment Tools and Risk Factors

GOAL: "Identify at risk individuals needing prevention and the specific factors placing them at risk.

Bed- and chair-bound individuals or those with impaired ability to reposition should be assessed for additional factors that increase risk for developing pressure ulcers. These factors include immobility, incontinence, nutritional factors such as inadequate dietary intake and impaired nutritional status, and altered level of consciousness. Individuals should be assessed on admission to acute care and rehabilitation hospitals, nursing homes, home care programs, and other health care facilities. A systematic risk assessment can be accomplished by using a validated risk assessment tool such as the Braden Scale or Norton Scale. Pressure ulcer risk should be reassessed at periodic intervals. All assessments of risk should be documented.

Rationale: To prevent pressure ulcers, individuals at risk must be identified so that risk factors can be reduced through intervention. The primary risk factors for pressure ulcers are immobility and limited activity levels (Allman, compiled, 1991; Berlowitz & Wilking, 1989; Norton, McLaren, & Exton-Smith, 1975; Okamoto, Lamers, & Shurtleff, 1983). Therefore, persons with impaired ability to reposition themselves or those whose activity is limited to bed or any chair should be assessed for their risk of developing a pressure ulcer. To determine the magnitude of risk, the degree to which mobility and activity levels are limited can be quantified. Both the Norton Scale (Norton et al., 1975) and the Braden Scale (Braden & Bergstrom, 1987; Bergstrom, Braden, Laguzza, & Holman, 1987) assess these factors. . . .

continued

Other risk factors for pressure ulcer development include incontinence, impaired nutritional status, and altered level of consciousness. Incontinence is assessed by the Moisture subscale of the Braden Scale (Braden & Bergstrom, 1987) and the Incontinence component of the Norton Scale. . . . Nutritional factors are considered indirectly in the General Condition component of the Norton Scale (Norton, 1989) and the Nutritional Status subscale of the Braden Scale. . . . Altered level of consciousness is assessed by the Norton Scale's Mental Condition subscale and the Braden Scale's Sensory Perception subscale.

Numerous risk assessment tools exist; however, only the Braden Scale and the Norton Scale (original and modified) have been tested extensively. The Braden Scale has been evaluated in diverse sites that include medical-surgical units, intensive care units, and nursing homes. The Norton Scale has been tested with elderly subjects in hospital settings.

The reported sensitivity and specificity of these risk assessment tools have varied greatly. This variability probably reflects differences in study settings, populations, and outcome measures. . . . The degree to which preventative interventions have been implemented in response to the findings of the risk assessments in these studies may have also contributed to the variability in their reported performance. . . .

Despite the limitations of the Norton and Braden scales, their use ensures systematic evaluation of individual risk factors. No information is currently available to suggest that adaptations of these risk assessment tools or the assessment of any single risk factor or a combination of risk factors predict risk as well as the overall scores obtained by the tools.

The condition of an individual admitted to a health care facility is not static; consequently, pressure ulcer risk requires routine reexamination. The frequency with which such reevaluations need to be done is unknown. However, if an individual becomes bed- or chair-bound or develops difficulty with repositioning, pressure ulcer risk needs to be assessed. Accurate and complete documentation of all risk assessments ensures continuity of care and may be used as a foundation for the skin care plan." (Panel for the Prediction and Prevention of Pressure Ulcers in Adults, 1992, pp. 13–15)

Once you have read and summarized the research literature, you need to decide whether there is adequate knowledge to make a change in clinical practice. For example, what changes would you make in your practice after reading the summary of research literature on risk assessment tools and risk factors for prevention of pressure ulcers? Research has shown that the Braden and Norton scales are effective in assessing patients at risk for developing pressure ulcers. In addition, both scales have been effective in assessing pressure ulcer risk in the elderly. You might submit both scales to your agency so that the administration and staff might select one for use in practice. The next step _involves developing a plan to change practice based on research. The process for using research findings in practice is the focus of Chapter 13.

SUMMARY

The review of literature in a research report is a summary of current knowledge about a particular practice problem and includes what is known and not known about this problem. The literature is reviewed to summarize knowledge for use in practice or to provide a basis for conducting a study. To increase your understanding of the literature reviews presented in published studies, the following areas are addressed: (1) the sources included in a literature review and (2) the purposes of the literature review in quantitative and qualitative studies. A literature review often includes theoretical literature (concept analyses, maps or models, and theories) and empirical literature (studies) that support the research problem and purpose studied. Usually primary sources are cited versus secondary sources. The purpose of the literature review in quantitative research is to direct the development and implementation of the study and is the same for the different types of studies (descriptive, correlational, quasi-experimental, and experimental). In qualitative research, the purpose and timing of the literature review vary based on the type of study to be conducted. The purposes for conducting literature reviews for phenomenology, grounded theory, ethnographic, and historical research are addressed.

This chapter also provides guidelines for critiquing the literature review section in a published study. Questions are identified to help you determine the quality of a study's literature review. The literature review from Vyhlidal et al. (1997) on the effects of mattress surfaces on the incidence of pressure ulcers is presented as an example, and a critique of this literature review is provided.

A literature review is conducted to generate a picture of the current knowledge about a problem and to determine whether the knowledge is ready for use in practice. The steps for reviewing the literature include (1) using the library, (2) identifying relevant research sources, and (3) locating research sources. Academic and special libraries have a variety of sources and resources that facilitate the literature review process. To identify relevant sources, conduct a brief manual search of the literature and then a computer search. A manual search involves examining library sources, such as catalog listings and indexes, by hand to identify relevant sources for an area of interest. Most manual searches are conducted to clarify and narrow the research topic and provide direction for a computer search. Through the advancement of technology, computer searches can be conducted to scan the citations in different databases and identify sources relevant to a research topic. Locating research sources involves organizing a list of sources, searching the library for these sources, and systematically recording the references.

The final step in the literature review process is summarizing relevant studies to determine the current body of knowledge. Summarizing research literature involves the selection of relevant studies, synthesis of the study findings, and the mechanics of writing the review.

A comprehensive, scholarly synthesis of the literature is evident in published integrative reviews of research. These reviews are conducted to identify, analyze, and synthesize the results from independent studies to determine the current knowledge in a particular area. The literature review usually begins with an introduction, includes empirical sources, and concludes with a summary of current knowledge. A brief summary of the research literature related to prevention of pressure ulcers in adults is presented as an example.

REFERENCES

Allman, R. M. (1991). Pressure ulcers among bedridden hospitalized elderly. Division of Gerontology/Geriatrics, University of Alabama at Birmingham. Unpublished data compiled.

American Psychological Association. (1994). *Publication manual of the American Psychological Association* (4th ed.). Washington, DC: American Psychological Association.

Barnsteiner, J. H. (1994). The online *Journal of Knowledge Synthesis for Nursing. Reflections, 20*(2), 10–11.

Beck, C. T. (1994). Replication strategies for nursing research. *Image: Journal of Nursing Scholarship, 26*(3), 191–194.

Bergstrom, N., Braden, B. J., Laguzza, A., & Holman, V. (1987). The Braden Scale for predicting pressure sore risk. *Nursing Research, 36*(4), 205–210.

Berlowitz, D. R., & Wilking, S. V. (1989). Risk factors for pressure sores. A comparison of cross-sectional and cohort-derived data. *Journal of the American Geriatric Society, 37*(11), 1043–1050.

Braden, B., & Bergstrom, N. (1987). A conceptual schema for the study of the etiology of pressure sores. *Rehabilitation Nursing, 12*(1), 8–12.

Burns, N., & Grove, S. K. (1997). *The practice of nursing research: Conduct, critique, and utilization* (3rd ed.). Philadelphia: Saunders.

Carlson, C. E., & King, R. B. (1990). Prevention of pressure sores. In J. J. Fitzpatrick, R. L. Taunton, & J. O. Benoliel (Eds.), *Annual review of nursing research* (Vol. 8, pp. 35–56). New York: Springer.

Cooper, D. M. (1987). Pressure ulcers: Unpublished research 1976–1986: Process to outcome. *Nursing Clinics of North America, 22*(2), 475–492.

Cooper, H. M. (1984). *The integrative research review: A systematic approach.* Beverly Hills, CA: Sage.

Damrosch, S., & Damrosch, G. D. (1996). Methodology corner. Avoiding common mistakes in APA style: The briefest of guidelines. *Nursing Research, 45*(6), 331–333.

Ganong, L. H. (1987). Integrative reviews of nursing research. *Research in Nursing & Health, 10*(1), 1–11.

Gunter, L. (1981). Literature review. In S. D. Krampitz & N. Pavlovich (Eds.), *Readings for nursing research* (pp. 11–16). St. Louis: Mosby.

Haller, K. B., & Reynolds, M. A. (1986). Using research in practice: A case for replication in nursing—part two. *Western Journal of Nursing Research, 8*(2), 249–252.

Harrison, M. B., Wells, G., Fisher, A., & Prince, M. (1996). Practice guidelines for the prediction and prevention of pressure ulcers: Evaluating the evidence. *Applied Nursing Research, 9*(1), 9–17.

Hebda, T., Czar, P., & Mascara, C. (1998). *Handbook of informatics for nurses and health care professionals.* Menlo Park, CA: Addison-Wesley.

Hedrick-Thompson, J., Halloran, T., Strader, T., & McSweeney, M. (1993). Pressure-reduction products: Making appropriate choices. *Journal of ET Nursing, 20*(6), 239–244.

Husain, T. (1953). An experimental study of some pressure effects on tissues with reference to the bed sore problem. *Journal of Pathology and Bacteriology, 66,* 347–358.

Jester, J., & Weaver, V. (1990). A report of clinical investigation of various tissue support surfaces used for the prevention, early intervention, and management of pressure ulcers. *Ostomy/Wound Management, 26,* 39–45.

Kemp, M., Kopanke, D., Tordeciella, L., Fogg, L., Shott, S., Matthiesen, V., & Johnson, B. (1993). The role of support surfaces and patient attributes in preventing pressure ulcers in elderly patients. *Research in Nursing & Health, 16*(2), 89–96.

Kosiak, M. (1959). Etiology and pathology of decubitus ulcers. *Archives of Physical Medicine and Rehabilitation, 42,* 19–29.

Krouskop, T., Williams, R., Krebs, M., Herszkowicz, I., & Garber, S. (1985). Effectiveness of mattress overlays in reducing interface pressures during recumbency. *Journal of Rehabilitation Research and Development, 22*(3), 7–10.

Kubler-Ross, E. (1969). *On death and dying.* New York: Macmillan.

Landis, E. (1930). Micro-injection studies of capillary blood pressure in human skin, *Heart, 15,* 209–278.

Martin, P. A. (1995). More replication studies needed. *Applied Nursing Research, 8*(2), 102–103.

Martin, P. A. (1997). Ask an expert: Writing a useful literature review for a quantitative research project. *Applied Nursing Research, 10*(3), 159–162.

Mills, M. E., Romano, C. A., & Heller, B. R. (1996). *Information management in nursing and health care.* Springhouse, PA: Springhouse.

Munhall, P. L., & Oiler, C. J. (1993). *Nursing research: A qualitative perspective* (2nd ed.). New York: National League for Nursing.

Naisbitt, J., & Aburdene, P. (1990). *Megatrends 2000: Ten new directions for the 1990's.* New York: Morrow.

Nicoll, L. H. (1993). The practical computer: Keeping abreast of the literature electronically. *Nursing Research, 42*(5), 315–317.

Nicoll, L. H., & Ouellette, T. H. (1997). *Computers in nursing: Nurses' guide to the Internet.* Philadelphia: Lippincott.

Norton, D. (1989). Calculating the risk: Reflections on the Norton Scale. *Decubitus, 2*(3), 24–31.

Norton, D., McLaren, R., & Exton-Smith, A. N. (1975). *An investigation of geriatric nursing problems in hospital.* London: Churchill Livingstone.

Okamoto, G. A., Lamers, J. V., & Shurtleff, D. B. (1983). Skin breakdown in patients with myelomeningocele. *Archives of Physical Medicine Rehabilitation, 64*(1), 20–23.

Panel for the Prediction and Prevention of Pressure Ulcers in Adults. (1992). *Pressure ulcers in adults: Prediction and prevention. Clinical practice guidelines.* AHCPR Publication No. 92–0047. Rockville, MD: Agency for Health Care Policy and Research, Public Health Service, U.S. Department of Health and Human Services.

Pinch, W. J. (1995). Synthesis: Implementing a complex process. *Nurse Educator, 20*(1), 34–40.

Smith, M. C., & Stullenbarger, E. (1991). A prototype for integrative review and meta-analysis of nursing research. *Journal of Advanced Nursing, 16*(11), 1272–1283.

Stoneberg, C., Pitcock, N., & Myton, C. (1986). Pressure sores in the homebound: One solution. *American Journal of Nursing, 86*(4), 426–428.

Strauch, K., Linton, R., & Cohen, C. (1989). *Library research guide to nursing: Illustrated search strategy and sources.* Ann Arbor, MI: Pierian Press.

Taunton, R. L. (1989). Replication: Key to research application. *Dimensions of Critical Care Nursing, 8*(3), 156–158.

Vyhlidal, S. K., Moxness, D., Bosak, K. S., Van Meter, F. G., & Bergstrom, N. (1997). Mattress replacement or foam overlay? Prospective study on the incidence of pressure ulcers. *Applied Nursing Research, 10*(3), 111–120.

Whitney, J., Fellows, B., & Larson, E. (1984). Do mattresses make a difference? *Journal of Gerontological Nursing, 10*(10), 20–25.

Williams, A. (1972). A study of factors contributing to skin breakdown. *Nursing Research, 21*(3), 238–243.

Understanding Theory and Research Frameworks

Completing this chapter should enable you to:

1. *Explain the purpose of the framework of a study.*
2. *Describe the elements of a framework (concept, relational statement, conceptual model, theory, and conceptual map).*
3. *Identify the framework of a published study and develop a conceptual map of the framework.*
4. *Discuss the relationship of concepts and variables in research.*
5. *Examine the relationship between theory and research.*
6. *Critique a study framework.*

Abstract
Concept
Conceptual definition
Conceptual map
Conceptual model
Constructs
Existence statement
Framework

Hypothesis
Phenomenon (Phenomena)
Philosophy
Proposition
Relational statement
Statement
Theory
Variables

*R*esearch is based on theory; that is, the ideas that lead the researcher to develop a particular study have their roots in theory. The researcher has a theory about what the study outcomes are expected to be and why. This theory is expressed as the study framework. By performing the study, the researcher can answer the question "Was my theory correct?" Thus, a study tests the accuracy of theoretical ideas. When a study is completed, the researcher is expected to interpret the meaning of the findings in relation to the theoretical framework. Understanding the theory on which the study is based will help you determine whether or not it is appropriate to apply the study findings to your practice. But first, it is important that you identify and evaluate the framework as a part of critiquing the quality of the study. To assist you, this chapter discusses the nature of theories and theory testing, frameworks for theory testing, strategies for identifying the framework in a published study, and the critique of frameworks.

What Is a Theory?

We use theories to organize what we know about a phenomenon. Formally, a *theory* is defined as an integrated set of defined concepts and statements that present a view of a phenomenon and can be used to describe, explain, predict, and/or control that phenomenon. In Chapter 1, we indicated that the purpose of research can be either theory generation or theory testing. Most quantitative research is designed for theory testing. Theories are tested through research to determine the correctness of their descriptions, explanations, predictions, and strategies to control outcomes. Theories may be generated through qualitative research.

Theories Guide Nursing Practice

Theories have been developed in nursing to explain phenomena important to clinical practice. For example, we have a theory of uncertainty in illness (Mischel, 1988), a theory of health promotion behavior (Pender & Pender, 1996), and a theory of mother-infant attachment (Walker, 1992). Sometimes we use theories developed in other disciplines, such as psychology, and apply them to nursing situations. Although we use these theories to guide our practice, in many cases we have not tested them to determine whether or not the nursing actions proposed by the theory actually have the effects claimed.

A theory of mother-infant bonding proposed that bonding between a mother and her newborn child occurred within hours or days of birth (Klaus & Kennell, 1976). The theory proposed that if physical contact between mother and child did not occur during this short time frame, bonding would not occur and the relationship between mother and child would be permanently impaired. Nurses leaped on this idea and focused intensely on ensuring that physical contact between mother and newborn occurred. However, research testing this theoretical notion demonstrated that it was not true (Walker, 1992). Mother and newborn, kept apart because of illness or other circumstances, were able to bond. A theory of attachment, based on long-term studies of mothers and infants, emerged. These studies found that development of an attachment between mother and child was indeed critical but that the process occurred over a period of months rather than days. These findings, expressed as the theory of attachment, guide nurses in their care of mothers and their children.

Theories Are Abstract

Theories are abstract rather than concrete. *Abstract* means that the theory is the expression of an idea apart from any specific instance. An abstract idea focuses on more general things. Concrete ideas are concerned with realities or actual instances; they are particular rather than general. For example, the word "anxiety" represents an abstract idea; a family member pacing in an intensive care waiting room is a particular reality and thus is concrete. The abstract ideas in theories can be tested through research to verify that they hold true in a concrete reality. The abstract idea of the mother bonding with her newborn infant within a few hours or days did not hold true in a concrete reality. In some cases, theories are generated as a result of research. The specific instances discovered during the study are used by the researcher to develop more abstract (or general) ideas about the phenomenon of interest. Selye's (1976) theory of stress was developed through specific instances demonstrated in multiple studies. The specific instances discovered during a qualitative study are often used to generate theory. Critical thinking is required to generate theory, to test theory, or to relate concrete realities to abstract ideas.

Conceptual Models

Conceptual models are similar to theories and are sometimes referred to as theories. However, conceptual models are even more abstract than theories. A *conceptual model* broadly explains phenomena of interest, expresses assumptions, and reflects a philosophical stance. A *phenomenon* (the pleural form is *phenomena*) is an occurrence or a circumstance that is observed, something that impresses the observer as extraordinary, or a thing that appears to and is constructed by the mind. Caring is a phenomenon. Assumptions are statements that are taken for granted or considered true, even though they have not been scientifically tested. For example, we might assume that people who are poor feel poor. *Philosophies* are rational intellectual explorations of truths, principles of being, knowledge, or conduct. A *philosophical stance* is a specific philosophical view held by a person or group of individuals. For example, a philosophical stance might hold that there is no single reality, that reality is different for each individual. Although conceptual models vary in their level of abstraction and in the breadth of phenomena they explain, they all provide a broad overall picture of the phenomena they explain. Conceptual models are not generally considered testable through research. However, theories derived from a conceptual model can be tested.

Most disciplines have several conceptual models, each with a distinctive vocabulary. A number of conceptual models have been developed in nursing. For example, Roy's model describes adaptation as the primary phenomenon of interest to nursing (Roy & Andrews, 1998). Her model identifies the elements she considers essential to adaptation and describes how they interact to produce adaptation. Orem (1995) considers self-care to be the phenomenon central to nursing. Her model explains how nurses facilitate the self-care of clients. Rogers sees human beings as the central phenomenon of interest to nursing, and her model is designed to explain the nature of human beings (Rogers, Malinski, & Barrett, 1994). A conceptual model may use the same or similar terms as other models but define them in different ways. For example, Roy, Orem, and Rogers all may use the term "health" but define it in different ways.

Framework

A *framework* is a brief explanation of a theory or those portions of a theory to be tested in a study. Every study has a framework. This is true whether the study is physiologic or psychosocial. A clearly expressed framework is one indication of a well-developed study. Perhaps the researcher expects one variable to cause the other. In a well-thought-out study, the researcher would explain abstractly in the framework why one variable is expected to cause the other. Concretely, the idea would be expressed as a hypothesis to be tested through the study methodology.

Unfortunately, in some studies, the ideas that compose the framework remain nebulous and vaguely expressed. Although the researcher believes that the variables being studied are related in some fashion, this notion is expressed only in concrete terms. The researcher may make little attempt to explain why the variables are thought to be related. However, the rudiment of a framework is the expectation (perhaps not directly expressed) that there may be an important link(s) among the study variables. Sometimes rudimentary ideas for the framework are expressed in the introduction or literature review, in which linkages among variables found in previous studies are discussed, but then the researcher stops without fully developing the ideas as a framework. These are referred to as "implicit frameworks." In most cases, a careful reader can extract an implicit framework from the text. Unfortunately, many nursing studies have implicit frameworks; 49% of nursing practice studies published between 1977 and 1986 had no identifiable theoretical perspective (Moody, Wilson, Smyth, Schwartz, Tittle, & Van Cott, 1988).

As the body of knowledge related to a phenomenon increases, the development of a framework to express the knowledge becomes easier. Therefore, frameworks for quasi-experimental and experimental studies, which usually have a background of descriptive and correlational studies, should be more easily and fully developed than frameworks for descriptive studies. Descriptive studies often examine multiple factors to understand a phenomenon not previously well studied. Theoretical work related to the phenomenon may be tentative or nonexistent. Therefore, the framework may not be as well developed.

In some studies, the framework is derived from a well-tested theory that has been used as the framework for many studies. Most theories used as nursing research frameworks are from other fields and are based on theoretical works from psychology (e.g., the theory of stress and coping; Lazarus & Folkman, 1984), physiology (e.g., the theory of biological rhythms; Luce, 1970), and sociology (e.g., the theory of internal versus external control; Rotter, 1966). However, few nursing studies actually test statements from existing theory. Rather, the theory has been used somewhat shallowly to provide an overall orientation for the study. Thus, the framework is disconnected and does not guide the research process. In other words, it does not influence the statement of hypotheses, the design of the study, or the interpretation of findings.

In other studies, the framework is developed from newly proposed theory.

Newly proposed theories in nursing often emerge from questions related to identified nursing problems or from the clinical insight that a relationship exists between or among elements important to desired nursing outcomes. These situations tend to be concrete and require that the researcher, using critical reasoning, express these concrete ideas in abstract language. New theories may also be developed from elements of existing theories not previously related or from conceptual models.

The Elements of Theory

The first step in understanding theories is to become familiar with the elements related to theoretical ideas and their application. These elements include the concepts, relational statements, and conceptual map.

Concept

The concept is the basic element of a theory. A published study should include identification of all of the concepts important to the framework and definitions of these concepts. Two terms closely related to concept are construct and variable. The linkages among constructs, concepts, and variables are illustrated following.

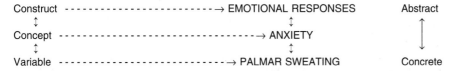

A *concept* is a term that abstractly describes and names an object or phenomenon, thus providing it with a separate identity or meaning. For example, the term "anxiety" is a concept. In conceptual models, concepts have very general meanings and are sometimes referred to as *constructs*. A construct associated with the concept of anxiety might be "emotional responses." At a more concrete level, terms are referred to as variables and are narrow in their definition. A *variable* is more specific than a concept and implies that the term is defined so that it is measurable. The word "variable" means that numerical values of the term vary from one instance to another. A variable related to anxiety might be "palmar sweating" because a specific method exists for assigning numerical values to varying amounts of palmar sweat.

Defining Concepts

Defining concepts allows consistency in the way the term is used. A *conceptual definition* differs from the dictionary definition of a word. A conceptual definition is more comprehensive than a denotative (or dictionary) definition and includes associated meanings the word may have. For example, a conceptual definition of "fireplace" might include the senses of hospitality and warm comfort that are often associated with fireplaces, while the dictionary definition is more narrow and specific. Many terms commonly used in nursing language have not been clearly defined. The use of these terms in theory or research requires thoughtful exploration of the meanings the terms have within nursing and a clear statement of their meaning within the particular theory or study.

The importance of going beyond the dictionary definition of a concept is illustrated in a study designed to explore the meaning of the concept "caring" (Morse, Solberg, Neander, Bottorff, & Johnson, 1990) that was funded by the National Center for Nursing Research. The questions posed by these researchers illustrate the critical thought that must precede the development of a conceptual definition. Although the concept of caring is central to nursing, efforts to define it have been difficult. For example, the terms "caring," "care," and "nursing care" have different meanings. Caring may be an action such as "taking care of" or a concern such as "caring about." Caring may be viewed from the perspective of the nurse or the patient. The authors identified five categories of caring: (1) caring as a human trait, (2) caring as a moral imperative (ethically, one is obligated to provide it), (3) caring as an affect (feeling), (4) caring as an interpersonal relationship, and (5) caring as a therapeutic intervention. Caring has an effect on the subjective experience of the patient and the physical response of the patient.

There are a number of questions about caring that need to be answered: (1) "Is caring a constant and uniform characteristic, or may caring be present in various degrees within individuals?" (2) "Is caring an emotional state that can be depleted?" (3) "Can caring be nontherapeutic? Can a nurse care too much?" (4) "Can cure occur without caring? Can a nurse provide safe practice without caring?" (5) "What difference does caring make to the patient?" (Morse et al., 1990, pp. 9–11). The authors' conclusion was that a clear conceptual definition of caring did not yet exist. The work of these authors generated considerable effort by others to develop further the conceptual definition of caring.

A related concept, "direct caregiving," has been carefully examined and defined by Swanson, Jensen, Specht, Johnson, and Maas (1997) to be "provision by a family care provider of appropriate personal and health care for a family member or significant other" (pp. 68–69). Caregiving addresses the care recipient's emotional, social, and physical needs. In order for direct caregiving to occur, the caregiver must have "a sense of responsibility, filial obligation, adequate financial resources, good health, and family and marital support. Social skills, spiritual support, the history of the relationship between caregiver and care recipient, and role acceptance have also been identified as important antecedents to direct caregiving" (p. 69).

Because of the significance of conceptual definitions, it is important that you identify the researcher's conceptual definitions of terms when you critique a study. Each variable in the study should be associated with a concept, a conceptual definition, and a method of measurement. You need to determine links among the conceptual definitions, the variables in the study, and the related measurement methods. (These linkages are discussed in Chapter 3.)

TO CRITIQUE a framework, use your critical thinking skills to seek answers to the following questions about the concepts, conceptual definitions, variables, and measurement methods.

1. *What are the concepts in the framework?*
2. *How are the concepts defined?*
3. *Are the conceptual definitions clear and adequate?*
4. *What are the variables in the study?*
5. *Is each study variable associated with a concept and its definition?*
6. *What measurement methods are used in the study?*
7. *Is each measurement method consistent with its associated concept and conceptual definition?*

Critiquing a framework requires that you go beyond the framework itself to examine its linkages to other components of the study. To answer the questions above, you must first extract the concepts and conceptual definitions from written text in the literature review or discussion of the framework. Then you must judge the adequacy of the definitions and the linkages of concepts to variables and their measurement.

Example—How to Extract Concepts and Conceptual Definitions from a Published Framework

The following framework was obtained from a study by Scherer and Schmeider (1996) of the role of self-efficacy in assisting patients with chronic obstructive pulmonary disease to manage breathing difficulty. The study was published in *Clinical Nursing Research*. Concepts have been circled and conceptual definitions have been underlined to show you how to identify and mark them in published studies.

concept
conceptual
definition

concept

concept
conceptual
definitions

"Perceived self-efficacy is defined as individuals' perceptions that they will be capable of performing a given behavior to produce a certain outcome (Bandura, 1977). Self-efficacy theory postulates that two types of expectancies influence behavior: outcome and efficacy. Outcome expectancy refers to the conviction that certain behaviors will lead to certain outcomes. Efficacy expectancy is the conviction that one can successfully execute the behavior required to produce the outcome. According to Bandura (1977), the strength of individuals' convictions about their ability to produce a specific outcome determines whether or not they attempt to deal with a difficult situation. Thus self-efficacy judgments play a part in determining which activities or situations a person will perform or avoid.

concept

conceptual
definition

Expectations of personal self-efficacy are based on four sources of information: performance accomplishments, vicarious experiences, verbal persuasion, and emotional/physical arousal. Performance accomplishments refer to successful mastery that results from personal experience. Successful mastery of a task tends to increase perceived self-efficacy (Bandura, 1977). Performance accomplishments can be fostered through encouragement of patient goal setting. Target behaviors are then divided into easily managed tasks that proceed in a stepwise manner to facilitate success. Success will increase perceived self-efficacy.

concept

conceptual
definition

Vicarious experiences are fostered by exposing individuals to persons of similar capabilities who have successfully performed the behavior. Such observations enhance individuals' expectation of mastery. Examples of vicarious experiences include the use of videos, peer groups, tapes, books, and pamphlets.

concept

conceptual
definition

Verbal persuasion is used to convince people, through discussion, that they can perform an activity. Verbal persuasion is readily provided through praise and encouragement. Emotional/physiological arousal can also influence self-efficacy expectations.

concept

No clear
conceptual
definition

Individuals rely on physiological feedback to judge their capabilities. Individuals perceive anxiety, fatigue, and other symptoms as signs of physical inefficacy. Interpreting symptoms, and using stress management techniques to reduce anxiety, can improve efficacy expectations and performance.

concept

conceptual
definition

In addition, self-efficacy expectations vary on several dimensions that have an important effect on performance and these include magnitude, generality, and strength (Bandura, 1977, 1986). Magnitude refers to the level of difficulty of the task. Some individuals feel capable of performing only simple tasks (i.e., low-magnitude expectation). (Generality) refers to the extent that a domain of behavior can be generalized to other situations. For example, if patients with COPD are successful in performing an activity (such as stair climbing) when supervised, they may anticipate being successful when performing the activity unsupervised. (Strength) refers to the confidence individuals have in the accomplishment of a specific task." (Scherer & Schmeider, 1996, pp. 344–346)

— concept
conceptual
definition
— concept
conceptual
definition

Statements

Statements express claims that are important to the theory. An *existence statement* declares that a given concept exists or that a given relationship between concepts occurs. For example, an existence statement might claim that a condition referred to as "stress" exists and that there is a relationship between the concept of stress and the concept of health. A *relational statement* clarifies the type of relationship that exists between or among concepts. For example, one relational statement might propose that high levels of stress are related to declining levels of health. Another relational statement might propose that exercise is related to weight. It is the statements of a theory that are tested through research, not the theory itself. Testing a theory involves determining the truth of each relational statement in the theory. However, a single study might test only one relational statement. As more studies examine a single relational statement, increasing evidence of the truth or falsity of that statement is confirmed. Many studies are required to validate all the statements in a theory.

In theories, *propositions* or relational statements can be expressed at various levels of abstraction. The statements found in conceptual models (general propositions) are at a high level of abstraction. Statements found in theories (specific propositions) are at a moderate level of abstraction. Hypotheses are at a low level of abstraction and are specific. As statements are expressed in a less abstract way, they become more narrow in scope (Fawcett & Downs, 1992), as shown below.

General Propositions

↕

Specific Propositions

↕

Hypotheses

Statements at varying levels of abstraction that express relationships between or among the same conceptual ideas can be arranged in hierarchical form, from general to specific. This will allow the reader to see the logical links among the various levels of abstraction.

1. *What statements are expressed within the publication?*
2. *Are all of the study concepts included within the statements?*
3. *Are the statements expressed as both propositions and hypotheses (or research questions)?*
4. *Are one or more statements being tested by the study design?*

Extracting Statements from a Published Framework

In some studies, the statements are implied rather than clearly stated, and sometimes they are located within the introduction or literature review rather than within a clearly expressed framework. If the statements are only implied, use your critical reasoning to extract them from the text and express them as statements. To begin, search through the introduction, the background and significance, the literature review, and the framework for sentences that seem to express relationships between concepts included in the study. Write down a single sentence from the text that seems to be a relational statement. Express it graphically. For example the statement "exercise is related to weight" could be expressed as

exercise ↔ weight

Move to the next statement you can identify and express it graphically. Continue until you have graphically expressed all of the statements related to the selected concepts. Examine the linkages among the graphic statements you have developed. The theoretical ideas embedded in the text will gradually become clearer.

The extraction of statements from text in a published study is illustrated in Scherer and Schmieder's (1996) study. Note that all of the concepts previously identified are included in these statements. General propositions are underlined, specific propositions are underlined with a wavy line, and hypotheses are underlined with a double rule. If you were marking text in an article, you might use a variety of colored highlighters to differentiate these various types of statements. You might also write in the margins.

general proposition ⟨ "Perceived self-efficacy is defined as individuals' perceptions that they will be capable of performing a given behavior to produce a certain outcome (Bandura, 1977). Self-efficacy theory postulates that two types of expectancies influence behavior: outcome and efficacy. Outcome expectancy refers to the conviction that certain behaviors will lead to certain outcomes. Efficacy expectancy is the conviction that one can successfully execute the behavior required to produce the outcome. According to Bandura (1977), the strength of individuals' convictions about their ability to produce a specific outcome determines whether or not they attempt to deal with a difficult situation. Thus self-efficacy judgments play a part in determining which activities or situations a person will perform or avoid. *[specific proposition]*

Expectations of personal self-efficacy are based on four sources of information: performance accomplishments, vicarious experiences, verbal persuasion, and emotional/physical arousal. *[general proposition]* Performance accomplishments refer to successful mastery that results from personal experience. Successful mastery of a task tends to increase perceived self-efficacy (Bandura, 1977). *[general proposition]* Performance accomplishments can be fostered through encouragement of patient goal setting. *[specific proposition]* Target behaviors are then divided into easily managed tasks that proceed in a stepwise manner to facilitate success. Success will increase perceived self-efficacy.

Vicarious experiences are fostered by exposing individuals to persons of similar capabilities who have successfully performed the behavior. Such observations enhance individuals' expectation of mastery. Examples of vicarious experiences include the use of videos, peer groups, tapes, books, and pamphlets.

Verbal persuasion is used to convince people, through discussion, that they can perform an activity. Verbal persuasion is readily provided through praise and encouragement. Emotional/physiological arousal can also influence self-efficacy expectations. Individuals rely on physiological feedback to judge their capabilities. Individuals perceive anxiety, fatigue, and other symptoms as signs of physical inefficacy. Interpreting symptoms, and using stress management techniques to reduce anxiety, can improve efficacy expectations and performance. *[specific proposition]*

In addition, self-efficacy expectations vary on several dimensions that have an important effect on performance and these include magnitude, generality, and strength (Bandura, 1977, 1986). *[general proposition]* Magnitude refers to the level of difficulty of the task. Some individuals feel capable of performing only simple tasks (i.e., low-magnitude expectation). Generality refers to the extent that a domain of behavior can be generalized to other situations. For example, if patients with COPD are successful in performing an activity (such as stair climbing) when supervised, they may anticipate being successful when performing the activity unsupervised. Strength refers to the confidence individuals have in the accomplishment of a specific task. Confidence regarding one's ability to manage or avoid breathing difficulties would increase following attendance at this [pulmonary rehabilitation] program [on self-efficacy expectations in patients with COPD]." (Scherer & Schmeider, 1996, p. 346) *[hypothesis]*

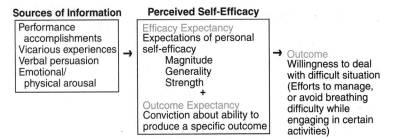

FIGURE 5-1

Conceptual map constructed from statements extracted from Scherer and Schmeider's (1996) study. (Data from Scherer, Y. K., & Schmeider, L. E. [1996]. The role of self-efficacy in assisting patients with chronic obstructive pulmonary disease to manage breathing difficulty. *Clinical Nursing Research, 5*[3], 343–355.)

Conceptual Map

One strategy for expressing a theory is a *conceptual map* that graphically shows the interrelationships of the concepts and statements (Artinian, 1982; Fawcett & Downs, 1992; Moody, 1989; Newman, 1979; Silva, 1981). A conceptual map is developed to explain which concepts contribute to or partially cause an outcome. The map should be supported by references from the literature. A conceptual map summarizes and integrates what is known about a phenomenon more succinctly and clearly than does a literary explanation and allows one to grasp the wholeness of a phenomenon.

A conceptual map includes all of the major concepts in a theory or framework. These concepts are linked by arrows expressing the proposed linkages between concepts. Each linkage shown by an arrow is a graphic illustration of a relational statement (proposition) of the theory. Mapping is useful in identifying gaps in the logic of the theory and reveals inconsistencies, incompleteness, and errors (Artinian, 1982). Scherer and Schmeider (1996) did not provide a conceptual map with their framework. The map in Figure 5-1 was constructed from the statements extracted from their published study.

IN CRITIQUING a conceptual map, use critical reasoning to seek answers to the following questions:

1. *Is the framework expressed as a conceptual map?*
2. *Are all of the concepts in the study included on the map?*
3. *Does the author provide conceptual definitions of each concept on the map?*
4. *Does the author provide statements for each linkage between concepts shown on the map?*
5. *Does the author provide references from the literature to support the linkages between concepts shown on the map?*
6. *Is it clear which linkages on the map are being tested by the published study? If no conceptual map is provided, develop a map that represents the study's framework and describe the map.*

Frameworks for Physiologic Studies

Until recently, physiologic studies tended not to have a clearly defined framework. Some physiologic researchers discounted the importance of the theoretical dimension of research. This was due, in part, to the emphasis in nursing on psychosocial theories and a tendency to discount biological knowledge. The theoretical basis for physiologic studies is derived from physics, physiology, and pathophysiology and may not be considered theory by some. The knowledge in these areas is well tested through research, and theoretical relationships are often referred to as "laws" and "principles." They may be considered facts rather than theories. However, propositions can be developed and tested using these laws and principles and applying them to nursing problems. Developing a framework to clearly express the logic on which the study is based is helpful both to the researcher and to those reading the published study. The critique of a physiologic framework is no different from that of other frameworks. However, concepts and conceptual definitions may be less abstract than those of many psychosocial studies. Concepts in physiologic studies might be terms such as "cardiac output," "dyspnea," "wound healing," "blood pressure," "tissue hypoxia," "metabolism," and "functional status."

Timmerman and Stevenson (1996) developed a physiologic framework for a study of the relationship between binge eating severity and body fat in non-purge binge eating women. Following is their description of their framework.

"The conceptual framework for this study was the set point theory of energy regulation in which body fat is regulated within specific parameters or a set point. In defense of the body's set point, variations in food intake are counteracted by adjustments in the level of energy expended. The body responds to increased consumption by increasing the energy expended and to decreased consumption by reducing the energy expended (Keesey, 1986). This theory explains why weight gains and losses cannot be predicted solely on changes in caloric intake. Obesity occurs when body fat is regulated at an elevated set point. Although further research is needed on how the set point becomes elevated, consumption of long-term, high fat diets is one factor identified as potentially increasing the set point (Hill, Dorton, Sykes, & Digirolamo, 1989).

According to the set point theory, the body would defend its set point against intermittent binge episodes by increasing energy expenditure. However, when severity of binge eating increases (larger amounts ingested and binges more frequent), the body's set point would be elevated. A long history of habitual binge eating may contribute to [the] degree of obesity by progressively elevating the set point. Thus, individuals with different levels of binge eating

continued

severity should, hypothetically, have different amounts of body fat."
(p. 390)

"The purpose of this study was to clarify the relationship between binge eating severity and degree of body fat by using more precise measurements of binge eating severity (caloric intake) and body fat (underwater weight) than [those] used in previous studies. In addition, length of binge eating history was measured as a separate variable to determine its role in the accumulation of body fat. Other factors identified from the literature (total caloric intake, age, parity, weight cycling, activity level, genetic predisposition to obesity, and age of obesity onset) also were measured in order to examine their influence on degree of body fat in the nonpurge binge eating population.

The research questions were: (a) What is the relationship between binge eating severity and body fat (percent of body fat and BMI) in non-purge binge eating women? and (b) What are the best predictors for body fat (percent of body fat and BMI [body mass index]) among nonpurge binge eating women?" (p. 391)

Frameworks Including Conceptual Nursing Models

Relatively few nursing studies have frameworks that include a conceptual nursing model. Moody and colleagues (1988), who examined nursing practice research from 1977 to 1986, found an increase in studies using a nursing model as a framework from 8% in the first half of the decade under study to 13% in the second half. The most frequently used models were those of Orem, Rogers, and Roy. Silva (1986), who studied the extent to which five nursing models (those of Johnson, Roy, Orem, Rogers, and Newman) had been used as frameworks for nursing research, found 62 studies between 1952 and 1985 that used these models. However, only nine of these studies met her specified criteria as actually testing nursing theory. Only in these nine studies were statements from the nursing theory extracted and tested by the study design.

Building a body of knowledge related to a particular conceptual model requires an organized program of research. This program of research is referred to as a "research tradition." A group of scholars dedicated to conducting research related to the model develop theories compatible with the model, including propositions for testing. An organized plan for testing these propositions is agreed upon. Researchers conducting studies consistent with a particular research tradition often maintain a network of communication regarding their work. In some cases, annual conferences focused on the model are held to share research findings, explore theoretical ideas, and maintain network contacts. Conceptual models of nursing do not have well-established research tradi-

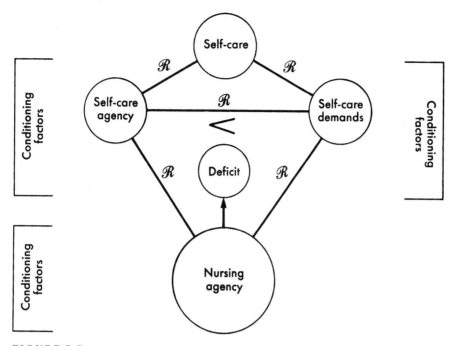

FIGURE 5-2

A conceptual framework for nursing (R = relationship; < = deficit relationship, current or projected). (From Orem, D. E. [1995]. *Nursing: Concepts of practice* [5th ed.]. St. Louis: Mosby-Year Book, with permission.)

tions (Fawcett, 1989). However, research traditions are developing for some nursing models.

One example of a nursing model with an emerging research tradition is Orem's (1995) model of self-care. This model focuses on the domain of nursing practice and on what nurses actually do when they practice nursing. Orem proposes that individuals generally know how to take care of themselves (self-care). If they are dependent in some way (by being a child, aged, or handicapped, for example), family members take on this responsibility (dependent care). If individuals are ill or have some defect (such as diabetes or a colostomy), they or their family members acquire special skills to provide that care (therapeutic self-care). An individual's capacity to provide self-care is referred to as "self-care agency." A self-care deficit occurs when self-care demand exceeds self-care agency. These ideas are expressed graphically in Figure 5-2.

Nursing care is provided only when there is a deficit in the self-care or dependent care that the individual and the family cannot provide (self-care deficit). In this case, the nurse (or nurses) develops a nursing system to provide the needed care. This system involves prescribing, designing, and providing the needed care. The goal of nursing care is to facilitate resumption of self-care by the person and/or family. There are three types of nursing systems: wholly compensatory, partly compensatory, and supportive-educative. Selection of one of these systems is based on the capacity of the person to perform self-care.

The notion of self-care as an important construct for nursing has drawn nurse researchers to Orem's work. Multiple studies have been performed examining self-care in a variety of nursing situations. Instruments, consistent with Orem's model, have been developed to measure some of Orem's concepts. Orem (1995) has developed three theories related to her model: the Theory of Self-Care Deficits, the Theory of Self-Care, and the Theory of Nursing Systems (also referred to as the General Theory of Nursing). However, few propositions emerging from Orem's theories have been tested.

For a number of years, Dodd and colleagues have been conducting studies based on Orem's model (Dodd, 1982a,b, 1983a,b, 1984a–c, 1987a,b, 1988a,b, 1991, 1996; Dodd & Dibble, 1993; Dodd, Dibble, & Thomas, 1992a,b; Dodd et al., 1986–1990, 1996; Dodd et al., 1988–1992; Dodd, Lindsay, et al., 1992; Dodd, Lovejoy, et al., 1992; Dodd & Moody, 1981; Dodd, Thomas, & Dibble, 1991; Facione & Dodd, 1995; Musci & Dodd, 1990). Many of these studies have been funded through the National Institutes of Health (NIH). This is an important example of the carefully planned programs of research that are necessary to validate the usefulness of a nursing theory in guiding nursing practice.

In 1996, Dodd, Larson, Dibble, Miaskowski, Greenspan, MacPhail, Hauch, Paul, Ignoffo, and Shiba conducted a National Cancer Institute-funded study to test the effectiveness of a nurse-initiated systematic oral hygiene teaching program in preventing chemotherapy-induced oral mucositis. In previous studies (Dodd et al., 1986–1990; 1988–1992), Dodd and colleagues had found that nursing management of mucositis in patients receiving chemotherapy for cancer was "in disarray." Because most patients are receiving chemotherapy on an outpatient basis, it is not possible to monitor closely the condition of the patient's mouth.

> "Many patients were told that they might experience oral problems because of their chemotherapy, but they were not instructed in any type of preventive mouth care. Therefore, most patients who experienced mouth problems initially tried to self-manage using a trial-and-error approach. When patients sought assistance from their physicians or nurses, they were offered a variety of remedies with instructions to 'swish and spit.' Many patients indicated that this approach was not only ineffective, it actually increased their discomfort and mouth problems." (Dodd et al., 1996, p. 922)

Basing her claims on Orem's theory of self-care agency, Dodd proposed that a nurse-initiated systematic oral hygiene teaching program [PRO-SELF©: Mouth Aware (PSMA) Program] offered prior to the development of mucositis would enhance the patient's self-care agency, resulting in a decrease in the incidence and severity of mucositis (see Fig. 5-3). The Oral Assessment Guide

Mouth Care

Each day you MUST:

1. **Look** at your whole mouth, including your lips and tongue *every morning* before brushing, flossing, and rinsing. **Check** for problems listed below.
2. **Brush** your teeth for 90 seconds *twice a day*– after breakfast and before bedtime.
3. **Floss** your teeth at least *once a day*.
4. **Rinse** your mouth with one capful of the medicated mouthwash for 30 seconds *twice a day*–after breakfast and before bedtime. Swish thoroughly and spit out. DO NOT SWALLOW. **Do not use any other mouthwash.***
5. **Do NOT eat or drink ANYTHING, including WATER, FOR 30 MINUTES** after using the medicated mouthwash.
6. **Avoid** smoking, alcoholic beverages, and spicy foods.

Mouth Problems to Check for Daily

*If you have any of the following **problems**,* you must call your nurse AS SOON AS POSSIBLE.

1. **Sores** in your mouth
2. **White spots** in your mouth
3. **Pain** in your mouth
4. **Difficulty** eating or drinking
5. Unusual amount of **bleeding**

Nurse's name _____

Phone number _____

* Specific instructions for denture wearers were provided.

FIGURE 5-3

PRO-SELF© Mouth Aware Prevention Program for Non-Denture Wearers. (From Dodd, et al. [1996]. Randomized clinical trial of chlorhexidine versus placebo for prevention of oral mucositis in patients receiving chemotherapy. *Oncology Nursing Forum, 23*[6], 921, with permission.)

(Eilers, Berger, & Peterson, 1988) was used to guide clinician ratings of chemotherapy-related changes in the oral mucosa. The study developed to validate this proposition also tested the effectiveness of two mouthwashes used in the mouth care protocol: chlorhexidine and a placebo control (sterile water). The findings of the study validated Orem's concept of self-care agency. "The PSMA program provided patients with the knowledge and skills needed to perform the systematic oral hygiene protocol. Evidence exists that the patients used the PSMA program as instructed. . . . Data from this study suggest that the use of a systematic oral hygiene program prescribed in the PSMA program may have reduced the incidence of chemotherapy-induced mucositis from an a priori estimate of 44% to less than 26%" (p. 926). No significant difference was found in the effectiveness of the two mouthwashes used in the study. Thus, Dodd and colleagues recommend the use of water in implementing the PSMA program. This study was selected for the 1996 Oncology Nursing Society (ONS)/Schering Corporation Excellence in Cancer Nursing Research Award.

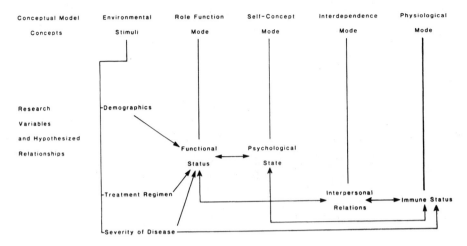

FIGURE 5-4
Conceptual map including a conceptual nursing model (Roy) and a tentative theory: framework for studying functional status after diagnosis of breast cancer. (From Tulman, L., & Fawcett, J. [1990]. A framework for studying functional status after diagnosis of breast cancer. *Cancer Nursing, 13*[2], 98, with permission.)

Critiquing a framework that includes both a conceptual model and a theory is more complex than critiquing a framework based only on a theory. You need to identify constructs and their definitions, as well as concepts and their definitions. Both general and specific propositions need to be identified and linked to the hypotheses or research questions. Including a conceptual model as well as a theory in a framework is a relatively new idea in nursing. Therefore, few published studies have frameworks that include a conceptual model, a theory, and a conceptual map illustrating the linkage between the model and the theory. The map for such a framework must include both the conceptual model and a testable theory. Figure 5-4 shows an example of a map including both. This map was developed by Tulman and Fawcett (1990) to illustrate a framework designed to study functional status after diagnosis of breast cancer and is based on Roy's Model of Adaptation.

Critiquing a Framework

A FRAMEWORK must be critiqued within the context of the overall study. There-fore, in addition to critiquing the logical structure of the framework itself, you need to use critical reasoning to address the following questions:

1. Did the framework guide the methodology of the study? To determine this, use the following criteria.
   a. The concepts are linked with variables that are measured.

    b. The concepts are represented in hypotheses, research questions, or objectives.

    c. The study hypotheses, research questions, or objectives emerge from propositions in the framework.

    d. The hypotheses, research questions, or objectives are tested statistically.

2. *Were the study findings related to the framework? Examine the discussion of findings. Look for comments connecting the findings to specific elements of the framework. The author may discuss the adequacy of the variables and measurements as reflections of the concepts. Search for comments discussing the implications of the findings in terms of the truth or falsity of framework propositions. The author may make evaluative statements about the overall framework or suggest modifications based on study findings.*

3. *a. Are the findings for each hypothesis, question, or objective consistent with those proposed by the framework?*

    Judge the truth or falsity of the framework propositions based on the study findings.

    b. What do the findings tell you about the usefulness of the framework for clinical practice and future studies?

4. *If the findings are not consistent with the framework, was the methodology adequate to test the hypothesis, research question, or objective?*

    This question will need to be answered individually for each hypothesis, research question, or objective. You will need to become familiar with the content of Chapters 7 (research designs), 8 (sampling), 9 (measurement), and 10 (statistical analysis) to answer this question adequately.

5. *Are the findings consistent with those of other studies using the same framework (or testing the same propositions)?*

    Your ability to answer this question is dependent upon the author's providing information in the published study of other studies that have tested the same propositions.

SUMMARY

Research is based on theory. We use theories to organize what we know about a phenomenon. A theory is defined as an integrated set of defined concepts and statements that present a view of a phenomenon and can be used to describe, explain, predict, and/or control that phenomenon. Theories are abstract rather than concrete. Abstract means the theory is the expression of an idea apart from any specific instance. Concrete ideas are concerned with realities or actual instances. Conceptual models are similar to theories and are sometimes referred to as theories. Conceptual models are even more abstract than theories. A conceptual model broadly explains phenomena of interest, expresses assumptions, and reflects a philosophical stance. A framework is a brief explanation of a theory or those portions of a theory to be tested in a study. Every study has a framework, although some frameworks are poorly expressed. The framework must identify and define the concepts and the relational statements being tested. Because frameworks are important in the conduct of research, an essential element of critiquing a study is to identify and evaluate the framework. To critique a framework, you need to understand the structure of theories and the logic on which they are based.

The first step in understanding theories is to become familiar with the terms related to theoretical ideas and their application. These terms include concept, relational statement, and conceptual map. A concept is a term that abstractly describes and names an object or a phenomenon, thus providing it with a separate identity or meaning. Defining a concept allows consistency in the way the term is used. A statement expresses a claim that is important to the theory. Existence statements declare that a given concept exists or that a given relationship occurs. Relational statements clarify the type of relationship that exists between or among concepts. Statements can be expressed at various levels of abstraction. The statements found in conceptual models (general propositions) are at a high level of abstraction. Statements found in theories (specific propositions) are at a moderate level of abstraction. Hypotheses are at a low level of abstraction and are specific. One strategy for expressing a theory is a conceptual map that diagrammati-

cally shows the interrelationships of the concepts and statements. A conceptual map includes all of the major concepts in the theory. These concepts are linked together by arrows that indicate the proposed linkages between concepts. Testing a theory involves determining the truth of each relational statement in the theory. Critiquing a framework requires the identification and evaluation of the concepts, their definitions, and the statements linking the concepts. Questions are provided throughout the chapter to assist you in this process. Examples of the critiques of published studies are included to illustrate the critique process.

Relatively few nursing studies have frameworks that include a conceptual nursing model. An organized program of research is important for building a body of knowledge related to the phenomena explained by a particular conceptual model. This program of research is referred to as a research tradition. One example of a nursing model with an emerging research tradition is Orem's model of self-care. An example of a framework that includes Roy's model is presented to illustrate the development of a framework with both a model and a theory.

REFERENCES

Artinian, B. (1982). Conceptual mapping. Development of the strategy. *Western Journal of Nursing Research, 4*(4), 379–393.

Bandura, A. (1977). Self-efficacy: Toward a unifying theory of behavior and change. *Psychological Review, 84*(2), 191–215.

Bandura, A. (1986). *Social foundations of thought and action: A social cognitive theory.* Englewood Cliffs, NJ: Prentice Hall.

Dodd, M. J. (1982a). Chemotherapy knowledge in patients with cancer: Assessment and informational interventions. *Oncology Nursing Forum, 9*(3), 39–44.

Dodd, M. J. (1982b). Assessing patient self-care for side effects of cancer chemotherapy—Part I. *Cancer Nursing, 5*(6), 447–451.

Dodd, M. J. (1983a). Assessing patient self-care for side ef-

fects of cancer chemotherapy—Part II. *Cancer Nursing, 5*(6), 63–67.

Dodd, M. J. (1983b). Self-care for side effects of cancer chemotherapy: An assessment of nursing interventions. *Cancer Nursing, 6*(1), 63–67.

Dodd, M. J. (1984a). Patterns of self-care in cancer patients receiving radiation therapy. *Oncology Nursing Forum, 10*(3), 23–27.

Dodd, M. J. (1984b). Self-care for patients with breast cancer to prevent side effects of chemotherapy: A concern for public health nursing. *Public Health Nursing, 1*(4), 202–209.

Dodd, M. (1984c). Measuring informational intervention for chemotherapy knowledge and self-care behavior. *Research in Nursing & Health, 7*(1), 43–50.

Dodd, M. J. (1987a). *Managing side effects of chemotherapy and radiation therapy: A guide for patients and nurses.* Norwich, CT: Appleton & Lange.

Dodd, M. J. (1987b). Efficacy of proactive information on self-care in radiation therapy patients. *Heart & Lung, 16*(5), 538–544.

Dodd, M. J. (1988a). Efficacy of proactive information on self-care in chemotherapy patients. *Patient Education and Counseling, 11*(3), 215–225.

Dodd, M. J. (1988b). Patterns of self-care in patients with breast cancer. *Western Journal of Nursing Research, 10*(1), 7–14.

Dodd, M. J. (1991). *Managing the side effects of chemotherapy and radiation: A guide for patients and their families* (2nd ed.). Englewood Cliffs, NJ: Prentice Hall.

Dodd, M. J. (1996). *Managing the side effects of chemotherapy and radiation therapy: A guide for patients and their families* (3rd ed.). San Francisco: University of California, San Francisco, School of Nursing Press.

Dodd, M. J., & Dibble, S. L. (1993). Predictors of self-care: A test of Orem's model. *Oncology Nursing Forum, 20*(6), 895–901.

Dodd, M. J., Dibble, S. L., & Thomas, M. L. (1992a). Outpatient chemotherapy: Patients' and family members' concerns and coping strategies. *Journal of Public Health Nursing, 9*(1), 37–44.

Dodd, M. J., Dibble, S. L., & Thomas, M. L. (1992b). Self-care for patients experiencing cancer chemotherapy side effects: A concern for home care nurses. *Home Healthcare Nurse, 9*(1), 21–26.

Dodd, M. J., Larson, P. J., Dibble, S. L., Miaskowski, C., Greenspan, D., MacPhail, L., Hauch, W. W., Paul, St. M., Ignoffo, R., & Shiba, G. (1996). Randomized clinical trial of chlorhexidine versus placebo for prevention of oral mucositis in patients receiving chemotherapy. *Oncology Nursing Forum, 23*(6), 921–927.

Dodd, M. J., Lindsey, A. M., Larson, P., Musci, E., Thomas, M., Dibble, S. L., Hudes, M., & Hauck, W. (1986–1990). *Coping and self-care of cancer families: Nurse prospectus* (Final report). Funded by the National Institutes of Health, R01 CA 1440.

Dodd, M. J., Lindsey, A. M., Stetz, K., Lewis, B., Holzemer, W., Larson, P., Musci, E., Lovejoy, N., Dibble, S. L., Paul, S., & Hauck, W. (1988–1992). *Self-care interventions to decrease chemotherapy morbidity* (Final Report). Funded by the National Institutes of Health and the National Cancer Institute, R01 CA 48312.

Dodd, M. J., Lovejoy, N., Larson, P., Stetz, K., Lewis, B., Holzemer, W., Hauck, W., Paul, S., Lindsey, A., & Jusci, E. (1992). *Self-care intervention to decrease chemotherapy morbidity*. Invited paper presented at the Seventeenth Annual Congress of the Oncology Nursing Society, San Diego, CA.

Dodd, M. J., & Mood, D. W. (1981). Chemotherapy: Retention and review of information. *Cancer Nursing, 4*, 311–318.

Dodd, M. J., Thomas, M. L., & Dibble, S. L. (1991). Self-care for patients experiencing cancer chemotherapy side effects: A concern for home care nurses. *Home Healthcare Nurse, 9*(6), 21–26.

Eilers, J., Berger, A. M., & Peterson, M. C. (1988). Development, testing, and application of the oral assessment guide. *Oncology Nursing Forum, 15*(3), 325–330.

Facione, N., & Dodd, M. J. (1995). Women's narratives of help seeking for breast cancer. *Cancer Practice, 3*(4), 219–225.

Fawcett, J. (1989). *Analysis and evaluation of conceptual models of nursing* (2nd ed.). Philadelphia: Davis.

Fawcett, H., & Downs, F. (1992). *The relationship of theory and research* (2nd ed.). Norwalk, CT: Appleton-Century-Crofts.

Hill, J., Dorton, J., Sykes, M., & Digirolamo, M. (1989). Reversal of dietary obesity is influenced by its duration and severity. *International Journal of Obesity, 13*(5), 711–722.

Keesey, R. (1986). A set point theory of obesity. In K. Brownell & J. Foreyt (Eds.). *Handbook of eating disorders* (pp. 63–87). New York: Basic Books.

Klaus, M. H., & Kennell, J. H. (1976). *Maternal–infant bonding: The impact of early separation or loss on family development*. St. Louis: Mosby.

Lazarus, R., & Folkman, S. (1984). *Stress appraisal and coping*. New York: Springer.

Luce, G. (1970). *Biological rhythms in psychiatry and medicine*. Washington, DC: U.S. Public Health Service.

Mischel, M. H. (1988). Uncertainty in illness. *Image: Journal of Nursing Scholarship, 20*(4), 225–232.

Moody, L. E. (1989). Building a conceptual map to guide research. *Florida Nursing Review, 4*(1), 1–5.

Moody, L. E., Wilson, M. E., Smyth, K., Schwartz, R., Tittle, M., & Van Cott, M. L. (1988). Analysis of a decade of nursing practice research: 1977–1986. *Nursing Research, 37*(6), 374–379.

Morse, J. M., Solberg, S. M., Neander, W. L., Bottorff, J. L., & Johnson, J. L. (1990). Concepts of caring and caring as a concept. *Advances in Nursing Science, 13*(1), 1–14.

Musci, I., & Dodd, M. (1990). Predicting self-care with patients and family members' affective states and family function. *Oncology Nursing Forum, 17*(3), 394–400.

Newman, M. A. (1979). *Theory development in nursing*. Philadelphia: Davis.

Orem, D. E. (1995). *Nursing: Concepts of practice* (5th ed.). St. Louis: Mosby-Year Book.

Pender, N. J., & Pender, A. R. (1996). *Health promotion in nursing practice* (3rd ed.), Norwalk, CT: Appleton & Lange.

Rogers, M. E., Malinski, V. M., & Barrett, E. A. M. (1994). *Martha E. Rogers: Her life and her work*. Philadelphia: Davis.

Rotter, J. (1966). Generalized expectancies for internal versus external control of reinforcement. *Psychological Monographs, 80*(1), 1–28.

Roy, C., & Andrews, H. A. (1998). *Roy adaptation model.* Norwalk, CT: Appleton & Lange.

Scherer, Y. K., & Schmeider, L. E. (1996). The role of self-efficacy in assisting patients with chronic obstructive pulmonary disease to manage breathing difficulty. *Clinical Nursing Research, 5*(3), 343–355.

Selye, H. (1976). *The stress of life.* New York: McGraw-Hill.

Silva, M. C. (1981). Selection of a theoretical framework. In S. D. Krampitz & N. Pavlovich (Eds.). *Readings for nursing research* (pp. 17–28). St. Louis: Mosby.

Silva, M. C. (1986). Research testing nursing theory: State of the art. *Advances in Nursing Science, 9*(1), 1–11.

Swanson, E. A., Jensen, D. P., Specht, J., Johnson, M. L., & Maas, M. (1997). Caregiving: Concept analysis and outcomes. *Scholarly Inquiry for Nursing Practice: An International Journal, 11*(1), 65–79.

Timmerman, G. M., & Stevenson, J. S. (1996). The relationship between binge eating severity and body fat in non-purge binge eating women. *Research in Nursing & Health, 19*(5), 389–398.

Tulman, L., & Fawcett, J. (1990). A framework for studying functional status after diagnosis of breast cancer. *Cancer Nursing, 13*(2), 95–99.

Walker, L. O. (1992). *Parent-infant nursing science: Paradigms, phenomena, methods.* Philadelphia: Davis.

Examining Ethics
in Nursing Research

Completing this chapter should enable you to:

1. *Identify the historical events influencing the development of ethical codes and regulations for research.*
2. *Describe three ethical principles that are important in conducting research on human subjects.*
3. *Discuss the human rights that require protection in research.*
4. *Describe the informed consent process.*
5. *Evaluate the consent process in a research project.*
6. *Describe the functions of institutional review boards in research.*
7. *Examine the benefit-risk ratio of studies conducted in clinical agencies.*
8. *Describe the types of scientific misconduct that are occurring in the conduct, reporting, and publication of research today.*
9. *Discuss the use of animals in research.*
10. *Critique the ethical information provided in a published study.*

Anonymity

Autonomous agents

Benefit-risk ratio

Breach of confidentiality

Coercion

Confidentiality

Consent form

Covert data collection

Deception

Diminished autonomy

Discomfort and harm from a study

Ethical principles

Human rights

Informed consent

Institutional review

   Complete review

   Exempt from review

   Expedited review

Invasion of privacy

Minimal risk

Nontherapeutic research

Privacy

Scientific misconduct

Therapeutic research

Voluntary consent

*W*hat is unethical research? Are unethical studies that violate subjects' rights or involve scientific misconduct conducted today? One would like to believe that unethical research, such as the Nazi experiments of World War II, is a thing of the past. However, this is not the case, since studies continue to include evidence of scientific misconduct with the violation of subjects' rights and the publication of inaccurate scientific information (Beecher, 1966; Rankin & Esteves, 1997).

Scientific misconduct or fraud involves such practices as fabrication, falsi-fication, or forging of data; dishonest manipulation of the design or methods with protocol violations; misrepresentation of findings; and plagiarism (Rankin & Esteves, 1997). Scientific misconduct produces unethical research and can occur during the conduct, reporting, and publication of studies. This is a severe problem, with over half of the top 50 research institutions in the United States having fraud investigations (Chop & Silva, 1991). Thus, the ethical aspects of published studies and of research conducted in clinical agencies need to be critiqued. Most published studies include ethical information about subject selection and the data collection process in the methods section of the report. Studies conducted in clinical agencies need to be reviewed by an institutional review board to determine whether they are ethical.

To provide you with a background for examining ethical aspects of studies, this chapter includes some historical events, ethical codes, and regulations that influence the conduct of research. The following elements of ethical research are detailed: (1) protecting subjects' rights, (2) balancing the benefits and risks in a study, (3) obtaining informed consent, and (4) obtaining institutional approval for research. Your role as a patient advocate when research is conducted in your agency is also discussed. Two timely ethical issues of scientific misconduct and the use of animals in research are discussed. The chapter concludes with critique guidelines to assist you in determining whether a study is ethical or unethical.

Historical Events Influencing the Development of Ethical Codes and Regulations

Since the 1940s, four experimental projects have been highly publicized for their unethical treatment of human subjects: the Nazi medical experiments, the Tuskegee Syphilis Study, the Willowbrook Study, and the Jewish Chronic Disease Hospital Study (Berger, 1990; Levine, 1986). Although these were biomedical studies and the primary investigators were physicians, there is evidence that nurses were aware of the research, identified potential research subjects, delivered treatments to the subjects, and served as data collectors. These unethical studies demonstrate the importance of ethical conduct when one is reviewing, participating in, or conducting nursing or biomedical research (Carico & Harrison, 1990). These studies also influenced the formulation of ethical codes and regulations that currently direct the conduct of research.

Nazi Medical Experiments

From 1933 to 1945, atrocious unethical medical activities were performed by the Third Reich in Europe. The programs of the Nazi regime included sterilization, euthanasia, and numerous medical experiments to produce a population of racially pure Germans that were destined to rule the world. The medical experiments were conducted on prisoners of war and persons considered to be racially valueless, such as Jews, who had been confined in concentration camps. The experiments involved exposing subjects to high altitudes, freezing temperatures, malaria, poisons, spotted fever (typhus), and untested drugs and operations, usually without any form of anesthesia. Extensive examination of the records from some of these studies indicated that they were poorly conceived and conducted. Thus, little if any useful scientific knowledge was generated by this research (Berger, 1990; Steinfels & Levine, 1976).

The Nazi experiments violated numerous rights of the research subjects. The selection of subjects for these studies was racially based and unfair, and the subjects had no choice; they were prisoners who were forced to participate. As a result of these experiments, subjects were frequently killed, or they sustained permanent physical, mental, and social damage (Levine, 1986).

Nuremberg Code

Those involved in the Nazi experiments were brought to trial before the Nuremberg Tribunals, and their unethical research received international attention. The mistreatment of human subjects in these studies led to the development of the Nuremberg Code in 1949 (Table 6-1). This code includes guidelines that will help you evaluate the consent process, the protection of subjects from harm, and the balance of benefits and risks in a study.

Declaration of Helsinki

The Nuremberg Code provided the basis for the development of the Declaration of Helsinki, which was adopted in 1964 and revised in 1975 by the World Medical Assembly (Levine, 1986). This document differentiated therapeutic research from nontherapeutic research. *Therapeutic research* provides patients with an opportunity to receive an experimental treatment that might have beneficial results. *Nontherapeutic research* is conducted to generate knowledge for a discipline; the results of the study might benefit future patients but will probably not benefit those acting as research subjects. The Declaration of Helsinki stated that (1) greater care should be exercised to protect subjects from harm in nontherapeutic research, (2) strong, independent justification is required for exposing a healthy volunteer to substantial risk of harm just to gain new scientific information, and (3) the investigator must protect the life and health of the research subject (Oddi & Cassidy, 1990). Most of the institutions involved in clinical research adopted the Nuremberg Code and Declaration of Helsinki; however, these regulations did not prevent the conduct of unethical research.

Tuskegee Syphilis Study

In 1932, the U.S. Public Health Service initiated a study of syphilis in African-American men in the small rural town of Tuskegee, Alabama (Levine, 1986; Rothman, 1982). The study, which continued for 40 years, was conducted to

TABLE 6-1. **The Nuremberg Code**

1. The voluntary consent of the human subject is absolutely essential. . . .
2. The experiment should be such as to yield fruitful results for the good of society, unprocurable by other methods or means of study, and not random and unnecessary in nature.
3. The experiment should be so designed and based on the results of animal experimentation and a knowledge of the natural history of the disease or other problem under study that the anticipated results will justify the performance of the experiment.
4. The experiment should be so conducted as to avoid all unnecessary physical and mental suffering and injury.
5. No experiment should be conducted where there is an *a priori* reason to believe that death or disabling injury will occur, except, perhaps, in those experiments where the experimental physicians also serve as subjects.
6. The degree of risk to be taken should never exceed that determined by the humanitarian importance of the problem to be solved by the experiment.
7. Proper preparations should be made and adequate facilities provided to protect the experimental subject against even remote possibilities of injury, disability, or death.
8. The experiment should be conducted only by scientifically qualified persons. The highest degree of skill and care should be required through all stages of the experiment of those who conduct or engage in the experiment.
9. During the course of the experiment the human subject should be at liberty to bring the experiment to an end if he has reached the physical or mental state where continuation of the experiment seems to him to be impossible.
10. During the course of the experiment the scientist in charge must be prepared to terminate the experiment at any stage, if he has probable cause to believe, in the exercise of the good faith, superior skill and careful judgment required of him that a continuation of the experiment is likely to result in injury, disability, or death to the experimental subject. . . .

From The Nuremberg Code, 1949, pp. 285–286.

determine the natural course of syphilis in the adult African-American male. Many of the subjects who consented to participate in the study were not informed about the purpose and procedures of the research. Some were unaware that they were subjects in a study. By 1936, it was apparent that the men with syphilis had developed more complications than the control group. Ten years later, the death rate among those with syphilis was twice as high as it was for the control group. The subjects were examined periodically but did not receive treatment for syphilis, even when penicillin was determined to be an effective treatment for the disease in the 1940s. Information about an effective treatment for syphilis was withheld from the subjects, and deliberate steps were taken to keep them from receiving treatment (Brandt, 1978).

Published reports of the Tuskegee Syphilis Study started appearing in 1936, and additional papers were published every 4 to 6 years. No effort was made to stop the study; in fact, in 1969, the Centers for Disease Control and Prevention (then called the Center for Disease Control) decided that the study should continue. In 1972, an account of the study in the *Washington Star* sparked public outrage; only then did the Department of Health, Education, and Welfare stop the study. The study was investigated and found to be ethically unjustified (Brandt, 1978).

Willowbrook Study

From the mid-1950s to the early 1970s, research on hepatitis was conducted by Dr. Saul Krugman at Willowbrook, an institution for the mentally retarded in Staten Island, New York (Rothman, 1982). The subjects were children who were deliberately infected with the hepatitis virus. During the 20-year study, Willowbrook closed its doors to new inmates because of overcrowded conditions. However, the research ward continued to admit new inmates, and parents had to give permission for their child to be in the study in order to gain the child's admission to the institution (Levine, 1986).

From the late 1950s to the early 1970s, Krugman's research team published several articles describing the study protocol and findings. In 1966, the Willowbrook Study was cited by Beecher (1966) as an example of unethical research in the *New England Journal of Medicine.* The investigators defended injecting the children with the virus because they believed most of them would acquire the infection upon admission to the institution. They also stressed the benefits the subjects received, which were a cleaner environment, better supervision, and a higher nurse-patient ratio on the research ward (Rothman, 1982). Despite the controversy, this unethical study continued until the early 1970s.

Jewish Chronic Disease Hospital Study

Another highly publicized unethical study was conducted at the Jewish Chronic Disease Hospital in New York in the 1960s. The purpose of this study was to determine patients' rejection responses to live cancer cells. Twenty-two patients were injected with a suspension containing live cancer cells that had been generated from human cancer tissue (Levine, 1986). The rights of these patients were not protected in that they were not informed that they were taking part in research or that the injections they received were live cancer cells. In addition, the study was never presented for review to the research committee of the Jewish Chronic Disease Hospital, and the physicians caring for the patients were unaware that the study was being conducted. The physician directing the research was an employee of the Sloan-Kettering Institute for Cancer Research, and there was no indication that this institution had conducted a review of the research project (Hershey & Miller, 1976). This unethical study was conducted without the informed consent of the subjects and without institutional review and had the potential to cause the human subjects injury, disability, or even death.

Department of Health, Education, and Welfare Regulations

The continued conduct of harmful, unethical research made additional controls necessary. In 1973, the Department of Health, Education, and Welfare (DHEW) published its first set of regulations for the protection of human research subjects. These regulations also provided protection for persons having limited capacity to consent, such as the ill, mentally impaired, and dying (Levine, 1986). According to the DHEW regulations, all research involving human subjects had to undergo full institutional review, which increased the protection of human subjects. However, reviewing all studies, without regard for the degree of risk involved, greatly increased the time required for approval to conduct research.

National Commission for the Protection of Human Subjects of Biomedical and Behavioral Research

Because the issue of protecting human subjects in research was not resolved by the DHEW regulations, the National Commission for the Protection of Human Subjects of Biomedical and Behavioral Research (1978) was formed. This commission was established by the National Research Act (Public Law 93-348) passed in 1974. The commission identified three *ethical principles* that are relevant to the conduct of research involving human subjects: respect for persons, beneficence, and justice. The principle of respect for persons indicates that persons have the right to self-determination and the freedom to participate or not participate in research. The principle of beneficence encourages the researcher to do good and, above all, to do no harm. The principle of justice states that human subjects should be treated fairly.

In response to the commission's recommendations, the Department of Health and Human Services (DHHS) developed a set of regulations that were much more reasonable than those proposed in 1973. The DHHS regulations include (1) general requirements for informed consent, (2) documentation of informed consent, (3) criteria for Institutional Review Board (IRB) review of research, (4) exempt and expedited review procedures for certain kinds of research, (5) criteria for IRB approval of research, and (6) directives for dealing with and reporting of scientific misconduct (DHHS, 1981, 1983, 1989, 1991). These DHHS regulations remain the established guidelines for evaluating the ethical aspects of research today.

Protecting Human Rights

What are human rights? How are these rights protected during research? *Human rights* are claims and demands that have been justified in the eyes of an individual or by the consensus of a group of individuals. If you critique published studies, review research for conduct in your agency, or assist with data collection for a study, you have an ethical responsibility to determine whether the rights of the research subjects are protected. The human rights that require protection in research include the rights to (1) self-determination, (2) privacy, (3) anonymity and confidentiality, (4) fair treatment, and (5) protection from discomfort and harm (American Nurses Association, 1976, 1985; American Psychological Association, 1982).

Right to Self-Determination

The right to self-determination is based on the ethical principle of respect for persons and indicates that humans are capable of controlling their own destiny. Thus, humans should be treated as *autonomous agents,* who have the freedom to conduct their lives as they choose without external controls. Subjects are treated as autonomous agents in a study if the researcher (1) informed them about the study, (2) allowed them to choose to participate or not participate, and (3) allowed them to withdraw from the study at any time without penalty (Levine, 1986). Flynn (1997) studied the health practices of homeless women and documented that her subjects were treated as autonomous agents.

> "The study was approved by the university's Institutional Review Board for the protection of human subjects. To ensure protection of human rights, all prospective participants were informed, both verbally and in writing, of the maintenance of confidentiality, their right to refuse to participate, and [that] the refusal to participate would in no way affect their status or services received at the shelter." (p. 74)

Flynn obtained informed consent from her subjects to participate in the study and indicated that subjects would not be penalized for refusing to participate or withdrawing from the study.

Violation of the Right to Self-Determination

A subject's right to self-determination can be violated through the use of coercion, covert data collection, and deception. *Coercion* occurs when an overt threat of harm or an excessive reward is intentionally presented by one person to another to obtain compliance. Some subjects are coerced to participate in research because they fear harm or discomfort if they do not participate. For example, some patients feel that their medical and nursing care will be negatively affected if they do not agree to be research subjects. Other subjects are coerced to participate in studies because they believe that they cannot refuse the excessive rewards offered, such as large sums of money, special privileges, or jobs (Rudy, Estok, Kerr, & Menzel, 1994).

With *covert data collection,* subjects are unaware that research data are being collected (Reynolds, 1979). For example, in the Jewish Chronic Disease Hospital Study, most of the patients and their physicians were unaware of the study. The subjects were informed that they were receiving an injection of cells, but the word "cancer" was omitted (Beecher, 1966).

The use of *deception* (the actual misinforming of subjects for research purposes) (Kelman, 1967) can also violate a subject's right to self-determination. A classic example of deception is the Milgram (1963) study, in which the subjects thought they were administering electric shocks to another person, but the person was really a professional actor who pretended to feel the shocks. If deception is used in a study, the research report needs to indicate how the subjects were deceived and the fact that the subjects were informed of the actual research activities and the findings at the end of the study.

Persons with Diminished Autonomy

Some persons have *diminished autonomy* or are vulnerable and less advantaged because of legal or mental incompetence, terminal illness, or confinement to an institution (DHHS, 1991; Levine, 1986). These persons require additional protection of their right to self-determination because of their decreased ability or inability to give informed consent. In addition, these persons are vulnerable to coercion and deception. The research report needs to include justification for the use of subjects with diminished autonomy, and the need for justification increases as the subject's risk and vulnerability increase.

Legally and Mentally Incompetent Subjects. Children (minors), the mentally impaired, and unconscious patients are legally and mentally incompetent to give informed consent. These individuals often lack the ability to comprehend information about a study and to make decisions regarding participation in or withdrawal from the study. These persons have a range of vulnerability from minimal to absolute. The use of persons with diminished autonomy as research subjects is more acceptable if (1) the research is therapeutic, that is, the subjects might benefit from the experimental process; (2) the researcher is willing to use both vulnerable and nonvulnerable individuals as subjects; and (3) the risk is minimized, and the consent process is strictly followed to ensure the rights of the prospective subjects (Levine, 1986; Watson, 1982).

Children. The laws defining the minor status of a child are statutory and vary from state to state. Often a child's competence to give consent is operationalized by age, with incompetence being nonrefutable up to age 7 (Broome & Stieglitz, 1992; Thompson, 1987). However, by age 7, children are capable of concrete operations of thought and are capable of providing meaningful assent

TABLE 6-2. Guide to Obtaining Informed Consent, Based on the Relationship Between a Child's Level of Competence, the Therapeutic Nature of the Research, and Risk versus Benefits

	Nontherapeutic		Therapeutic	
	MMR-LB	*MR-LB*	*MR-HB*	*MMR-HB*
Child, incompetent (generally 0–7 yr)				
Parents' consent	Necessary	Necessary	Sufficient*	Sufficient
Child's assent	Optional†	Optional†	Optional	Optional
Child, relatively competent (7 yr and older)				
Parents' consent	Necessary	Necessary	Sufficient‡	Recommended
Child's assent	Necessary	Necessary	Sufficient§	Sufficient

Key; MMR, more than minimal risk; MR, minimal risk; LB, low benefit; HB, high benefit.
*A parent's refusal can be superseded by the principle that a parent has no power to forbid the saving of a child's life.
†Children making a "deliberate objection" would be precluded from participation by most researchers.
‡In cases not involving the privacy rights of a "mature minor."
§In cases involving the privacy rights of a "mature minor."
From Thompson, P. J. (1987). Protection of the rights of children as subjects for research. *Journal of Pediatric Nursing, 2*(6), 397, with permission.

to participation as research subjects (Thompson, 1987). With advancing age and maturity, the child should play a stronger role in the consent process.

The DHHS regulations require "soliciting the assent of the children (when capable) and the permission of their parents or guardians. Assent means a child's affirmative agreement to participate in research. . . . Permission means the agreement of parent(s) or guardian to the participation of their child or ward in research" (DHHS, 1991, Section 46.402). Using children as research subjects is also influenced by the therapeutic nature of the research and the risks versus benefits. Thompson (1987) developed a guide for obtaining informed consent based on the child's level of competence, the therapeutic nature of the research, and the risks versus benefits (Table 6-2).

Bournaki (1997) studied the pain-related responses of school-age children to venipunctures. The procedure section of the article documented the consent of the parents and the assent of the children to participate in the study. "All subjects were recruited before their clinic appointments. Participation in the study was voluntary, and informed consent from female caregivers and children's assents were obtained in accordance with the institution's committee for Protection of Human Subjects" (p. 150).

Adults. Certain adults, due to mental illness, cognitive impairment, or a comatose state, are incompetent and incapable of giving informed consent. Persons are said to be incompetent if, in the judgment of a qualified clinician, they have those attributes that ordinarily provide the grounds for adjudicating in-competence (Levine, 1986). Incompetence can be temporary (e.g., inebria-tion), permanent (e.g., advanced senile dementia), or subjective or transitory (e.g., behavior or symptoms of psychosis). If an individual is judged incompe-tent and incapable of giving consent, the researcher must seek approval from the prospective subject and his or her legally authorized representative. A le-gally authorized representative is an individual or another body authorized un-der applicable law to consent on behalf of a prospective subject to the subject's participation in the procedure(s) involved in the research (DHHS, 1991, Section 46.102). However, individuals can be judged incompetent and can still assent to participate in certain minimal-risk research if they are able to understand what they are being asked to do (Levine, 1986).

Dansky, Dellasega, Shellenbarger, and Russo (1996) studied the home health services provided a group of elderly patients after hospitalization. These authors described the ethical procedures they used to obtain informed consent from their subjects:

> ". . . Before patients left the hospital, a research assistant (a regis-tered nurse with a master's degree in medical-surgical nursing) con-tacted each potential subject, explained the purposes of the study, and asked the patient to participate. Interested patients receive a written explanation of the study and then completed the consent form. If necessary, legal guardians provided consent, and the same procedure was followed." (p. 188)

Terminally Ill Subjects. Participating in research could have increased risks and minimal or no benefits for terminally ill subjects. In addition, the dying subject's condition could affect the study results and lead the researcher to misinterpret the results (Watson, 1982). For example, cancer patients have become an overstudied population, in whom it is not unusual for the majority of blood work, bone marrow scans, lumbar punctures, and biopsies to be conducted for purposes of research to fulfill protocol requirements (Strauman & Cotanch, 1988). These biomedical research treatments can easily compromise the care of these individuals, which poses ethical dilemmas for clinical nurses. More and more nurses will be responsible for ensuring adherence to ethical standards in research as they participate in institutional review of research and serve as patient advocates in the clinical setting (Carico & Harrison, 1990; Davis, 1989).

McCorkle, Robinson, Nuamah, Lev, and Benoliel (1998) studied the "ef-fects of home nursing care for patients during terminal illness on the bereaved's psychological distress" (p. 2). The investigators were cautious in obtaining per-mission from the patients and their spouses to participate in the study. The patients were contacted by their physician or his or her designee to determine if the patient was willing to participate. Only those patients who agreed to be contacted were called by the investigators and asked to participate in the study. Only 100 of the 127 patients contacted agreed to participate. The spouses of these patients were also asked to participate; only 91 completed the study because some chose to withdraw after the death of their spouse. Studying the terminally ill is important to generate essential knowledge for their care, but the rights of these individuals need to be closely guarded during the conduct of a study.

Subjects Confined to Institutions. Hospitalized patients and prisoners are individuals confined to institutions who are perceived to have diminished autonomy. Hospitalized patients have diminished autonomy because they are ill and are confined in settings that are controlled by health care personnel. Some hospitalized patients feel obligated to be research subjects because they want to assist a particular nurse or physician with his or her research. Others feel coerced to participate because they fear that their care will be adversely affected if they refuse. Prison inmates have diminished autonomy in research projects because of their confinement. They might feel coerced to participate in research because they fear harm or desire the benefits of early release, special treatment, or monetary gain (Levine, 1986).

IN CRITIQUING studies, you need to evaluate the subjects' capacity for self-determination and assess whether the rights of subjects with diminished autonomy were protected. The following questions will assist you in critiquing studies.

1. Were the subjects informed about the research project?
2. Did the subjects voluntarily give their consent to be in the study?
3. Did the subjects have the freedom to withdraw from the study?
4. Did the subjects have diminished autonomy because of legal or mental incompetence, terminal illness, or confinement to an institution? If they did, were special precautions taken in obtaining consent from these subjects and their parents or guardians?

Right to Privacy

Privacy is the freedom an individual has to determine the time, extent, and general circumstances under which private information will be shared with or withheld from others. Private information includes one's attitudes, beliefs, behaviors, opinions, and records. The research subject's privacy is protected if the subject is informed and consents to participate in a study and voluntarily shares private information with a researcher (Levine, 1986).

Invasion of Privacy

An *invasion of privacy* occurs when private information is shared without an individual's knowledge or against his or her will. The invasion of subjects' right to privacy brought about the Privacy Act of 1974. As a result of this act, individuals have the right to provide or prevent access of others to their records (Levine, 1986). A research report will often indicate that the subjects' privacy was protected and might include the details of how this was accomplished.

Right to Anonymity and Confidentiality

Based on the right to privacy, the research subject has the right to anonymity and the right to assume that the data collected will be kept confidential. Complete *anonymity* exists if the subject's identity cannot be linked, even by the researcher, with his or her individual responses (American Nurses Association, 1985). For example, Mullins (1996) promised her subjects anonymity when she studied nurse caring behaviors desired by patients with acquired immunodeficiency syndrome (AIDS) or human immunodeficiency virus (HIV).

> "A letter explaining the study, the CBA (Caring Behavior Assessment) tool, a letter to participants, and the demographic sheet were sent to administrators of health care agencies. . . . After access to agency clients was obtained, potential subjects who met the sampling criteria were asked if they would like to participate in the study. Those potential subjects who expressed interest in the study were given a packet containing the CBSA tool, a letter describing the study, and a demographic sheet. . . . By completing the CBA tool and the demographic sheet, the subject agreed to participate in the study. Subjects did not indicate their names or addresses on the tools or demographic sheets, thus allowing participants to be anonymous. Tools and demographic sheets were not coded in any way to link them with agencies or subjects." (p. 20)

In most studies, researchers know the identity of their subjects, and they promise them that their identity will be kept anonymous from others and that the research data will be kept confidential. *Confidentiality* is the researcher's management of private information shared by a subject. The researcher must refrain from sharing that information without the authorization of the subject. Confidentiality is grounded in the following premises: "(1) Individuals can share personal information to the extent they wish and are entitled to have secrets; (2) one can choose with whom to share personal information; (3) those accepting information in confidence have an obligation to maintain confidentiality; and (4) professionals, such as researchers, have a duty to maintain confidentiality that goes beyond ordinary loyalty" (Levine, 1986, p. 164).

A *breach of confidentiality* can occur when a researcher, by accident or direct action, allows an unauthorized person to gain access to raw data of a study. Confidentiality can also be breached in reporting or publishing a study if a subject's identity is accidentally revealed, violating the subject's right to anonymity (Ramos, 1989). This is of special concern in qualitative studies that have few subjects and involve the reporting of long quotes made by the subjects. These long quotes might reveal the identity of a subject to others, resulting in a breach of confidentiality (Sandelowski, 1994). Breaches of confidentiality that can be especially harmful to subjects include those regarding religious preferences; sexual practices; income; racial prejudices; drug use; child abuse; and personal attributes such as intelligence, honesty, and courage.

You need to examine the research report for evidence that subject confidentiality was maintained during data collection and analysis. In addition, the research findings need to be reported so that a subject or group of subjects cannot be identified by their responses. Czar and Engler (1997) protected their subjects' rights to privacy and self-determination in their study of the learning needs of patients with coronary artery disease.

"The study was reviewed by the Committee on Human Research at the University of California, San Francisco. Subjects were selected from the admission log of the CCU, the transition care unit, or both. Each chart was reviewed for inclusion and exclusion criteria. Subjects fulfilling the criteria were approached when their condition was considered stable and they were pain free (verbal denial of pain symptoms). The purpose of the study was explained, and a written consent was obtained. Subjects were assured confidentiality of responses to both the questionnaire and the personal data sheet. Subjects were asked not to write their name on the questionnaire but were provided a code number." (p. 112)

In this study, data were analyzed as a group for the sample of 28 subjects, and the results were presented in such a way that individual subjects could not be identified by their responses.

IN CRITIQUING a published study, you might examine whether the subjects' right to anonymity and confidentiality was protected by addressing the following questions:

1. Were the subjects' identities kept anonymous?

2. Were the subjects ensured confidentiality or anonymity by the researchers?

3. Were the research data kept confidential?

4. Were the data analyzed and the findings presented in a way to ensure the anonymity of the subjects in the research report?

Right to Fair Treatment

The right to fair treatment is based on the ethical principle of justice. According to this principle, people should be treated fairly and should receive what they are due or owed. The research report needs to indicate that the selection of subjects and their treatment during the study were fair.

Fair Selection and Treatment of Subjects

In the past, injustice in subject selection resulted from social, cultural, racial, and sexual biases in society. For many years, research was conducted on categories of individuals who were thought to be especially suitable as research subjects, such as poor people, charity patients, prisoners, slaves, peasants, dying persons, and others who were considered undesirable (Reynolds, 1979). Researchers often treated these subjects carelessly and had little regard for the harm and discomfort they experienced. The Nazi medical experiments, the Tuskegee Syphilis Study, the Willowbrook Study, and the Jewish Chronic Disease Hospital Study all exemplify unfair subject selection.

Another concern with subject selection is that some researchers select subjects because they like them and want them to receive the specific benefits of a study. Other researchers have been swayed by power or money to make certain individuals subjects so that they can receive potentially beneficial treatments. Random selection of subjects can eliminate some of the researcher's biases that might influence subject selection.

Researchers and subjects should have a specific agreement regarding the subject's participation and the researcher's role in a study (American Psychological Association, 1982). While conducting the study, the researcher should treat the subjects fairly and respect that agreement. For example, the activities or procedures that the subject is to perform should not be changed without the subject's consent. The benefits promised the subjects should be provided. In addition, subjects who participate in studies should receive equal benefits regardless of age, race, or socioeconomic level.

The research report needs to indicate that the selection and treatment of the subjects were fair. Subjects should have been selected for reasons directly related to the problem being studied and not for their easy availability, compromised position, manipulability, or friendship with the researcher (National Commission for the Protection of Human Subjects of Biomedical and Behavioral Research, 1978). In addition, the procedures section of the research report needs to indicate fair and equal treatment of the subjects during data collection. The Mullins (1996) study of nursing care behaviors desired by patients with AIDS or HIV introduced earlier in this chapter demonstrates fair selection and treatment of subjects.

". . . The sample for this study included persons with a diagnosis of AIDS/HIV who agreed to participate in the study and met specific criteria for the sample's subjects. . . . Criteria for this study were as follows. Subjects in the sample were at least 18 years of age and had the diagnosis of either AIDS or HIV-seropositive status. Subjects had to be alert and could not be confused to be able to give reliable responses. . . . Patients who were initially diagnosed as having AIDS or as HIV-seropositive during the present hospitalization or clinic visit were not included in the sample. This criterion was included to allow the patient newly diagnosed with AIDS/HIV time to begin to accept the reality of being diagnosed with a fatal disease." (pp. 19–20)

Mullins (1996) demonstrated fair selection of subjects by allowing any potential subject the option of participating or not in the study. The cognitively impaired and those with a new diagnosis of AIDS/HIV were excluded, which indicates that the researcher was attempting to protect the individuals with diminished autonomy by not including them in the study. The subjects were treated the same way throughout the study and were only asked to complete a demographic sheet and a study scale.

Right to Protection from Discomfort and Harm

The right to protection from *discomfort and harm from a study* is based on the ethical principle of beneficence, which states that one should do good and, above all, do no harm. According to this principle, members of society should take an active role in preventing discomfort and harm and promoting good in the world around them. In research, discomfort and harm can be physical, emotional, social, and/or economic. Reynolds (1972) identified five categories of studies based on levels of discomfort and harm: no anticipated effects, temporary discomfort, unusual levels of temporary discomfort, risk of permanent damage, and certainty of permanent damage.

No Anticipated Effects

In some studies, no positive or negative effects are expected for the subjects. For example, studies that involve reviewing patients' records, students' files, pathology reports, or other documents have no anticipated effects on the research subjects. In this type of study, the researcher does not interact directly with the subjects; however, there is still a potential risk of invading a subject's privacy.

Temporary Discomfort

Studies that cause temporary discomfort are described as minimal-risk studies, in which the discomfort is similar to what the subject would encounter in his or her daily life and ceases with the termination of the experiment (DHHS, 1991). Many nursing studies require the completion of questionnaires or participation in interviews, which usually involve minimal risk or are a mere inconvenience for the subjects. The physical discomfort might include fatigue, headache, or muscle tension. The emotional and social risks might include anxiety or embarrassment associated with answering certain questions. The economic risks might include the time commitment required or travel costs to the study site.

Most clinical nursing studies examining the effect of a treatment involve minimal risk. For example, a study might involve examining the effects of exercise on the blood glucose levels of diabetics. For the study, the subjects would be asked to test their blood glucose level one extra time per day. Discomfort occurs when the blood is drawn, and there is a potential risk of physical changes that might occur with exercise. The subjects might also feel anxiety and fear associated with the additional blood testing, and the testing could be an added expense. The diabetic subjects in this study would encounter similar discomforts in their daily lives, and the discomfort would cease with the termination of the study.

Unusual Levels of Temporary Discomfort

In studies that involve unusual levels of temporary discomfort, subjects frequently have discomfort both during the study and after it has been completed. For example, subjects might have prolonged muscle weakness, joint pain, and dizziness after participating in a study that required them to be confined to bed for 10 days to determine the effects of immobility. Studies that require subjects to experience failure, extreme fear, or threats to their identity or to act in unnatural ways involve unusual levels of temporary discomfort. In some qualitative studies, subjects are asked questions that open old wounds or involve reliving traumatic events (Ford & Reutter, 1990). For example, asking subjects to describe their rape experience could precipitate feelings of extreme anger, fear, and/or sadness. In such studies, investigators should indicate in their research report that they were vigilant in assessing the subjects' discomfort and referred them as necessary for appropriate professional intervention.

Risk of Permanent Damage

In some studies, subjects might sustain permanent damage; this is more common in biomedical research than in nursing research. For example, medical studies of new drugs and surgical procedures have the potential to cause subjects permanent physical damage. Some topics investigated by nurses have the potential to permanently damage subjects emotionally and socially. Studies examining sensitive information, such as sexual behavior, child abuse, AIDS/HIV status, or drug use, can be very risky for subjects. These types of studies have the potential to cause permanent damage to a subject's personality or reputation. There are also potential economic risks, such as less efficient job performance or loss of employment.

Certainty of Permanent Damage

In some research, such as the Nazi medical experiments and the Tuskegee Syphilis Study, the subjects experienced permanent damage. Conducting research that will permanently damage subjects is highly questionable, regardless of the benefits that will be gained. Frequently, the benefits gained are for other individuals but not for the research subjects. Studies causing permanent damage to subjects violate the fifth principle of the Nuremberg Code (see Table 6-1).

IN CRITIQUING a published study, you need to determine the level of discomfort and harm experienced by the subjects.

1. What was the level of risk of the study? Was the risk no anticipated effects, temporary discomfort, unusual levels of temporary discomfort, risk of permanent damage, or certainty of permanent damage?

2. Was this level of risk reasonable for the study based on the potential benefit of the knowledge generated?

3. Should the study have been revised or not conducted because the risk level was too great? If revision is suggested, how might the study have been revised?

Understanding Informed Consent

What is informed consent? How is informed consent obtained from research subjects? Informing is the transmission of essential ideas and content from the investigator to the prospective subject. Consent is the prospective subject's agreement to participate in a study as a subject. Every prospective subject, to the degree that he or she is capable, should have the opportunity to choose whether to participate in research (Brent, 1990; Cassidy & Oddi, 1986). *Informed consent* includes four elements: (1) disclosure to the subject of essential study information, (2) comprehension of this information by the subject, (3) competence of the subject to give consent, and (4) voluntary consent of the subject to participate in the study.

Essential Information for Consent

Informed consent requires the researcher to disclose specific information to each prospective subject. The following information is identified as essential for informed consent in research (DHHS, 1991; Levine, 1986).

1. *Introduction of research activities.* The initial information presented to the prospective subject clearly indicates that a study is to be conducted and that the individual is being asked to participate as a subject.
2. *Statement of the research purpose.* The researcher states the immediate purpose of the research and any long-range goals related to the study.
3. *Selection of research subjects.* The researcher explains to prospective subjects why they were selected as possible subjects.
4. *Explanation of procedures.* Prospective subjects receive a complete description of the procedures to be followed and identification of any procedures that are experimental in the study (DHHS, 1991, Section 46.116a).
5. *Description of risks and discomforts.* Prospective subjects are informed of any reasonably foreseeable risks or discomforts (physical, emotional, social, and/or economic) that might result from the study (DHHS, 1991, Section 46.116a).
6. *Description of benefits.* The investigator describes any benefits to the subject or to others that may reasonably be expected from the research (DHHS, 1991, Section 46.116a), including any financial advantages or other rewards for participating in the study.
7. *Disclosure of alternatives.* The investigator discloses the appropriate alternative procedures or courses of treatment, if any, that might be advantageous to the subject (DHHS, 1991, Section 46.116a). For example, the researchers of the Tuskegee Syphilis Study should have informed the subjects with syphilis that penicillin was an effective treatment for the disease.
8. *Assurance of anonymity and confidentiality.* Prospective subjects need to know the extent to which their responses and records will be kept confidential. Subjects are promised that their identity will remain anonymous in reports and publications of the study.
9. *Offer to answer questions.* The researcher offers to answer any questions the prospective subjects may have.
10. *Noncoercive disclaimer.* Subjects are asked to sign a noncoercive disclaimer, which is a statement that participation is voluntary and that refusal to participate will involve no penalty or loss of benefits to which the subject is otherwise entitled (DHHS, 1991, Section 46.116a).
11. *Option to withdraw.* Subjects are informed that they may discontinue participation (withdraw from a study) at any time without penalty or loss of benefits (DHHS, 1991, Section 46.116a).
12. *Consent to incomplete disclosure.* In some studies, subjects are not completely informed of the study purpose because that knowledge would alter their actions. However, prospective subjects must be told when certain information is being withheld deliberately.

A *consent form* is a written document that includes the elements of informed consent required by the DHHS Regulations (1991, Section 46.116). In addition, a consent form might include other information required by the institution where the study is to be conducted or by the agency funding the study. An example of a consent form is presented in Figure 6-1; descriptors indicate the essential consent information.

Comprehension of Consent Information

Informed consent implies not only the imparting of information by the researcher but also the comprehension of that information by the prospective subjects. The researcher needs to take the time to teach the subjects about the study. The amount of information to be taught depends on the subjects' knowledge of research and the specific research topic. The benefits and risks of a study need to be discussed in detail, with examples that the potential subject can understand. As a patient advocate in a clinical agency, you need to assess whether patients involved in research understand the purpose and the potential risks and benefits of their participation in a study.

Competence to Give Consent

Autonomous individuals, who are capable of understanding the benefits and risks of a proposed study, are competent to give consent. Persons with diminished autonomy because of legal or mental incompetence, terminal illness, or confinement to an institution are frequently not legally competent to consent to participate in research (see the section "Right to Self-Determination" earlier in this chapter). The competence of the subject is often determined by the researcher (Douglas & Larson, 1986). In the research report, the investigator will often indicate the competence of the subjects and the process that was used for obtaining informed consent.

Voluntary Consent

Voluntary consent means the prospective subject has decided to take part in a study of his or her own volition without coercion or any undue influence (Douglas & Larson, 1986). Voluntary consent is obtained after the prospective subject has been given the essential information about the study and has shown comprehension of this information.

A research report will often discuss the consent process and identify some of the essential consent information that was provided to the potential subjects. All research reports should have some mention of the consent process for that

CONSENT FORM

Study Title: The Needs of Family Members of Critically Ill Adults
Investigator: Linda L. Norris, R.N.

Ms. Norris is a registered nurse studying the emotional and social needs of family members of patients in the Intensive Care Units (**research purpose**). Although the study will not benefit you directly, it will provide information that might enable nurses to identify family members' needs and to assist family members with those needs (**potential benefits**).

The study and its procedures have been approved by the appropriate people and review boards at The University of Texas at Arlington and X hospital (**IRB approval**). The study procedures involve no foreseeable risks or harm to you or your family (**potential risks**). The procedures include: (1) responding to a questionnaire about the needs of family members of critically ill patients and (2) completing a demographic data sheet (**explanation of procedures**). Participation in this study will take approximately 20 minutes (**time commitment**). You are free to ask any questions about the study or about being a subject and you may call Ms. Norris at (999) 999-9999 (work) or (111) 111-1111 (home) if you have further questions (**offer to answer questions**).

Your participation in this study is voluntary; you are under no obligation to participate (**voluntary consent**). You have the right to withdraw at any time and the care of your family member and your relationship with the health care team will not be affected (**option to withdraw**).

The study data will be coded so it will not be linked to your name. Your identity will not be revealed while the study is being conducted or when the study is reported or published. All study data will be collected by Ms. Norris, stored in a secure place and not shared with any other person without your permission (**assurance of anonymity and confidentiality**).

I have read this consent form and voluntarily consent to participate in this study.

	(If appropriate)
Subject's Signature Date	Legal Representative Date

Relationship to Subject

I have explained this study to the above subject and have sought his/her understanding for informed consent.

Investigator's Signature   Date

FIGURE 6-1
Sample consent form.

study, but the depth of the discussion will vary based on the research purpose and the types of subjects included in the study. Logan and Jenny (1997) studied patients' work during mechanical ventilation and weaning and clearly described the consent process in the following sections of their article.

> SAMPLE AND SETTING. "After approval by the hospital research ethics committee, patients were recruited from a 14-bed multispecialty intensive care unit (ICU) of a 740-bed urban university teaching hospital. The patient inclusion criteria were an ability to recall their ventilator weaning experience, lack of cognitive impairment, sufficient alertness to discuss their experiences, and stable physical status as determined by the attending nurse. . . .
>
> PROCEDURE. Patients were invited to participate in the study after discharge from the ICU. A master's-prepared nurse research assistant explained the purpose, risks and benefits, confidentiality, voluntary participation, and research procedures to the participants, and a signed consent was obtained from each of them." (p. 141)

In the Logan and Jenny (1997) study, the subjects seemed competent to give consent because they were adults who lacked cognitive impairment and were alert enough to discuss their experiences. The attending nurse also indicated that the patients were physically stable. The subjects received detailed information about the study to promote their comprehension regarding participation. In addition, they were invited to participate in the study and were informed that participation was voluntary. A written consent form (with essential consent information) was presented to and signed by the subjects. This indicates that the four aspects of informed consent were addressed: essential information for consent, comprehension of consent information, competence to give consent, and voluntary consent.

A CRITIQUE of a research report requires examining the ethics of the consent process. You might use the following questions to direct your critique.

1. *Was the essential information for consent provided?*
2. *Were the subjects capable of comprehending the information?*
3. *Did the researcher take any action to ensure that the subjects comprehended the consent information?*
4. *Were the subjects competent to give consent?*
5. *If the subjects were not competent to give consent, who acted as their legally authorized representatives?*
6. *Did it seem that the subjects participated voluntarily in the study?*

Understanding Institutional Review

In *institutional review,* a committee of peers called an institutional review board (IRB) examines studies for ethical concerns. You might be part of an IRB that examines studies in your agency. Thus, you need to know the activities of an IRB and the guidelines used in determining the ethical acceptability of a study.

The functions of an IRB involve reviewing research to determine whether (1) the rights and welfare of the subjects were protected, (2) the methods used to secure informed consent were appropriate, and (3) the potential benefits of the study were greater than the risks (Martin, 1996). The DHHS Regulations (1991) identify three levels of review: exempt from review, expedited review, and complete review. The level of the review required for each study is decided by the IRB chairperson and/or the committee, not by the researcher.

Studies are usually *exempt from review* if they involve no apparent risks for the research subjects. Research qualifying for exemption from review by the DHHS (1991, Section 46.101b) is described in Table 6-3. Nursing studies that have no foreseeable risks or are a mere inconvenience for subjects are usually identified as exempt from review by the chairperson of the IRB. Studies with risks that are considered minimal are expedited in the review process. *Minimal risk* means that the risks of harm anticipated in the proposed research are no greater, in probability and magnitude, than those ordinarily encountered in daily life or during the performance of routine physical or psychological examinations or tests (DHHS, 1991, Section 46.102i). Under *expedited review* procedures, the review may be carried out by the IRB chairperson or by one or more experienced IRB reviewers designated by the chairperson. Table 6-4 describes research that qualifies for expedited review.

Studies that have greater than minimal risks must receive a *complete review* by an IRB. To obtain IRB approval, researchers need to ensure that (1) risks to subjects are minimized, (2) risks to subjects are reasonable in relation to anticipated benefits, (3) selection of subjects is equitable, (4) informed consent is sought from each prospective subject or the subject's legally authorized representative, (5) informed consent is appropriately documented, (6) the research plan makes adequate provision for monitoring data collection for subjects' safety, and (7) adequate provisions are made to protect the privacy of subjects and maintain the confidentiality of data (DHHS, 1991, Section 46.111a).

In a research report, the investigator will usually indicate that the study was approved by the appropriate IRB(s). Menzel (1997) detailed the institutional review process in her study of patients' communication-related responses during intubation and after extubation.

> PROCEDURE. "The study was approved by the institutional review boards of Case Western Reserve University and the medical center where the data were collected. Staff nurses and unit directors in the critical care units were informed about the study and were frequently instrumental in alerting me to potential subjects. . . ." (p. 366)

TABLE 6-3. Research Qualifying for Exemption from IRB Review

Unless otherwise required by department or agency heads, research activities in which the only involvement of human subjects will be in one or more of the following categories are exempt from review.

(1) Research conducted in established or commonly accepted educational settings, involving normal educational practices, such as (i) research on regular and special education instructional strategies, or (ii) research on the effectiveness of or the comparison among instructional techniques, curricula, or classroom management methods.

(2) Research involving the use of educational tests (cognitive, diagnostic, aptitude, achievement), survey procedures, interview procedures or observation of public behavior, unless:

(i) information obtained is recorded in such a manner that human subjects can be identified, directly or through identifiers linked to the subjects; and (ii) any disclosure of the human subjects' responses outside the research could reasonably place the subjects at risk of criminal or civil liability or be damaging to the subjects' financial standing, employability, or reputation.

(3) Research involving the use of educational tests (cognitive, diagnostic, aptitude, achievement), survey procedures, interview procedures, or observation of public behavior that is not exempt under paragraph (b)(2) of this section, if:

(i) the human subjects are elected or appointed public officials or candidates for public office; or (ii) Federal statute(s) require(s) without exception that the confidentiality of the personally identifiable information will be maintained throughout the research and thereafter.

(4) Research involving the collection or study of existing data, documents, records, pathological specimens, or diagnostic specimens, if these sources are publicly available or if the information is recorded by the investigator in such a manner that subjects cannot be identified, directly or through identifiers linked to the subjects.

(5) Research and demonstration projects which are conducted by or subject to the approval of Department or Agency heads, and which are designed to study, evaluate, or otherwise examine:

(i) Public benefit or service programs; (ii) procedures for obtaining benefits or services under those programs; (iii) possible changes in or alternatives to those programs or procedures; or (iv) possible changes in methods or levels of payment for benefits or services under those programs.

(6) Taste and food quality evaluation and consumer acceptance studies, (i) if wholesome foods without additives are consumed or (ii) if a good is consumed that contains a food ingredient at or below the level and for a use found to be safe, or agricultural chemical or environmental contaminent at or below the level found to be safe, by the Food and Drug Administration or approved by the Environmental Protection Agency or the Food Safety and Inspection Service of the U.S. Department of Agriculture.

Excerpted from *Federal Register* of June 18, 1991 (DHHS, 1991, Section 46.101b).

TABLE 6-4. Research Qualifying for Expedited IRB Review

Expedited review (by committee chairpersons or designated members) for the following research involving no more than minimal risk is authorized:

1. Collection of hair and nail clippings, in a nondisfiguring manner; deciduous teeth and permanent teeth if patient care indicates a need for extraction.
2. Collection of excreta and external secretions including sweat, uncannulated saliva, placenta removed at delivery, and amniotic fluid at the time of rupture of the membrane prior to or during labor.
3. Recording of data from subjects 18 years of age or older using noninvasive procedures routinely employed in clinical practice. This includes the use of physical sensors that are applied either to the surface of the body or at a distance and do not involve input of matter or significant amounts of energy into the subject or an invasion of the subject's privacy. It also includes such procedures as weighing, testing sensory acuity, electrocardiography, electroencephalography, thermography, detection of naturally occurring radioactivity, diagnostic echography, and electroretinography. It does not include exposure to electromagnetic radiation outside the visible range (for example, x-rays, microwaves).
4. Collection of blood samples by venipuncture, in amounts not exceeding 450 milliliters in an eight-week period and no more than two times per week, from subjects 18 years of age or older and who are in good health and not pregnant.
5. Collection of both supra- and subgingival dental plaque and calculus, provided the procedure is not more invasive than routine prophylactic scaling of the teeth and the process is accomplished in accordance with accepted prophylactic techniques.
6. Voice recordings made for research purposes such as investigations of speech defects.
7. Moderate exercise by healthy volunteers.
8. The study of existing data, documents, records, pathological specimens, or diagnostic specimens.
9. Research on individual or group behavior or characteristics of individual, such as studies of perception, cognition, game theory, or test development, where the investigator does not manipulate subjects' behavior and research will not involve stress to subjects.
10. Research on drugs or devices for which an investigational new drug exemption or an investigational device exemption is not required.

Excerpted from the *Federal Register* of June 18, 1991 (DHHS, 1991, Section 46.110). Additional regulations that apply to research involving fetuses, pregnant women, human in vitro fertilization, and prisoners are available in the *Federal Register*, 1991, part 46.

Examining the Benefit-risk Ratio of a Study

If you serve on an IRB for your agency, act as a patient advocate when research is conducted in your agency, or are asked to collect data for a study, you will need to examine the balance of benefits and risks in studies. To determine this balance, or *benefit-risk ratio*, you need to assess the benefits and risks of the sampling method, consent process, procedures, and potential outcomes of the

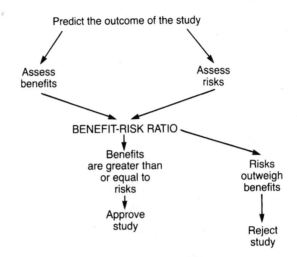

FIGURE 6-2
Balancing benefits and risks for a study.

study (Fig. 6-2). Informed consent must be obtained from subjects, and selection and treatment of subjects during the study must be fair. An important outcome of research is the development and refinement of knowledge. You need to assess what type of knowledge might be developed from the study and who will be influenced by the knowledge.

The type of research conducted (therapeutic or nontherapeutic) affects the potential benefits for the subjects. In therapeutic research, subjects might benefit from the study procedures in areas such as skin care, range of motion, touch, and other nursing interventions. The benefits might include improved physical condition, which could facilitate emotional and social benefits. Some researchers have noted that participation in descriptive research has encouraged subjects to process and disclose thoughts regarding life-altering events and that these actions have been beneficial to their health and well-being (Carpenter, 1998). Nontherapeutic nursing research does not benefit subjects directly but is important because it generates and refines nursing knowledge. By participating in research, subjects can increase their understanding of the research process and know the findings from a particular study.

Examining the benefit-risk ratio also involves assessing the type, degree, and number of risks subjects might encounter while participating in a study. The risks involved depend on the purpose of the study and the procedures used to conduct the study. Risks can be physical, emotional, social, and economic and can range from no risk or mere inconvenience to the risk of permanent damage (see the "Right to Protection from Discomfort and Harm" section earlier in this chapter) (Levine, 1986; Reynolds, 1972). If the risks outweigh the benefits, the study is probably unethical and should not be conducted. If the benefits outweigh the risks, the study is probably ethical and has the potential to add to nursing's knowledge base (see Figure 6-2).

Let us examine the benefit-risk ratio for a study that focused on the effects of an exercise and diet program on the subjects' serum lipid values and cardiovascular (CV) risk level. The serum lipid levels examined were serum cholesterol, low-density lipoprotein, and high-density lipoprotein. The subjects voluntarily agreed to participate in the study and signed a consent form. All subjects were treated fairly during subject selection and data collection. The potential benefits to the participants included (1) exercise and diet instruction, (2) information on serum lipid values and CV risk level at the start of the program and 1 year later, (3) improved serum lipid values, (4) lowered CV risk level, and (5) improved exercise and diet habits. The risks included the discomfort of having blood drawn twice and the time spent participating in the study (Bruce, 1991; Bruce & Grove, 1994). These discomforts were temporary and no more than what subjects would experience in their daily lives and ceased with the termination of the study. The subjects' time spent participating in the study was minimized through efficient organization and precise scheduling of research activities.

In examining the benefit-risk ratio, we note that the benefits appear to be greater in number and importance than the risks; the risks are temporary and can be minimized by the researcher. The researcher received institutional approval to conduct the study, and informed consent was obtained from each subject. The informed consent process involved (1) providing each subject with essential information about the study orally and in writing, (2) giving each subject the choice to participate or not participate in the study, (3) and having each subject read and sign a consent form. Thus, this study was ethical, and provided benefits both to the subjects and their families and to the development of nursing knowledge regarding the effects of exercise and diet on serum lipid levels and CV risk level.

If you were a member of the IRB that reviewed this study, you and the other committee members would probably recommend approving the study for implementation in your agency. Because the risks of the study are minimal, the review process would probably be expedited. If you were a patient advocate, you would examine the risks and benefits, determine whether the study had received IRB approval, and examine the appropriateness of the informed consent process. Because the study meets ethical guidelines, you would probably encourage patients to be subjects in this study so that they might receive the identified benefits. You would also probably be willing to identify potential subjects or collect data for the researcher.

Critiquing the Ethics of a Study

THE ETHICAL ASPECTS of a study include having the research project approved by the IRB for the setting and obtaining informed consent from the subjects. This information should be included in published studies. You might use the following questions to critique the ethical aspects of a study.

1. *Was the study approved by the appropriate IRB?*
2. *Was informed consent obtained from the subjects?*
3. *If the subjects were legally or mentally incompetent, terminally ill, or confined to an institution, were special precautions taken in obtaining their consent? Did the incompetent subjects assent to participate in the study? Did their legally authorized representative give permission for them to participate in the study?*
4. *Were the rights of the subjects protected during sampling, data collection, and data analysis?*
5. *Was the privacy of the subjects protected during the study and in the research report?*
6. *Was the benefit-risk ratio of the study acceptable? Did the benefits outweigh the risks?*

Understanding Scientific Misconduct

The goal of research is to generate sound scientific knowledge, which is possible only through the honest conduct, reporting, and publication of quality research. However, during the last 15 years, an increasing number of fraudulent studies have been published in prestigious scientific journals. In the late 1980s, scientific misconduct was deemed a serious problem that was investigated by the DHHS. In a final ruling in 1989, the DHHS defined *scientific misconduct* or fraud as "fabrication, falsification, plagiarism, or other practices that seriously deviate from those that are commonly accepted within the scientific community for proposing, conducting, or reporting research. It does not include honest error or honest differences in interpretation or judgments of data" (p. 32449). Thus, scientific fraud includes intentional, not unintentional, misconduct.

In 1989, two new federal agencies were organized for reporting and investigating scientific misconduct. The Office of Scientific Integrity Review (OSIR) was established to manage scientific misconduct by grant recipients. The Office of Scientific Integrity (OSI) supervises the implementation of the rules and regulations related to scientific misconduct and manages any investigations (DHHS, 1989; Hawley & Jeffers, 1992). The investigations by these federal agencies revealed a variety of fraudulent behaviors. In some situations, the fraudulent studies were never conducted, and the data and results were fabricated by the researchers. In other cases, the findings were consciously distorted. Some of

TABLE 6-5. Dishonesty in Research	
Type	*Description*
Fabrication, falsification, or forging	Deliberate invention of nonexistent information
Manipulation of design or methods	Intentional planning of the study design or data collection methods so that the results will be biased toward the research hypothesis
Selective retaining or manipulation of data	Choosing only data that are consistent with the research hypothesis and discarding the rest
Plagiarism	Intentional representation of the work or ideas of others as one's own, or rewording one's own work to produce a new paper based on the same data; abuse of confidentiality of information from others
Irresponsible collaboration	Failure to participate appropriately in an investigative team or fulfill responsibilities as a coauthor

From Larson, E. (1989). Maintaining quality in clinical research and evaluation: When corrective action is necessary. Reprinted from the *Journal of Nursing Care Quality, 3*(4), 30, with permission of Aspen Publishers, Inc., © 1989.

the common types of dishonest or fraudulent research are identified and described in Table 6-5.

An example of scientific misconduct was evident in the publications of Dr. Robert Slutsky, a heart specialist at the University of California, San Diego, School of Medicine. He resigned in 1986 when confronted with inconsistencies in his research publications. His publications contained "statistical anomalies that raised the question of data fabrication" (Friedman, 1990, p. 1416). In 6 years Slutsky published 161 articles, and at one time he was completing an article every 10 days. Eighteen of the articles were found to be fraudulent and have retraction notations, and 60 articles were questionable (Friedman, 1990).

Stephen Breuning, a psychologist at the University of Pittsburgh, engaged in deceptive and misleading practices in reporting his research on retarded children. He used his fraudulent research to obtain more than $300,000 in federal grants. In 1988, he was criminally charged with research fraud, pleaded guilty, was fined $20,000, and faced up to 10 years in prison (Chop & Silva, 1991).

More recently, Dr. Roger Poisson, principal investigator at St. Luc Hospital in Montreal, was found guilty of scientific misconduct by the OSI due to his actions during breast-cancer trials. The first evidence of misconduct was noted in 1990 but was not confirmed until 1993. The data from Dr. Poisson's setting were removed and the remaining data were reanalyzed, with similar results: that a lumpectomy was as effective as a mastectomy in the treatment of early breast cancer. There was a significant delay in the identification of the scientific misconduct and the publication of the reanalyzed results in 1994 (Angell &

Kassirer, 1994). Further investigation has now absolved Dr. Poisson of the charge of scientific misconduct, and lumpectomy is considered an effective treatment for early breast cancer.

The publication of fraudulent research is a major concern in medicine and a growing concern in nursing. The decreased funds available for research and the increased emphasis on research publications could lead to an increased incidence in fraudulent publications (Hawley & Jeffers, 1992). A study by Rankin and Esteves (1997) documented that scientific misconduct, such as plagiarism, cheating on data collection, misrepresentation of findings, protocol violations, violations of missing data, falsification of bibliographies, and questions about authorship, were perceived as occurring in many of the institutions by the respondents. All nursing professionals need to clearly understand the difference between ethical and unethical research practice and promote ethical behavior in research. Scientific misconduct must be identified and reported to maintain the quality of nursing research (Burns & Grove, 1997).

Examining the Use of Animals in Research

The use of animals as research subjects is a controversial issue of growing concern to nurse researchers (Burns & Grove, 1997). A small but increasing number of nurse scientists are conducting physiological studies that require the use of animals. Many scientists, especially physicians, believe the current animal-rights movement could threaten the future of health research. These groups are active in antiresearch campaigns and are backed by massive resources, with a treasury that was estimated at $50 million in 1988 (Pardes, West, & Pincus, 1991). Some of the animal-rights groups are trying to raise the consciousness of researchers and society to ensure that animals are used wisely in the conduct of research and treated humanely.

Two important questions need to be addressed: (1) Should animals be used as subjects in research? (2) If animals are used in research, what mechanisms ensure that they are treated humanely? The type of research project developed influences the selection of subjects. Animals are just one of a variety of subjects used in research; others include human beings, plants, and computer data sets. If possible, most researchers use nonanimal subjects because they are generally less expensive. If the studies are low risk, which most nursing studies are, human beings are frequently used as subjects. However, some studies require the use of animals to answer the research question. Approximately 17 to 22 million animals are used in research each year and 90 percent of them are rodents, with the combined percentage of dogs and cats being only 1–2% (Pardes et al., 1991).

Since animals are deemed valuable subjects for selected research projects, what mechanisms ensure that they are treated humanely? At least five separate types of regulations exist to protect research animals from mistreatment. In addition, over 700 institutions conducting health-related research have sought accreditation by the American Association for Accreditation of Laboratory Animal Care (AAALAC), which was developed to ensure the humane treatment of animals in research (Pardes et al., 1991). In conducting research, the type of subject needs to be carefully selected; and if animals are used as subjects, they require humane treatment.

SUMMARY

We would like to believe that unethical research, such as the Nazi experiments of World War II, is a thing of the past. However, this is not the case; published studies continue to include evidence that subjects' rights were violated. Thus, the ethical aspects of published studies and of research conducted in agencies must be critiqued. Historical events, ethical codes, and regulations are presented in this chapter to guide you in determining whether a study was conducted ethically.

Since the 1940s, four experimental projects have been highly publicized for their unethical treatment of human subjects: (1) the Nazi medical experiments, (2) the Tuskegee Syphilis Study, (3) the Willowbrook Study, and (4) the Jewish Chronic Disease Hospital Study. The unethical aspects of each are discussed. In response to these studies, a number of codes and regulations have been implemented. Two historical documents (the Nuremberg Code and the Declaration of Helsinki) have had a strong impact on the conduct of research. More recently, the DHHS (1981, 1983, 1991) passed regulations to promote ethical conduct in research, including (1) general requirements for informed consent and (2) guidelines for IRB review of research.

Conducting research ethically requires protection of the human rights of subjects. The rights that require protection in research include (1) self-determination, (2) privacy, (3) anonymity and confidentiality, (4) fair treatment, and (5) protection from discomfort and harm. You can help protect the rights of research subjects by (1) understanding the informed consent process, (2) being involved in the institutional review of research in your agency, and (3) examining the benefits and risks of studies conducted in your agency.

Informed consent involves the (1) transmission of essential study information, (2) comprehension of that information by the potential subject, (3) competence of the potential subject to give consent, and (4) voluntary consent by the potential subject to participate in the study. In institutional review, a study is examined for ethical concerns by a committee of peers (an IRB). The IRB conducts three levels of review: exempt, expedited, and complete. The chapter includes guidelines for obtaining informed consent and institutional review of research studies.

To balance the benefits and risks of a study, the type, degree, and number of risks are examined, and the potential benefits are identified. If possible, the risks should be minimized and the benefits maximized to achieve the best possible benefit-risk ratio. As a patient advocate, you need to determine that the research conducted on patients in your care is ethical. The chapter concludes with questions you might ask when you critique the ethical aspects of a research report. A serious ethical problem of the 1980s and 1990s is the conduct, reporting, and publication of fraudulent research. Researchers have fabricated data and research results for publication, distorted or incorrectly reported research findings, or mismanaged the implementation of study protocols. All disciplines need to be aware of the potential for scientific misconduct and to act responsibly in protecting the integrity of scientific knowledge. Another ethical concern in research is the use of animals as subjects. Some of the animal-right groups with their antire-search campaigns are threatening the future of health care research. Currently, animals are used infrequently in research, but if the study requires animals, they should be treated humanely.

REFERENCES

American Nurses Association. (1976). *Code for nurses with interpretive statements.* Kansas City, MO: American Nurses Association (Code No. G-56).

American Nurses Association. (1985). *Human rights guidelines for nurses in clinical and other research.* Kansas City, MO: American Nurses Association (Document No. D-46 5M).

American Psychological Association. (1982). *Ethical principles in the conduct of research with human participants.* Washington, DC: American Psychological Association.

Angell, M., & Kassirer, J. P. (1994). Setting the record straight in the breast-cancer trials. *New England Journal of Medicine, 330*(20), 1448–1449.

Beecher, H. K. (1966). Ethics and clinical research. *New England Journal of Medicine, 274*(24), 1354–1360.

Berger, R. L. (1990). Nazi science: The Dachau hypothermia experiments. *New England Journal of Medicine, 322*(20), 1435–1440.

Bournaki, M. (1997). Correlates of pain-related responses to venipunctures in school-age children. *Nursing Research, 46*(3), 147–154.

Brandt, A. M. (1978). Racism and research: The case of the Tuskegee syphilis study. *Hastings Center Report, 8*(6), 21–29.

Brent, N. J. (1990). Legal issues in research: Informed consent. *Journal of Neuroscience Nursing, 22*(3), 189–191.

Broome, M. E., & Stieglitz, K. A. (1992). The consent process and children. *Research in Nursing & Health, 15*(2), 147–152.

Bruce, S. L. (1991). *The effect of a coronary artery risk evaluation program on the serum lipid values of a selected military population.* Unpublished master's thesis, University of Texas at Arlington.

Bruce, S. L., & Grove, S. K. (1994). The effect of a coronary artery risk evaluation program on serum lipid values and cardiovascular risk levels. *Applied Nursing Research, 7*(2), 67–74.

Burns, N., & Grove, S. K. (1997). *The practice of nursing research: Conduct, critique, and utilization* (3rd ed.). Philadelphia: Saunders.

Carico, J. M., & Harrison, E. R. (1990). Ethical considerations for nurses in biomedical research. *Journal of Neuroscience Nursing, 22*(3), 160–163.

Carpenter, J. S. (1998). Methodology corner: Informing participants about the benefits of descriptive research. *Nursing Research, 47*(1), 63–64.

Cassidy, V. R., & Oddi, L. F. (1986). Legal and ethical aspects of informed consent: A nursing research perspective. *Journal of Professional Nursing, 2*(6), 343–349.

Chop, R. M., & Silva, M. C. (1991). Scientific fraud: Definitions, policies, and implications for nursing research. *Journal of Professional Nursing, 7*(3), 166–171.

Czar, M. L., & Engler, M. M. (1997). Perceived learning needs of patients with coronary artery disease using a questionnaire assessment tool. *Heart & Lung, 26*(2), 109–117.

Dansky, K. H., Dellasega, C., Shellenbarger, T., & Russo, P. C. (1996). After hospitalization: Home health care for elderly persons. *Clinical Nursing Research, 5*(2), 185–198.

Davis, A. J. (1989). Informed consent process in research protocols: Dilemmas for clinical nurses. *Western Journal of Nursing Research, 11*(4), 448–457.

Department of Health and Human Services (DHHS) (January 26, 1981). Final regulations amending basic HHS policy for the protection of human research subjects. *Code of Federal Regulations*, Title 45 Public Welfare, Part 46.

Department of Health and Human Services (DHHS) (March 8, 1983). Protection of human subjects. *Code of Federal Regulations*, Title 45 Public Welfare, Part 46.

Department of Health and Human Services (1989). Final rule: Responsibilities of awardee and applicant institutions for dealing with and reporting possible misconduct in science. *Federal Register*, 54, 32446–32451.

Department of Health and Human Services (DHHS) (June 18, 1991). Protection of human subjects. Code of Federal Regulations, Title 45 Public Welfare, Part 46.

Douglas, S., & Larson, E. (1986). There's more to informed consent than information. *Focus on Critical Care, 13*(2), 43–47.

Flynn, L. (1997). The health practices of homeless women: A causal model. *Nursing Research, 46*(2), 72–77.

Ford, J. S., & Reutter, L. I. (1990). Ethical dilemmas associated with small samples. *Journal of Advanced Nursing, 15*(2), 187–191.

Friedman, P. J. (1990). Correcting the literature following fraudulent publication. *Journal of the American Medical Association, 263*(10), 1416–1419.

Hawley, D. J., & Jeffers, J. M. (1992). Scientific misconduct as a dilemma for nursing. *Image: Journal of Nursing Scholarship, 24*(1), 51–55.

Hershey, N., & Miller, R. D. (1976). *Human experimentation and the law.* Germantown, MD: Aspen.

Kelman, H. C. (1967). Human use of human subjects: The problem of deception in social psychological experiments. *Psychological Bulletin, 67*(1), 1–11.

Levine, R. J. (1986). *Ethics and regulation of clinical research* (2nd ed.). Baltimore and Munich: Urban & Schwarzenberg.

Logan, J., & Jenny, J. (1997). Qualitative analysis of patients' work during mechanical ventilation and weaning. *Heart & Lung, 26*(2), 140–147.

Martin, P. A. (1996). Member responsibilities on a nursing research committee. *Applied Nursing Research, 9*(3), 154–157.

McCorkle, R., Robinson, L., Nuamah, I., Lev, E., & Benoliel, J. Q. (1998). The effects of home nursing care for patients during terminal illness on the bereaved's psychological distress. *Nursing Research, 47*(1), 2–10.

Menzel, L. K. (1997). A comparison of patients' communication-related responses during intubation and after extubation. *Heart & Lung, 26*(5), 363–371.

Milgram, S. (1963). Behavioral study of obedience. *Journal of Abnormal and Social Psychology, 67*(4), 371–378.

Mullins, I. L. (1996). Nurse caring behaviors for persons with acquired immunodeficiency syndrome/human immunodeficiency virus. *Applied Nursing Research, 9*(1), 18–23.

National Commission for the Protection of Human Subjects of Biomedical and Behavioral Research (1978). *Belmont report: Ethical principles and guidelines for research involving human subjects.* DHEW Publication No. (05) 78-0012. Washington, DC: U.S. Government Printing Office.

Nuremberg Code (1986). In R. J. Levine (Ed.), *Ethics and regulation of clinical research* (2nd ed., pp. 425–426). Baltimore and Munich: Urban & Schwarzenberg.

Oddi, L. F., & Cassidy, V. R. (1990). Nursing research in the United States: The protection of human subjects. *International Journal of Nursing Studies, 27*(1), 21–34.

Pardes, H., West, A., & Pincus, H. A. (1991). Physicians and the animal-rights movement. *New England Journal of Medicine, 324*(23), 1640–1643.

Ramos, M. C. (1989). Some ethical implications of qualitative research. *Research in Nursing & Health, 12*(1), 57–63.

Rankin, M., & Esteves, M. D. (1997). Perceptions of scientific misconduct in nursing. *Nursing Research, 46*(5), 270–275.

Reynolds, P. D. (1972). On the protection of human subjects and social science. *International Social Science Journal, 24*(4), 693–719.

Reynolds, P. D. (1979). *Ethical dilemmas and social science research.* San Francisco: Jossey-Bass.

Rothman, D. J. (1982). Were Tuskegee and Willowbrook studies in nature? *Hastings Center Report, 12*(2), 5–7.

Rudy, E. B., Estok, P. J., Kerr, M. E., & Menzel, L. (1994). Research incentives: Money versus gifts. *Nursing Research, 43*(4), 253–255.

Sandelowski, M. (1994). Focus on qualitative methods: The use of quotes in qualitative research. *Research in Nursing & Health, 17*(6), 479–482.

Steinfels, P., & Levine, C. (1976). Biomedical ethics and the shadow of Naziism. *Hastings Center Report, 6*(4), 1–20.

Strauman, J. J., & Cotanch, P. H. (1988). Oncology nurse research issues: Over studied populations. *Oncology Nursing Forum, 15*(5), 665–667.

Thompson, P. J. (1987). Protection of the rights of children as subjects for research. *Journal of Pediatric Nursing, 2*(6), 392–399.

Watson, A. B. (1982). Informed consent of special subjects. *Nursing Research, 31*(1), 43–47.

Clarifying Research Designs

Completing this chapter should enable you to:

1. *Identify the purpose of the research design.*
2. *Explain the relationships among the study framework; research objectives, questions, or hypotheses; and the study design.*
3. *Discuss the following concepts relevant to design: causality, multicausality, probability, bias, control, manipulation, and validity.*
4. *Describe the role of validity in conducting research.*
5. *Compare and contrast the four types of validity (statistical conclusion, internal, construct, and external).*
6. *Describe the threats to the four types of design validity.*
7. *Describe the elements of a good design (controlling the environment, controlling equivalence of subjects and groups, controlling the treatment, controlling measurement, and controlling extraneous variables).*
8. *Identify the designs of published studies.*
9. *Critique the quality of designs of quantitative nursing studies.*
10. *Explore the following study designs used in nursing research: descriptive, correlational, quasi-experimental, and experimental.*
11. *Model designs of published studies.*

Bias	*Homogeneity*
Carry-over effect	*Internal validity*
Causality	*Manipulation*
Construct validity	*Multicausality*
Control	*Probability*
Design validity	*Research design*
External validity	*Statistical conclusion validity*
Heterogeneity	

A research design is a blueprint for conducting a study that maximizes control over factors that could interfere with the validity of the findings. Just as the blueprint for a house must be individualized to the specific house being built, so must the design be made specific to a study. The control provided by the design increases the probability that the study results will be accurate reflections of reality. Skill in identifying the study design and in evaluating the threats to validity resulting from design flaws is an important part of critiquing studies.

Many published studies do not identify the design used in the study. Determining the design may require putting together bits of information from various parts of the research report. Clues to the design can be found in the purpose; framework; research objectives, questions, or hypotheses; and variables. Elements that must be identified to determine the study design include the presence or absence of a treatment, number of groups in the sample, number and timing of measurements to be performed, sampling methods, time frame for data collection, planned comparisons between variables or groups, and strategies used to control extraneous variables.

After you identify the design, you will need to critique its adequacy to accomplish the study purpose. To provide you with the information necessary to identify and critique the design of a published study, this chapter includes the concepts important to design, identifies some designs commonly used in nursing studies, and describes the elements of a good design.

Concepts Important to Design

Many terms used in discussing research design have special meanings within this context. Understanding the meanings of these concepts is critical to understanding the purpose of a specific design. Some of the major concepts used in relation to design are causality, multicausality, probability, bias, control, manipulation, and validity.

Causality

According to *causality* theory, things have causes, and causes lead to effects. The original criteria for causation required that a variable "cause" an identified "effect" each time the cause occurred. It was also assumed that each effect had a single cause. Although these assumptions may be true in the basic sciences, such as chemistry or physics, they are unlikely in the health sciences or social sciences. The term "causality" is currently defined with greater flexibility.

You may be able to determine whether the purpose of a study is to examine causality by examining the purpose statement and the propositions within the framework. For example, the purpose of a causal study might be to examine the effect of a specific preoperative education program on length of hospital stay. The proposition might state that preoperative teaching results in a decreased hospitalization period. Preoperative teaching is not the only factor affecting length of hospital stay. Other important factors include the diagnosis, type of surgery, patient's age, initial physical condition of the patient, and complications that occurred after surgery. However, from the perspective of causality, it is important to design the study so that the effect of a single cause (preoperative education program) can be examined apart from the other factors that affect length of hospital stay. The researcher using a causal perspective would design the study to include only a specific type of surgery, select only subjects who were initially in good physical condition and were within a narrow age range, and exclude patients who had complications after surgery. Multiple studies would be performed to examine the effects of different types of surgery, subjects in different physical conditions, or complications on length of hospital stay. Experimental or quasi-experimental designs are commonly used to examine causality. The independent variable in a study is expected to be the cause, and the dependent variable is expected to reflect the effect of the independent variable. Statistical analyses are likely to be bivariate—that is, examining differences between two groups on a single dependent variable using statistical procedures such as the *t*-test.

Multicausality

Multicausality, the recognition that a number of interrelating variables can be involved in causing a particular effect, is a more recent idea related to causality. Very few phenomena in nursing can be clearly pinned down to a single cause and a single effect. Because of the complexity of causal relationships, a theory is unlikely to identify every concept involved in causing a particular phenomenon. However, the greater the proportion of causal factors that can be identified and examined in a single study, the clearer the understanding of the overall phenomenon. This greater understanding is expected to increase the ability to predict and control. Thus, in examining the effect of preoperative teaching on length of hospital stay, researchers using the perspective of multicausality would design the study to include a broad range of diagnoses, patient ages, patient conditions, and complications after surgery. Studies developed from a multicausal perspective will include more variables than those using a strict causal orientation. Hypotheses or research questions are likely to be complex and to include more than two variables. Statistical analysis procedures will be selected to examine the combined effects of multiple independent variables on a single dependent variable.

Probability

Probability addresses relative rather than absolute causality. From the perspective of probability, a cause may not produce a specific effect each time that particular cause occurs. Using a probability orientation, the researcher will design the study to examine the probability that a given effect will occur under a defined set of circumstances or to examine the variations in a given effect based on the set of circumstances. The circumstances might be variations in multiple variables. For example, in examining the effect of multiple variables on length of hospitalization, the researcher might examine the probability of a given length of hospital stay under a variety of specific sets of circumstances. One specific set of circumstances might be that the patient had 15 minutes of preoperative teaching, a specific type of surgery, a certain age, a particular level of health before surgery, and a specific complication. One would expect the probability of a given length of hospital stay to vary as the set of circumstances varied. When examining probability, the researcher finds that hypotheses are complex, with multiple variables. Advanced statistical procedures would be used and might include regression analyses.

Bias

The term *bias* means a slant or deviation from the true or expected. Bias in a study distorts the findings from what the results would have been without the bias. Because studies are conducted to determine the real and the true, researchers place great value on identifying and removing sources of bias in their study or controlling their effects on the study findings. Designs are developed to reduce the possibility and effects of bias. Any component of a study that deviates or causes a deviation from a true measurement of the study variables leads to distorted findings. Many factors related to research can be biased: these include the researcher, the components of the environment in which the study is conducted, the individual subjects, the sample, the measurement tools, the data, and the statistics.

For example, in a preoperative teaching study, suppose one clerk added an additional day to the length of stay if the patient was still in the hospital at 10 A.M., while other clerks determined the length of stay by the date. If the patient went home before midnight, these clerks did not add a day to the patient's length of stay. Or suppose some of the subjects for the study were taken from a unit of the hospital in which the patients were participating in another study involving high-quality nursing care. Or suppose one nurse, selecting patients to include in the study, assigned those patients who were most interested in the study to the experimental group. Each of these situations introduces a bias to the study.

An important focus in critiquing a study is to identify possible sources of bias. This requires careful examination of the researcher's report of the study methods, including strategies for obtaining subjects and performing measurements. However, not all biases can be identified from the published report of a study. The article may not provide sufficient detail about the methods to detect all of the biases.

Control

One method of reducing bias is to increase the amount of control in the design. *Control* means having the power to direct or manipulate factors to achieve a desired outcome. For example, in a study of preoperative teaching, subjects might be randomly selected and then randomly assigned to the experimental or control group. The researcher might control the duration of preoperative teaching sessions, the content taught, the method of teaching, and who performed the teaching. The time that the teaching occurred in relation to surgery could be controlled, as well as the environment in which it occurred. Measurement of the length of hospital stay might be controlled by ensuring that the number of days was calculated exactly the same way for each subject. Limiting the characteristics of subjects in terms of diagnosis, age, type of surgery, and incidence of complications is a form of control. Control is particularly important in experimental and quasi-experimental studies. The greater the researcher's control over the study situation, the more credible (or valid) the study findings. The purpose of research designs is to maximize control factors in the study situation.

IN CRITIQUING a study, you need to identify the elements that were controlled and those that could have been controlled to improve the study design. The feasibility of controlling particular elements of the study needs to be considered. In addition, you need to consider the effect of not controlling elements specific to a particular study on the validity of the study findings.

Manipulation

One form of control is *manipulation*—moving around or controlling movement. Manipulation is used most commonly in experimental or quasi-experimental research. Controlling the treatment or intervention is the most commonly used manipulation. In a study of the effects of preoperative teaching, the situation might be manipulated so that one group of subjects received preoperative teaching and another did not. In a study on oral care, the frequency of care might be manipulated.

In nursing research, when experimental designs are used to explore causal relationships, the nurse must be free to manipulate the variables under study. If the freedom to manipulate a variable (e.g., the type, amount, or frequency of use of pain control measures) is under someone else's control (e.g., the physician or the staff nurses), a bias is introduced into the study. The treatment each subject receives will differ. The researcher will be, so to speak, comparing apples and oranges. In descriptive and correlational studies, little or no effort is made to manipulate factors in the situation. Instead, the purpose is to examine the situation as it exists. Thus, there is a greater possibility of biases influencing findings in these studies.

IN CRITIQUING a study, you need to determine which elements of the design were manipulated and how they were manipulated. You need to judge the adequacy of the manipulation and identify elements that should have been manipulated to improve the validity of the findings.

Validity

Design validity is the determination of whether the study provides a convincing test of the framework propositions. Critical analysis of research involves being able to think through any threats to validity and make judgments about how seriously these threats affect the integrity of the findings. Validity provides a major basis for deciding which findings are useful for patient care.

Cook and Campbell (1979) described four types of validity: statistical conclusion validity, internal validity, construct validity, and external validity. Each of these types of validity needs to be evaluated as a component of critiquing the study design. The following paragraphs discuss briefly each type of validity. For a more detailed discussion of the threats to design validity, see Burns and Grove (1997).

Statistical conclusion validity is concerned with whether the conclusions about relationships or differences drawn from statistical analyses are an accurate reflection of the real world. False conclusions can be reached in interpreting the results of statistical analyses. For example, a Type I error occurs when it is incorrectly concluded that a relationship or difference exists between variables or groups when in reality it does not. A Type II error occurs when it is concluded that no significant relationship or difference exists between variables or between groups when in reality it does. Researchers often examine the possibility of a Type II error in studies in which no significant difference or relationship was found by performing a power analysis.

A CRITIQUE of a study should identify conclusions that may be false. In nursing studies, there is a greater risk of a Type II than a Type I error. Therefore, in critiquing a study in which the findings indicate no statistically significant differences, you need to question the validity of those findings. Look for evidence that the researcher performed power analyses when no significant difference or relationship was found.

Internal validity is the extent to which the effects detected in the study are a true reflection of reality rather than the result of the effects of extraneous variables. Although internal validity should be a concern in all studies, it is addressed more frequently in relation to studies examining causality than in other studies. In studies examining causality, one needs to question whether the effect found in the study may have been caused by a third, often unmeasured, variable (an extraneous variable) rather than by the treatment. The possibility of an alternative explanation of cause is sometimes referred to as a "rival hypothesis." Any study can contain threats to internal validity, and these validity threats can lead to a false-positive or false-negative conclusion.

IN CRITIQUING a study, the following question needs to be considered: "Is there another reasonable (valid) explanation (rival hypothesis) for the finding other than that proposed by the researcher?"

Construct validity examines the fit between the conceptual definitions and operational definitions of variables. Concepts are defined within the framework (conceptual definitions). The conceptual definitions provide the basis for the development of operational definitions of the variables. Operational definitions (methods of measurement) need to reflect the concept. The threats to construct validity are related to the development and selection of measurement techniques.

IN CRITIQUING a study, you need to examine carefully the links between concepts, conceptual definitions, and methods of measurement for threats to construct validity.

External validity is concerned with the extent to which study findings can be generalized beyond the sample used in the study. The most serious threat would lead to the findings being meaningful only for the group being studied. To some extent, the significance of the study is dependent on the number of types of people and situations to which the findings can be generalized. Sometimes the factors influencing external validity are subtle and may not be reported in research papers. Generalization is usually more narrow for a single study than for multiple replications of a study using different samples (perhaps from different populations) in different settings.

IN CRITIQUING a study, you need to ask to which populations the findings can be generalized.

Designs for Nursing Studies

A wide variety of study designs are used in nursing research; the four types most commonly used are descriptive, correlational, quasi-experimental, and experimental. Descriptive and correlational studies examine variables in natural environments and do not include researcher-imposed treatments. Quasi-experimental and experimental studies are designed to examine cause and effect. These studies are conducted to examine differences in dependent variables thought to be caused by independent variables (treatments). The following discussion briefly describes the four types of designs and provides specific examples of each. For more detail on specific designs, see Burns and Grove (1997).

Use the algorithm shown in Figure 7-1 to determine the type of study design used in a published study. The algorithm includes a series of Yes/No responses to specific questions about the design. Begin with the question "Is there a treatment?" Your response will lead you to the next question. The four types of design are identified in the algorithm. You can then turn to a second algorithm

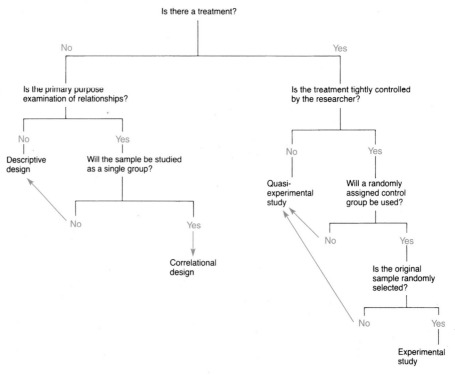

FIGURE 7-1
Algorithm for determining type of study design.

provided for each type of design to determine the specific design used in the study.

Descriptive Design

The descriptive study is designed to gain more information about characteristics within a particular field of study. Its purpose is to provide a picture of a situation as it naturally happens. A descriptive design may be used for the purpose of developing theory, identifying problems with current practice, justifying current practice, making judgments, or determining what others in similar situations are doing (Waltz & Bausell, 1981). No manipulation of variables is involved. Dependent and independent variables are not used within a descriptive design because no attempt is made to establish causality. In many aspects of nursing there is a need for a clearer picture of the phenomenon before causality can be examined. Protection against bias is achieved through (1) conceptual and operational definitions of variables, (2) sample selection and size, (3) valid and reliable instruments, and (4) data collection procedures that achieve some

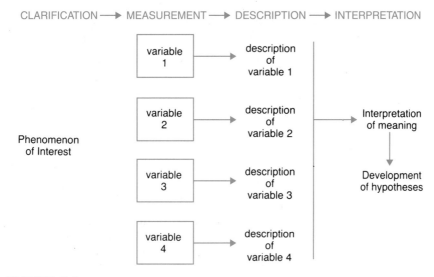

FIGURE 7-2
Typical descriptive design.

environmental control. Descriptive designs vary in level of complexity. Some contain only two variables; others may include multiple variables.

Typical Descriptive Design

The most commonly used design in the category of descriptive studies is presented in Figure 7-2. The design is used to examine characteristics of a single sample. The design includes identifying a phenomenon of interest, identifying the variables within the phenomenon, developing conceptual and operational definitions of the variables, and describing the variables. The description of the variables leads to an interpretation of the theoretical meaning of the findings and the development of hypotheses.

An example of a descriptive design is Troy and Dalgas-Pelish's (1997) study of postpartum fatigue. The following describes the design of the study.

"Postpartum fatigue has been described as a complex phenomenon related to physiologic, psychologic, and situational factors and experienced as feeling negative, uncomfortable, and less efficient (Pugh & Milligan, 1993). Fatigue has the potential to affect adversely the health of the new mother, her capacity to cope with parenting, and the developing mother-infant relationship (Gardner, 1991; Pugh & Milligan, 1993). Unrelieved postpartum fatigue has been

continued

identified as a factor in the development of postpartum depression (Affonso, Lovett, Paul, & Sheptak, 1990; Dunnihoo, 1990). Studies show that primiparous and multiparous women rank fatigue among the top five major concerns during the postpartum period (Gruis, 1977; Harrison & Hicks, 1983; Milligan, Parks, & Lenz, 1990; Smith, 1989; Tolbert, 1986)." (pp. 126–127)

METHODS. "Potential participants were recruited from childbirth education classes at several hospitals in a medium-sized city in the midwestern United States. If the criteria of being low-risk, primiparous, and vaginally delivering a healthy singleton infant were met by women who initially agreed to participate, a home visit was made within 1 week after delivery. At the home visit, the participant's required involvement was explained and a consent form was signed. Participants were asked to complete the 18-item Visual Analogue Scale (VAS-F), which measures fatigue, six times per week—three evenings and three mornings—during the 6-week period, beginning with Tuesday evenings and ending on Friday mornings. Research materials were returned by mail at the end of each week, and new copies of the research materials for the next week were mailed in an ongoing fashion. Reminder telephone calls were made twice weekly. Confidentiality was maintained through the use of code numbers and data storage in a locked office." (pp. 126–128)

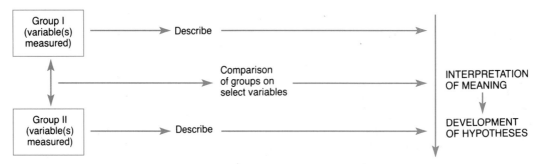

FIGURE 7-3
Comparative descriptive design.

Comparative Descriptive Design

The comparative descriptive design (Fig. 7-3) is used to describe variables and to examine differences in variables in two or more groups that occur naturally in a setting. Descriptive and inferential analyses may be used to examine differences between or among groups. The results obtained from these analyses are frequently not generalized to a population. An example of this design is Dansky, Dellasega, Shellenbarger, and Russo's (1996) study of home health care for elderly persons. Following are excerpts from the study.

"This exploratory study had the following objectives: to analyze the type and number of services used by elderly persons from the time of discharge to 2 weeks after discharge; to compare the postdischarge outcomes of individuals who receive home health services with [the outcomes of] those who do not receive [such] services; and to compare the postdischarge outcomes of individuals who suffer from cognitive impairment with [the outcomes of] those who are cognitively intact." (pp. 185–186)

"The population of interest was all persons age 65 and over who were inpatients on medical or surgical units at a medium-sized urban hospital in the United States. Not included in this study were those individuals in critical or intensive care units. Of 96 persons eligible to participate, 70 agreed to participate at the time of discharge, yielding a response rate of 73%. Those who refused to participate did so primarily because their families were opposed to their participation. This figure is, however, consistent with, or slightly higher than, [that in] previous studies of hospitalized elderly persons.

A discharge planner at the hospital provided the names of all patients who were 65 years or older and scheduled for discharge. Before patients left the hospital, a research assistant (a registered nurse with a master's degree in medical-surgical nursing) contacted each potential subject, explained the purposes of the study, and asked the patient to participate. Interested patients received a written explanation of the study and then completed the consent form. If necessary, legal guardians provided consent, and the same procedure was followed. Of the 70 volunteers, complete information was obtained from 51 subjects.

Before data collection began, the research assistant was trained in the administration of the study instruments. A pilot interview was conducted to establish interrater reliability between the research assistant and two registered nurses with clinical specialties

continued

in medical-surgical nursing. The level of agreement obtained was .90." (p. 188)

"Consenting participants were then screened on their discharge day. Measures of their cognitive and functional status were obtained. The Mini-Mental State Exam (MMSE; Folstein, Folstein, & McHugh, 1978) was used to test cognitive impairment. The Delirium Symptom Interview (DSI; Albert et al., 1992) was used as an additional measure of cognition, and the Everyday Problem Solving Test (EPT; Willis, 1993) was used to screen functional capacity." (pp. 188–189)

"The Resource Utilization Checklist (RUC), developed by Dellasega (1988) and revised for this study, was used to collect data on the use of health services and patient complications after hospital discharge. This checklist reflects information on the client's use of emergency services, visits to the physician, rehospitalization, and institutionalization in an extended-care facility." (p. 189)

"The research assistant conducted the initial predischarge assessment in the patient's hospital room, noted the postdischarge destination of each subject (home, nursing home, rehabilitation center, etc.), and obtained a follow-up telephone number. One week after discharge of a participating subject from the hospital, the research assistant called that subject. The purpose of this telephone interview was to collect data on the subject's cognitive status, as well as information on the use of health care services (both planned and emergency services). The identical procedure was followed for each patient 2 weeks after his or her hospital discharge. If a subject was unable to communicate, a significant other responded by proxy." (pp. 188–189)

Case Study Design

The case study design involves an intensive exploration of a single unit of study, such as a person, family, group, community, or institution, or a very small number of subjects who are examined intensively. Although the number of subjects tends to be small, the number of variables involved is usually large. In fact, it is important to examine all variables that might have an impact on the situation being studied.

Case studies were a commonly used design in nursing 30 years ago but appear in the literature less frequently today. Well-designed case studies are a good source of descriptive information and can be used as evidence to support or invalidate theories. Information from a variety of sources can be collected on each concept of interest using different data collection methods. This strategy can greatly expand the understanding of the phenomenon under study. Case studies are also useful in demonstrating the effectiveness of specific therapeutic techniques. In fact, the reporting of a case study can be the vehicle by which the technique is introduced to other practitioners. The case study design also has potential for revealing important findings that can generate new hypotheses for testing. Thus, the case study can lead to the design of large sample studies to examine factors identified by the case study.

The case study design is dependent on the circumstances of the case but usually includes an element of time. The subject's history and previous behavior patterns are usually explored in detail. As the case study proceeds, the researcher may become aware of components important to the phenomenon being examined that were not originally built into the study. Both quantitative and qualitative elements are likely to be incorporated into the case study design.

An example of a case study design is presented in Lillard and McFann's (1990) book, *A marital crisis: For better or worse.* The following is an excerpt from that book.

"A patient/family case history was selected for study based on the complexity of the marital relationship, an apparently unpredictable crisis occurring during a home visit by Hospice of Marin staff, and involvement of a maximum number of team members including nurses, chaplain, and counselor. Although there were adult children in the family constellation, the marital couple's relationship was pivotal and of major concern to the IDT [interdisciplinary team]. Consequently the study report focuses on the couple, presenting selected, relevant assessments and interventions that occurred during the course of hospice care. Names and demographics are changed in the report to assure family confidentiality." (p. 98)

To determine the type of descriptive design used in a published study, use the algorithm shown in Figure 7-4.

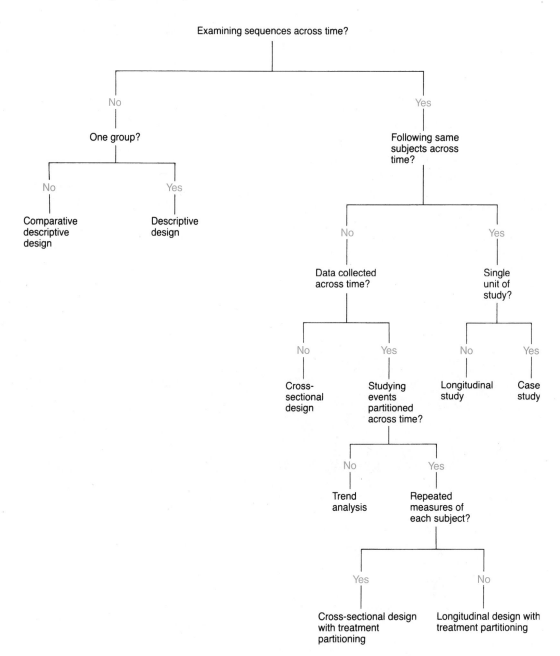

FIGURE 7-4
Algorithm for determining type of descriptive design.

Example Descriptive Study Design

Carty, Bradley, and Winslow (1996) conducted a study of "Women's perceptions of fatigue during pregnancy and postpartum: The impact of length of hospital stay." The following describes the purpose, methods, and sample characteristics for that study.

"The purpose of this article is to describe the experience of women with respect to rest, fatigue, and time spent on household duties during late pregnancy and the early postpartum period. The similarities and differences between women who were discharged at 3 days or less and those who were discharged on Day 4 or later were examined as part of a study evaluating early postpartum discharge in a community hospital on the west coast of Canada." (p. 68)

Method

STUDY DESIGN. "This was a descriptive, comparative study conducted in a community hospital on the west coast of Canada; all participants had the same medical and hospital insurance." (p. 71)

"The objective of this study was to access women's perception of fatigue during the pregnancy and postpartum periods as it related to time of discharge." (p. 70)

SAMPLE. "A convenience sample of 106 volunteer, low-risk pregnant women was studied. [Fifty-seven] women were discharged within 3 days or less (mean length of stay 1.79 days, SD = 1.15), and 49 women were discharged on the 4th day or later (mean length of stay 4.78 days, SD = 0.96). All women met the following inclusion criteria: they experienced a healthy pregnancy, and they had the ability to speak and write in English.

The mean age of the women was 29.85 years (SD = 4.25 years). About 25% of the sample had completed high school, whereas 73% had completed community college or university. Of the sample, 98% of the women were married or living with their partners and had been for an average of 6 years. About 75% of the women worked during their pregnancy, for a mean of 24.64 weeks (SD = 16.05). About 64% of the women were primiparous, and 36% were multiparous. The mean length of the gestation at the initial interview was 36.87 weeks (SD = 2.27). At the time of the initial interview, women were given the choice of staying in the hospital for a traditional length of stay (4 days) or being discharged early (in 3 days or less). About 40% ($n = 42$) of the women indicated they wanted early discharge." (p. 71)

continued

MEASURES. "A self-report Rest and Activity Questionnaire was developed for use in this study. The questionnaire was in three parts, comprising items related to women's perceptions of rest and sleep, feelings of fatigue, and activity levels. It was designed to be completed during the third trimester of pregnancy, at 1 week postpartum, and at 1 month postpartum. Data were collected on hours of sleep in a 24-hour period, number of times awake in the night and the reasons for waking, naps during the day, the ways in which being tired affected activities of daily living, perceptions of level of tiredness at each time period, and the kinds of activities that were being engaged in. The majority of questionnaire items were closed-ended, with ordered answer choices. The questionnaire was reviewed by perinatal nurses and pretested on a group of 30 women who had been discharged early prior to the beginning of the study." (pp. 71–72)

PROCEDURE. "Potential study participants were recruited from prenatal classes and hospital tours during the third trimester. The study coordinator visited the homes of the women who volunteered to participate to explain the study further, to obtain written consent, and to leave the Rest and Activity Questionnaire to be completed at the appropriate time and returned to the study coordinator. At the time of the initial home visit, the women indicated their preference for early or late discharge.

   Women who were discharged early received nursing visits in the home by hospital nurses on Days 2, 3, 5, and 10. Women who remained in the hospital received a visit from the public health nurse within 10 days of discharge. Women were reminded to return their Rest and Activity Questionnaires if they had not been received within 1 week of the expected date of return." (p. 72)

Critique of Example Descriptive Study Design

THIS INTERESTING study used a descriptive-comparative design and a convenience sample. It addresses an issue of concern related to the constraints imposed by managed care. The framework of the study, which must be extracted from the literature, is based on the findings of sleep research that describe two types of sleep: "NREM (non-rapid eye movement) sleep, which is divided into four stages, and REM (rapid eye movement) sleep (Kryger, Roth, & Dement, 1989; Moorcroft, 1989)" (Carty, Bradley, & Winslow, 1996, p. 68). We are not told what proportion of the women who were asked to participate agreed to do so. One must question whether women who chose not to participate were different in ways important to the study from those who participated. The study could have been strengthened by having equal numbers of primiparous and multiparous women. Characteristic of descriptive studies, the design has few control factors other than the requirement of having experienced a normal pregnancy. For example, there was no control indicated for the possibility of the birth of more than one child, (e.g., twins), which could affect the amount of fatigue experienced. Women who participated in the study were given a choice related to length of stay, which is a threat to the internal validity of the findings. This threat was identified by the authors as a limitation of the study and is a common threat in descriptive studies. The questionnaire used in the study has no documented validity other than validation by expert nurse clinicians. However, the authors wanted an instrument to gather specific data which may not have been available in existing instruments. The study might have been strengthened by inclusion of a valid instrument specifically designed to measure fatigue. The home visits made by nurses during the data collection period do not occur in the routine clinical setting and can further affect the ability to generalize the findings. The authors do not report a power analysis evaluating the adequacy of the sample size. Since the results reveal no significant differences in women discharged early and those with a longer stay, it is unclear whether this finding is an accurate reflection of the effect of length of hospitalization, or is a result of inadequate measurement of fatigue or of an inadequate sample size.

Correlational Design

The purpose of a correlational design is to examine relationships between or among two or more variables in a single group. This examination can occur at several levels. The researcher can seek to describe a relationship (descriptive correlational), predict relationships among variables (predictive correlational), or simultaneously test all the relationships proposed by a theory (model testing design). In correlational designs, a large variance in the variable scores is necessary to determine the existence of a relationship. Thus, the sample needs to reflect the full range of scores possible on the variables being measured. Some subjects need to have very high scores, others very low scores, and the rest distributed throughout the possible range of scores. Because of the need for wide variation on scores, correlational studies generally require large sample sizes. Subjects are not divided into groups because group differences are not being examined.

Descriptive Correlational Design

The purpose of a descriptive correlational design is to describe variables and examine relationships among these variables. Using this design will facilitate the identification of many interrelationships in a situation (Fig. 7-5). The study may examine variables in a situation that has already occurred or is currently occurring. No attempt is made to control or manipulate the situation. As with descriptive studies, variables must be clearly identified and defined.

An example of a descriptive correlational design is Medoff-Cooper and Gennaro's (1996) study of "The correlation of sucking behaviors and Bayley Scales of Infant Development at six months of age in VLBW [very low birth weight] infants."

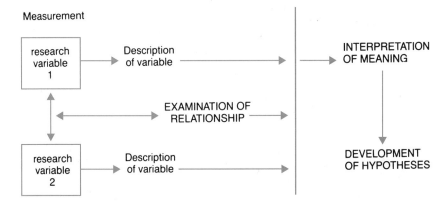

FIGURE 7-5
Descriptive correlational design.

"The purpose of this preliminary work was to explore the relationship between nutritive sucking patterns, as a developmental assessment technique in preterm infants, and psychomotor development at 6 months of age.

The conceptual framework of this study is the Als (1979) . . . synactive theory of infant development. . . . Als proposed (1979, 1991) that the behavioral organization displayed by an infant is a reflection of central nervous system integrity, defined as the potential for the brain to develop normally." (p. 291)

"Nutritive sucking is characterized by repetitive mouthing on a nursing nipple associated with negative intraoral pressure sufficient to deliver liquid from the nipple (Goldson, 1987). Compared with nonnutritive sucking, nutritive sucking requires greater coordination between suck, swallow, and respiratory effort (Harris, 1986)." (p. 293)

Sample. "All infants were born at a major teaching hospital. The sample consisted of 19 VLBW infants with a mean birth weight of 1,238.26 ± 413.5 g and a mean gestational age at birth of 29.1 ± 1.9 weeks." (p. 293)

Measures

"KRON NUTRITIVE SUCKING APPARATUS. The hardware of the Kron Nutritive Sucking Apparatus continuously measures negative pressure generated by the infant during sucking. The sucking apparatus incorporates a calibrated capillary tube for metering flow of nutrient into an ordinary nipple by embedding it in silicone rubber. A second tube embedded in the silicone measures the intraoral pressure and is connected to a Cobe pressure transducer.

"NEONATAL MORBIDITY SCALE. This scale (Minde, Whitelaw, Brown, & Fitzharding, 1983) was used to determine infant health status while the infant was still hospitalized." (p. 293)

"BAYLEY SCALES OF INFANT DEVELOPMENT (BSID). The BSID (Bayley, 1969) are composed of three distinct scales that measure mental acuities and abilities (Mental Scale), degree of control of body coordination and fine motor skills (Psychomotor Scale), and the child's social and objective orientation to the environment (Infant Behavior Record)." (p. 294)

"PROCEDURE. 'The sucking assessments were conducted when the infants were 34 weeks' PCA [post-conceptional age]. The Neonatal Morbidity Scale was scored on days 1 to 3 and 4 to 7 and then weekly until hospital discharge to determine an average hospital morbidity score. The BSID were completed at a 6-month follow-up visit' (p. 294). Correlational analysis was performed using all the values obtained from these measurements." (p. 194)

Predictive Correlational Design

The purpose of a predictive correlational design is to predict the value of one variable based on values obtained for another variable(s). Prediction is one approach to examining causal relationships between variables. Because causal phenomena are being examined, the terms "dependent" and "independent" are used to describe the variables. One variable is classified as the dependent variable and all other variables as independent variables. The aim of a predictive design (Fig. 7-6) is to predict the level of the dependent variable from the independent variables. The independent variables that are most effective in prediction are highly correlated with the dependent variable but not highly correlated with other independent variables used in the study. Predictive correlational designs require the development of a theory-based mathematical hypothesis proposing variables expected to effectively predict the dependent variable. The hypothesis is then tested using regression analysis.

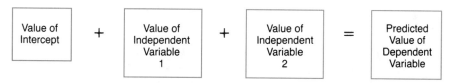

FIGURE 7-6
Predictive design.

Russell and Champion (1996) conducted a predictive correlational study of "Health beliefs and social influence in home safety practices of mothers with preschool children."

"The purpose of this study was to determine relationships among health beliefs, social influence, and home injury proofing-behavior in 140 low-income mothers with preschool children." (p. 59)

Variables in this study were perceptions of injury susceptibility and seriousness in relation to the child, perceived benefits and barriers to injury prevention, and self-efficacy and social influence in relation to performing injury-prevention behavior. The following hypotheses were developed for testing.

"a. The combination of injury experience, knowledge, demographic, health beliefs, and social influence variables will predict home hazard accessibility;

b. the combination of injury experience, knowledge, demographic, health beliefs, and social influence variables will predict home hazard frequency." (p. 60)

SAMPLE. "Study participants included 140 women residing in two inner city public housing complexes in a midwestern metropolitan city. . . . The children were 1 year to 3 years old and free of physical and mental handicapping conditions. Except for number of bedrooms and bathrooms per dwelling, the public housing units were identical in structure, scheduling of maintenance, and smoke-detector monitoring. Most of the sample was African-American (97.2%) with 2.1% White and 0.7% Hispanic. Their ages ranged from 15 to 41 years old with a mean age of 25.1 years (SD = 5.1). Most (82.1%) were never married, although 13.6% were divorced or separated, and 4.2% were married or lived with a male partner." (p. 60)

INSTRUMENTS. "The research instruments consisted of a questionnaire measuring health beliefs, social influence, and injury prevention-knowledge variables and an observational tool measuring the presence of hazards in the home. . . . Two observational scales, hazard accessibility and hazard frequency, were used to measure the presence of home-safety hazards." (pp. 60–61)

PROCEDURE. "Subjects were identified through door-to-door contact. A list of apartments with children ages 1 through 3 years old was obtained from the housing administration. Each residence on the list was visited. If mothers had more than one child between the ages of 1 through 3, a table of random numbers was used to determine which child would be the focus of the study. The study was approved by the institutional review board and informed consent was obtained.

A structured interview was administered to each subject in her home. Immediately upon completion of the interview, observations for safety hazards in the subject's home were made. As hazardous items were identified, they were pointed out to subjects. Information on corrective actions to take for eliminating each hazard was given each time a hazard was observed. Lastly, general childhood injury prevention materials and injury-related packets, consisting of soap, bandaids, and electric socket covers, were discussed and distributed. Bivariate and regression analyses were performed." (p. 61)

Model Testing Design

Some studies are designed specifically to test the accuracy of a hypothesized causal model. The design requires that all variables relevant to the model be measured. A large, heterogeneous sample is required. All the "paths" expressing relationships between concepts are identified, and a conceptual map is developed (Fig. 7-7). The analysis determines whether the data are consistent with the model.

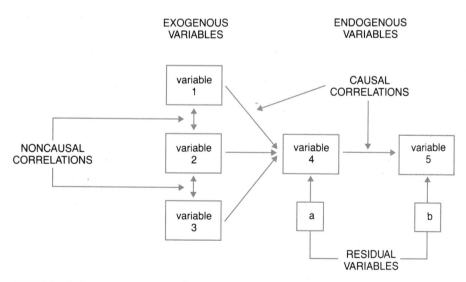

FIGURE 7-7
Model testing design.

Bailey (1996) used a model testing design to examine "Mediators of depression in adults with diabetes."

"The stress process model elaborated by Perlin, Lieberman, Menaghan, and Mullan (1981) was adapted for this study. The authors found that chronic life strains were strong predictors of depression, an indicator of distress. Chronic strains were related to depression because they diminished two aspects of the self: sense of mastery and feelings of self-esteem. Coping behaviors and social support were inversely related to depression, mediated by positive effects on sense of mastery and self-esteem." (pp. 28–29)

Figure 7-8 illustrates concepts from the stress process model applied to adults with diabetes.

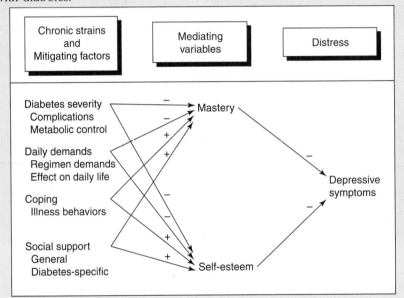

FIGURE 7-8

Conceptual framework for disease-related chronic strains, mitigating factors, mediating variables, and depression in diabetes. (From Bailey, B. J. [1996]. Mediators of depression in adults with diabetes. *Clinical Nursing Research, 5*[1], 30. ©1996. Reprinted by permission of Sage Publications, Inc.)

"The questions addressed by this study are:

1. Are disease-specific chronic strains related to depression in people with diabetes?
2. Do illness behaviors, as a type of problem-focused coping, or social support mitigate depression in people with diabetes?
3. Do mastery or self-esteem mediate any relationships between strains or mitigating factors and depression?" (p. 31)

METHOD. "To answer the research questions, a cross-sectional, correlational study was conducted, and tests of mediation were carried out as part of data analysis. A pilot study was conducted to pretest instruments." (p. 31)

PROCEDURES. "Following the pilot study, approval for the larger study was obtained from the Institutional Review Board. A convenience sample of adults with diabetes was recruited from a university medical center diabetes clinic, two health maintenance organizations, and two private medical practices in an urban area. Patients were invited to join the study when they came to clinic visits (university clinic) or were sent letters of invitation from their physicians (all other sites). Subjects had to be at least 21 years old, without a history of clinical depression, and without medications known to modify affect. All people recruited had to be insulin using, although they could have IDDM [insulin-dependent diabetes mellitus] or NIDDM [noninsulin dependent diabetes mellitus]. After consenting to participate, each subject completed a questionnaire and provided 5 ml of venous blood." (p. 33)

SAMPLE. "Of 373 people invited to participate in this study, 180 (48.2%) consented and provided complete data. Twenty subjects came from private medical practices; the remainder were evenly divided between the university medical center and the health maintenance organizations." (p. 33)

MEASURES. "The Diabetes Complication Scale is an inventory of 17 known complications of diabetes and the recency of diagnosis for each. Recently diagnosed complications are weighted more heavily, because people newly diagnosed with chronic health problems are known to be more distressed (Cassileth et al., 1984)." (p. 32)

"Metabolic control was defined as GHb [glucosylated hemoglobin], which is a measure of average blood glucose control for 8 weeks prior to sampling (Baynes et al., 1984). . . .

Regimen demands were measured with the Diabetes Regimen Demands Scale developed in the pilot study. Illness behaviors were assessed with the Diabetes Illness Behaviors Inventory. . . . General social support was measured by the Support Behaviors Inventory (SBI), (Brown, 1986), which addresses four types of support: esteem, appraisal, information, and instrumental. Higher scores indicate greater satisfaction with support. . . . Mastery, or control over one's life, was measured with a seven-item scale (Pearlin, Lieberman, Menaghen, & Mullan, 1981). Higher scores

continued

indicate that respondents feel greater control . . . the Rosenberg Self-Esteem Scale (Rosenberg, 1965) was used to measure feelings of self-worth. Higher scores on the 10-item scale indicate a more positive self-evaluation. . . . Depression was measured with the 20-item CES-D [Center for Epidemiologic Studies—Depression Scale] (Radloff, 1977). A score $\geq$ 16 indicates depression." (pp. 34–35)

"The 32.4% frequency of CES-D scores of 16 or greater corroborates previous findings of high prevalence of depression among people with diabetes. . . . Only one of the three mitigating factors proposed was related to depression. General social support was associated with fewer depressive symptoms, but neither diabetes-illness behaviors nor diabetes-specific social suspport achieved significance." (p. 37)

To determine the type of correlational design used in a published study, use the algorithm shown in Figure 7-9. For more detail on specific correlational designs referred to in this algorithm, see Burns and Grove (1997).

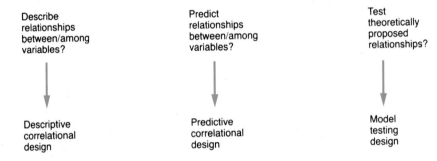

FIGURE 7-9
Algorithm for determining type of correlational design.

Critique of Example Correlational Study Design

IN CRITIQUING a correlational design, one searches for a large, representative sample with a wide range of values on the measured variables. Bailey's (1996) sample of 180 subjects is adequate to examine relationships among the variables identified in the research questions. Of the 373 individuals approached to participate in the study, 180 (48.2%) agreed to do so. It is likely that the time required to complete the instruments affects the willingness of individuals to participate. Of concern to the design is whether those individuals who declined were different elements of the population under study that was then not adequately represented in the sample. The majority (57.4%) were female, and 71.1% of the sample was white. The participants were more highly educated than could be expected of the general population, with a mean of

13.94 years of education. The range of education (3 years to postgraduate) appears to be relatively broad. In a correlational study, it is critical that there be a full range of scores for each of the variables included in the correlational analyses. The range and distribution of scores on the measures taken in the study are not reported; thus, it is not possible to judge the adequacy of the distribution of scores for the correlational analyses.

Testing Causality

Designs developed to test causality emerged in the early 1900s because of a need in agriculture to test the effectiveness of new methods designed to improve crop production (Fisher, 1935). The purpose of the experimental design is to provide the best method possible to obtain a true representation of cause and effect in the situation under study. This means providing the greatest amount of control possible in order to examine causality with the least error possible. To examine cause, the researcher must eliminate all factors influencing the dependent variable other than the cause (independent variable) being studied. The effects of some factors are eliminated by controlling them (e.g., sampling criteria). The study is designed to prevent other elements from intruding into the observation of the specific cause and effect that the researcher wishes to examine.

We consider the three essential elements of experimental research to be (1) random sampling; (2) researcher-controlled manipulation of the independent variable; and (3) researcher control of the experimental situation, including a control or comparison group. There is disagreement about whether random sampling is essential in labeling a study as experimental. Randomization, in which nonrandomly obtained subjects are randomly assigned to groups, is considered by some to be an acceptable substitute for random samples. Control of variance is considered by all to be essential in experimental designs. Sample criteria are explicit, the independent variable is provided in a precisely defined way, the dependent variables are carefully operationalized, and the environment in which the study is conducted is rigidly controlled to prevent the interference of unstudied factors from modifying the dynamics of the process being studied.

In nursing and medical research, as well as in research in other disciplines, such as education, achieving the control considered essential to an experimental design is difficult, and in some cases impossible. Clinical trials, from which much of the science used to guide clinical practice in nursing and medicine is derived, and which are critically reviewed and considered to have the best designs possible, use randomization but do not have random samples. Thus, clinical trials use comparison groups rather than control groups. There is a reduced probability of equivalence between the experimental group and the comparison group. We have been unable to locate experimental studies with random samples and control groups in the nursing literature to use as examples in this text.

Experimental Designs

A variety of experimental designs, some relatively simple and others very complex, have been developed for a variety of research questions. In some cases, researchers may combine characteristics of more than one design in order to meet the needs of their study. Names of designs vary from one textbook to another. In reading and critiquing a published study, you need to determine the author's name for the design (some authors do not name the design used) and read the description of the design in order to determine for yourself the type of design used in the study. To determine the type of experimental study design used in a published study, use the algorithm shown in Figure 7-10. For more detail on specific designs referred to in the figure, see Burns and Grove (1997).

Pretest–Post-test Design

The most common experimental design used in nursing studies is the pretest–post-test design. Multiple groups (both experimental and control) can be used to great advantage in this design. For example, one control group can receive no treatment, while another control group receives a placebo treatment. Multiple experimental groups can receive varying levels of the treatments, such as differing frequency, intensity, or length of nursing care measures. These additions greatly increase the generalizability of study findings.

Factorial Design

The factorial design is a complex, multivariate experimental design. In a factorial design, two or more characteristics, treatments, or events are independently varied within a single study. This design is a logical approach to examining multiple causality. The simplest arrangement is one in which two treatments or factors are involved, and within each factor, two levels are manipulated (e.g., the presence or absence of the treatment). This is referred to as a "2 × 2 factorial design." This design is illustrated in Figure 7-11, using the two independent variables of relaxation and distraction as means of pain relief.

A 2 × 2 factorial design produces a study with four cells. Each cell must contain an equivalent number of subjects. Cells B and C allow examination of each separate intervention. Cell D subjects receive no treatment and serve as a control group. Cell A allows examination of interaction between the two independent variables. The design can be used to control for confounding variables. The confounding variable is included as an independent variable, and interactions between it and the other independent variable are examined (Spector, 1981).

Randomized Clinical Trial

The randomized clinical trial has been used in medicine since 1945. However, until recently, it has not been used in nursing. The clinical trial uses large

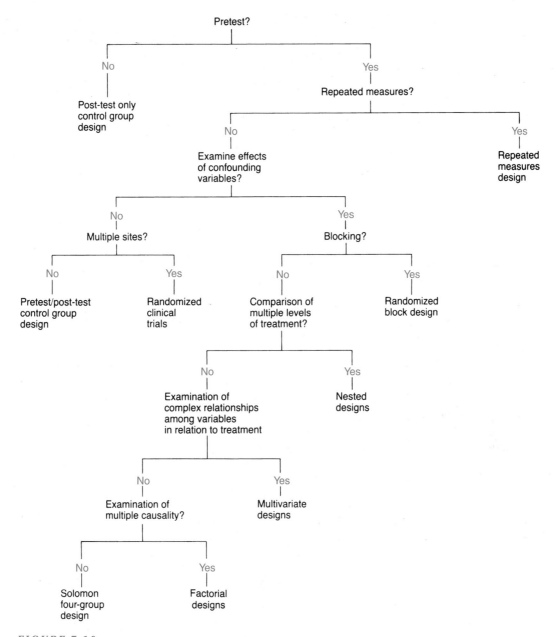

FIGURE 7-10
Algorithm for determining type of experimental design.

Level of Relaxation	Level of Distraction	
	Distraction	No Distraction
Relaxation	A	B
No Relaxation	C	D

FIGURE 7-11
Example of factorial design.

numbers of subjects to test the effects of a treatment and compare the results with those of a control group that has not received the treatment (or that has received a more traditional treatment). Subjects are drawn from a reference population, using clearly defined criteria, and are then randomly assigned to treatment or control groups. Baseline states must be comparable in all groups included in the study. The treatment must be equal and consistently applied, and outcomes need to be measured consistently. Care must be taken to ensure that randomization procedures are rigidly adhered to.

Because of the need to have large samples and to be able to generalize to a variety of clinical settings and patients, the study may be carried out simultaneously in multiple geographic locations coordinated by the primary researcher. Utilization of this design has the potential to greatly improve the scientific base for nursing practice (Fetter et al., 1989; Tyzenhouse, 1981).

Example Experimental Study Design

A study by Reese, Means, Hanrahan, Clearman, Colwill, and Dawson (1996) of "Diarrhea associated with nasogastric feedings" will be used as an example of an experimental study.

> PURPOSE/OBJECTIVES. "To determine the difference in the incidence of diarrhea among subjects given one of three formulas with varying fiber concentrations administered by nasogastric (NG) tube, variables affecting incidence of diarrhea, discomforts other than diarrhea associated with NG tube feedings, and effects of changing from continuous to interval feedings on incidence of diarrhea and discomforts." (p. 59)

Design. Prospective, double-blind, randomized study.

Setting. Midwestern tertiary care center otolaryngology nursing unit.

Sample. Eighty randomized subjects who were 18 years or older, English-speaking, and undergoing head and neck cancer surgery that required an NG tube postoperatively and who had no gastrointestinal (GI) illness within two weeks prior to surgery.

METHODS. "Subjects received continuous administration of formula containing no fiber, 7 gm/L of fiber, or 14 gm/L of fiber until they reached the caloric intake goal and then were advanced to interval feedings. Patients' medical records provided past medical history and information on medication administration. A bedside flow sheet was used for documenting incidence of diarrhea and other GI discomforts.

MAIN RESEARCH VARIABLES. Amount of fiber in the formula administered, patients' genders and prior food aversions, and antibiotics' effect on diarrhea and other GI discomforts.

FINDINGS. Multiple logistic regression showed significant odds ratios (ORs) for developing diarrhea in female subjects (OR = 7.96), subjects who had prior food aversions (OR = 2.67), and subjects receiving broad spectrum antibiotics (OR = 3.22). Diarrhea was four times more likely to occur in males who received fiber-free formula. Of all subjects, 70% experienced GI discomforts with continuous feedings, and 50% experienced discomforts when advanced to interval feedings.

CONCLUSIONS. Fiber formulas reduced the incidence of diarrhea in male subjects but not in female subjects. Antibiotics' effect on diarrhea paralleled the findings of other studies.

IMPLICATIONS FOR NURSING PRACTICE. Use formulas with fiber for males. Liquid stools do not require interruption of tube feeding; GI discomforts warrant interruption. Interval feeding schedules require monitoring similar to continuous feeding schedules." (p. 59)

Critique

This study, which was published in the *Oncology Nursing Forum,* was followed by a Commentary by Ropka (1996). It has become the policy of this journal to offer commentary for selected studies in order to promote research utilization. This strategy is an important contribution to the nursing body of knowledge. Selected text from Dr. Ropka's excellent commentary follows.

Study Evaluation for Application in Practice

"Reese et al. adequately present their study's purpose, as well as problems encountered, in their article. They identified pertinent and

continued

answerable questions by focusing on nutritional problems routinely experienced by patients with head and neck cancer, as identified by Goodwin and Byers (1993). The results of this study have potential practical clinical consequences, such as better wound healing or enhanced well-being and function because of improved nutritional status and greater tolerance of tube feedings.

PRIMARY QUESTION 1. Was the assignment of patients to treatments randomized? Reese et al.'s study used the strongest design available to answer questions of cause and effect—a prospective, randomized, controlled clinical trial. Subjects were randomly assigned to groups according to an independent variable—the amount of fiber in the formula received. The study also included a control group that received no fiber. Thus, the first key criterion of random assignment was met. However, the extent to which subjects in each treatment group received the treatment as assigned or achieved the treatment goal (i.e., the correct amount of fiber) is not reported.

PRIMARY QUESTION 2. Were all 23 female and 57 male patients who entered the trial properly accounted for and attributed at its conclusion? Were all measures taken on all subjects who began the trial known and reported at the end? Primary question 2 can be answered by addressing two additional questions. Was all follow-up complete? Results related to ascertainment of the primary outcome variable, diarrhea, are reported for all subjects. Minimal attrition from the study occurred because of discontinuation or loss-to-follow up. Were patients analyzed in the groups to which they were randomized? Data from subjects were initially analyzed in the three fiber groups to which they were randomly assigned. When the medium- and high-fiber groups experienced the same reported levels of outcome measure, diarrhea, they were combined in separate post hoc analyses. It might have been useful to ask some additional questions before deciding to combine the two fiber groups. Although subjects in both fiber groups experienced the same levels of diarrhea, differences in severity, frequency, and duration of diarrhea were not reported. Did subjects in one group experience different or more severe side effects, toxicities, or complications than subjects in the other group, making one fiber level preferable to the other? For example, subjects in all formula groups experienced equal incidences of constipation. Additional questions must be raised to determine whether either of the fiber formulas presented practical disadvantages, such as expense or inconvenience, or risks, such as greater incidence of contamination caused by necessary mixing of the medium-fiber supplement. Was tolerance of, and thus adherence to, therapy greater with one formula than the other, indicating that use of one would better improve nutritional status?" (p. 67)

"Secondary questions needed to determine study validity focus on several issues.

- Were patients, health workers, and study personnel "blind" to treatment? Presumably, patients did not know which formula they were receiving. In addition, one person prepared and administered the formulas, and a different person evaluated the occurrence of diarrhea. Thus, the evaluator presumably did not know which formula subjects had received. Unless there were apparent differences in the formulas' physical characteristics, the evaluator did conduct blind ascertainment of occurrence of diarrhea.
- Were the groups similar at the start of the trial? Based on clinical experience or prior research, investigators provided information regarding patient characteristics that they believed were potentially related to the primary outcome. Characteristics reported as similar at the start of the trial included subjects' age, gender, specific adult diseases, types of and duration of surgeries undergone, length of hospital stay, and weight loss experienced before admission.
- Aside from the experimental interventions, were the groups treated equally? Clinically relevant aspects of interventions performed in all groups are comparable, excluding the amount of fiber received. Aspects related to ascertaining the dependent variable (incidence of diarrhea) also were similar in all groups, including use of a standard definition of diarrhea and training of personnel administering enteral feedings about assessment parameters.

In summary, the strong study design suggests that the results are valid." (p. 67)

Will the Results Assist Nurses in Caring for Patients?

"One can decide whether to apply a study's results when caring for a patient only if the study's validity has been established. To gain a clear understanding of this study, readers of the article must understand the difference between random selection and random assignment of subjects to treatment groups. Subjects in this study presumably constitute a convenience sample of patients who met the study-eligibility criteria and were available in the established setting at that time. Therefore, these subjects were not randomly selected. Because of the potential sampling bias, generalization of findings to other patients with head and neck cancer should be limited." (p. 68)

Quasi-experimental Design

Quasi-experimental designs were developed to provide an alternative means for examining causality in situations that are not conducive to experimental controls. Quasi-experimental designs facilitate the search for knowledge and examination of causality in situations in which complete control is not possible. These designs were developed to control as many threats to validity as possible in a situation in which some of the components of true experimental design are lacking. A nonequivalent comparison group, one in which the control group is not selected by random means, is commonly used in quasi-experimental studies. Some groups are more nonequivalent than others. Although most quasi-experimental studies select experimental and comparison subjects from the same pool of potential subjects, some quasi-experimental designs involve using comparison and treatment groups that evolved naturally. For example, groups might include subjects who choose a treatment as the experimental group and subjects who chose not to receive a treatment as the comparison group. These groups cannot be considered equivalent because the individuals in the control group usually differ in important ways from those in the treatment group.

	Measurement of dependent variable(s)	Manipulation of independent variable	Measurement of dependent variable(s)
Experimental group	→ PRETEST	→ TREATMENT	→ POST-TEST
Nonequivalent control group	→ PRETEST		→ POST-TEST

Treatment—experimental group
           control group not treated

Control group—not randomly selected

Findings: • comparison of control and experimental pretest
           • comparison of pretest and post-test
           • comparison of control and experimental post-test

Example: Littlefield, Chang, & Adams (1990). Participation in alternative care: relationship to anxiety, depression, and hostility.

Uncontrolled • selection–maturation
threats   • instrumentation
to validity: • differential statistical regression
           • interaction of selection and history

FIGURE 7-12
Untreated comparison group design with pretest and post-test.

	Manipulation of independent variable	Measurement of dependent variable(s)
Experimental group ———→ TREATMENT	———————————→	**POST-TEST**
Nonequivalent control group	———————————————————→	**POST-TEST**

Treatment—often ex post facto
        may not be well defined

Experimental group—those who receive the treatment and the post-test

Pretest—inferred—norms of measures of dependent variable(s) of population from which
        pretreatment experimental group taken

Control group—not randomly selected—tend to be those who naturally in the situation do
        not receive the treatment

Findings: ● comparison of post-test scores of experimental and control groups
           ● comparison of post-test scores with norms

Example: Monahan (1991). Potential outcomes of clinical experience.

Uncontrolled   ● no link between treatment and change
threats   ● no pretest
to validity: ● selection

FIGURE 7-13
Post-test-only design with a comparison group.

Quasi-experimental study designs vary widely. The most frequently used design in social science research is the untreated control group design with pretest and posttest (Fig. 7-12). With this design, the researcher has an experimental group who receives the experimental treatment (or intervention) and a comparison group who receives no treatment (or, in some cases, the usual treatment [care] provided in the circumstances under study). Another commonly used design is the posttest-only design with a comparison group (Fig. 7-13). This design is used in situations in which a pretest is not possible. For example, if the researcher is examining differences in amount of pain during a painful procedure using a nursing intervention purported to reduce pain with the experimental group, it might not be possible (or meaningful) to pretest the amount of pain before the procedure. This design has a number of threats to validity because of the lack of a pretest and thus is sometimes referred to as a "preexperimental design." To determine the type of quasi-experimental study design used in a published study, use the algorithm shown in Figure 7-14. See Burns and Grove (1997) for more detail on specific designs identified in this algorithm.

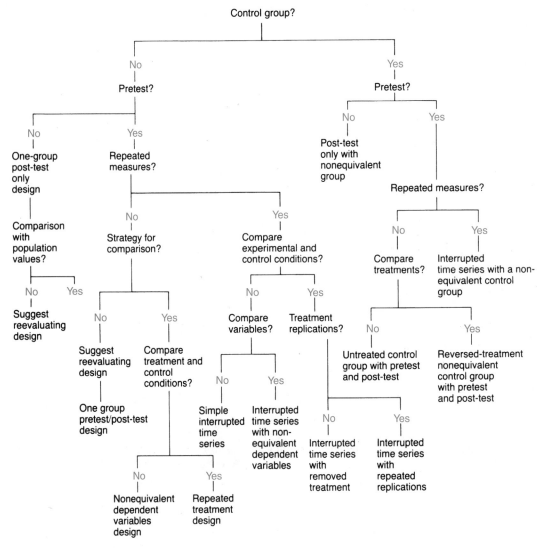

FIGURE 7-14
Algorithm for determining type of quasi-experimental design.

Example Quasi-experimental Study Design

Cason and Grissom (1997) conducted a quasi-experimental study to examine the effectiveness of a distraction intervention on subjects' perceptions of pain. They describe their methods as follows:

"This study evaluated a sensory based distraction intervention (kaleidoscope) on adults' perception of pain associated with phlebotomy." (p. 169)

"This study evaluated two hypotheses: (1) adults who engage in a distraction intervention during phlebotomy will have lower ratings of pain than adults who receive equivalent care but do not engage in a distraction intervention; and (2) measures of pain obtained from adults using the faces will correlate significantly with two valid and reliable measures (VAS [Visual Analogue Scale] and PPI [Present Pain Intensity scale]) of pain. A two group quasi-experimental design evaluated the hypotheses of the study. Before phlebotomy, subjects were randomly assigned to one of two groups. Subjects in the experimental group used the illusion kaleidoscope (Wildewood Creative Products, Sonora, CA) during phlebotomy . . . whereas subjects in the control group did not. . . . Data were collected on adults, 21 to 65 years old, scheduled for phlebotomy as part of a scheduled visit to a family practice clinic. . . . Subjects rated their perceptions of pain experience during phlebotomy (dependent variable) with each of three instruments: FACES, PPI, and VAS. To evaluate whether differences in the degree of pain anticipated by subjects influenced the effectiveness of the intervention, before phlebotomy subjects rated how painful they anticipated the phlebotomy would be on each of three instruments: FACES, PPI, and VAS. These measures served as covariables for purposes of analyses. After phlebotomy, subjects rated how painful phlebotomy was on the same instruments." (p. 170)

"Data were collected on 100 subjects. Data from four subjects were excluded, as successful phlebotomy required more than a single attempt. No significant differences emerged between the two groups on demographic variables (age, gender, education, and ethnicity) or on phlebotomy history (number of previous phlebotomies and most recent phlebotomy). Most subjects had blood drawn from the antecubital space (97%, $n = 93$) with a #21 needle with vacutainer (95%, $n = 91$). The average time for phlebotomy was 96 seconds (SD = 62), ranging from 22 to 442 seconds. Phlebotomy that took longer than average resulted from poor visualization of subjects' veins. Two technicians performed phlebotomy; however, there were no differences in subjects' phlebotomy experience or pain responses associated with which technician performed the phlebotomy. . . . Subjects in the control group had higher average ratings of experienced pain than did those in the experimental group." (pp. 171–172)

Mapping the Design

In quasi-experimental and experimental studies, the design can be mapped to clarify the points at which measurements are taken and treatments are provided for various groups in the study. Generally, the symbol **O** is used for an observation or a measurement. Several measurements or observations may be indicated by this symbol. The symbol **T** is used for a treatment. For example, in a study with two groups, experimental and control, who received a pretest and post-test (pretest–post-test control group design), the design could be mapped as follows.

	Pretest		Post-test
Experimental Group	**O**	**T**	**O**
Control Group	**O**		**O**

This design map could be used for a quasi-experimental or an experimental study. In the quasi-experimental study, the control group would be called the "comparison" (or "nonequivalent) group." Experimental design subjects are randomly selected and then randomly assigned to groups. If the study included several post-tests at monthly intervals, the design could be mapped as follows.

	Pretest		Post-test 1 mo.	2 mo.	3 mo.	4 mo.
Experimental Group	O_1	**T**	O_2	O_3	O_4	O_5
Control Group	O_1		O_2	O_3	O_4	O_5

Variations in the design map could be expressed for more than two groups (just add more rows), for repeated treatments (just place the **T** at each place the treatment is administered), or for multiple treatments. Multiple treatments could be labeled T_1, T_2, T_3, and so on.

Outcomes Research

Outcomes research is a relatively new approach to research design that focuses on the end results of patient care. Those promoting outcomes research demand that providers justify the selection of patient care interventions and systems of care based on evidence of improved patient lives and increased cost effectiveness. The strategies used in outcomes research are, to some degree, a departure from the accepted design strategies referred to as the "scientific method." Design methods for outcomes research have emerged from epidemiology, evaluation methods, and economic theory. Outcome studies provide rich opportunities to build a stronger scientific underpinning for nursing practice. Using the design strategies of outcomes research, nursing can document the impact of care provided by nurses. Some dimensions of nursing that lend themselves to outcome studies are the process through which nurses make decisions, nurse case management, outcomes of nurse practitioner care, and community health care. Hospitals are a major target of outcome research, and yet the patient outcomes are attributed either to the hospital as a whole or to physicians. Nursing practice in the hospital setting is invisible as a force influencing patient outcomes (Clark & Lang, 1992; Kelly, Huber, Johnson, McCloskey, & Maas, 1994).

Research designs and methodologies for outcomes studies are still emerging. The preferred methods of obtaining samples are different in outcomes studies; random sampling is not considered desirable and is seldom used. *Heterogeneous* (subjects with a wide variety of characteristics) rather than *homogeneous* (subjects with similar characteristics) samples are obtained. Rather than using sampling criteria that restrict subjects who are included in the study in order to decrease possible biases, outcome researchers seek large, heterogeneous samples that reflect as much as possible all patients who would be receiving care in the real world. Samples are expected to include, for example, patients with various comorbidities and patients with varying levels of health status. For further information on outcomes studies, see Burns and Grove (1997).

SUMMARY

A research design is a blueprint for conducting a study that maximizes control over factors that could interfere with the validity of the findings. Elements central to the study design include the presence or absence of a treatment, number of groups in the sample, number and timing of measurements to be performed, sampling method, time frame for data collection, planned comparisons, and control of extraneous variables.

Selecting a design requires an understanding of certain concepts: causality, multicausality, probability, bias, control, manipulation, and validity. In causality, there is an assumption that situations have causes and that causes lead to effects. Multicausality is the recognition that a number of interrelating variables can be involved in causing a particular effect. Probability deals with the likelihood that a specific effect will occur following a particular cause. Bias is of great concern in research because of the potential effect on the meaning of the study findings. Any component of the study that deviates or causes a deviation from the true measurement of variables leads to distorted findings. Manipulation is moving around or controlling the movement, such as manipulating the independent variable. If the freedom to manipulate a variable is under someone else's control, a bias is introduced into the study. Control means having the power to direct or manipulate factors to achieve a desired outcome. The greater the control the researcher has over the study situation, the more credible the study findings will be.

Validity is a measure of the truth or accuracy of a claim. When conducting a study, the researcher is confronted with major decisions regarding four types of validity: statistical conclusion validity, internal validity, construct validity, and external validity. Statistical conclusion validity is concerned with whether the conclusions about relationships drawn from statistical analysis are an accurate reflection of the real world. Internal validity is the extent to which the effects detected in the study are a true reflection of reality rather than a result of the effects of extraneous variables. Construct validity examines the fit between the conceptual and operational definitions of variables. External validity is concerned with the extent to which study findings can be generalized beyond the sample used in the study.

Four common types of quantitative designs are used in nursing: descriptive, correlational, quasi-experimental, and experimental.

Descriptive studies are designed to gain more information about variables within a particular field of study. Their purpose is to provide a picture of situations as they naturally happen. No manipulation of variables is involved. Descriptive designs vary in level of complexity; some contain only two variables, whereas others include multiple variables. Correlational studies examine relationships between variables. The researcher may seek to describe a relationship, predict relationships among variables, or test the relationships proposed by a theoretical proposition.

The purpose of quasi-experimental and experimental designs is to examine causality. The power of the design to accomplish this purpose is dependent on the degree to which the actual effects of the experimental treatment (the independent variable) can be detected by measurement of the dependent variable. Threats to validity are controlled through selection of subjects, manipulation of the treatment, and reliable measurement of variables. Experimental designs, with their strict control of variance, are the most powerful method of examining causality. Quasi-experimental designs were developed to provide alternative means for examining causality in situations not conducive to

experimental controls. The three essential elements of experimental research are (1) random sampling; (2) researcher-controlled manipulation of the independent variable; and (3) researcher control of the experimental situation, including a control or comparison group.

The purpose of design is to maximize the possibility of obtaining valid answers to research questions or hypotheses. In most studies, comparisons are the basis of obtaining valid answers. A good design provides the subjects, the setting, and the protocol within which these comparisons can be clearly examined. Critiquing a design involves examining the study's environment, sample, treatment, and measurement.

In critiquing the study, it is important to identify variables not included in the design (extraneous variables) that could explain some of the variance in measurement of the study variables. In a good design, the effect of these variables on variance is controlled. Outcomes research was developed to examine the end results of patient care. Those promoting outcomes research demand that providers justify the selection of patient care interventions and systems of care based on evidence of improved patient lives and increased cost effectiveness.

REFERENCES

Affonso, D. D., Lovett, S., Paul, S. M., & Sheptak, S. (1990). A standardized interview that differentiates pregnancy and postpartum symptoms from perinatal clinical depression. *Birth, 17*(3), 121–130.

Albert, M. S., Levkoff, S., Reilly, C., Liptzin, B., Pilgrin, D., Cleary, P., Evans, D., & Rowe, J. (1992). The delirium symptom interview: An interview for the detection of delirium symptoms in hospitalized patients. *Journal of Geriatric Psychiatry and Neurology, 5*, 14–21.

Als, H. (1979). Social interaction: Dynamic matrix for developing behavioral organization. In I. Uzgiris (Ed.), *New directions for child development* (pp. 21–41). San Francisco: Jossey-Bass.

Als, H. (1991). Neurobehavioral organization of the newborn: Opportunity for assessment and intervention. *NIDA Research Monographs, 114*, 106–116.

Bailey, B. J. (1996). Mediators of depression in adults with diabetes. *Clinical Nursing Research, 5*(1), 28–42.

Bayley, N. (1969). *Manual for the Bayley Scales of Infant Development*. New York: Psychological Corp.

Baynes, J. W., Bunn, J. F., Goldstein, D., Harris, M., Martin, D. B., Peterson, C., & Winterhalter, K. (1984). National Diabetes Data Group: Report of the expert committee on glucosylated hemoglobin. *Diabetes Care, 7*, 602–606.

Brown, M. A. (1986). Social support during pregnancy: A unidimensional or multidimensional construct? *Nursing Research, 35*(1), 4–9.

Burns, N., & Grove, S. K. (1997). *The practice of nursing research: Conduct, critique and utilization* (3rd ed.). Philadelphia: Saunders.

Carty, E. M., Bradley, C., & Winslow, W. (1996). Women's perceptions of fatigue during pregnancy and postpartum: The impact of length of hospital stay. *Clinical Nursing Research, 5*(1), 67–80.

Cason, C. L., & Grissom, N. L. (1997). Ameliorating adults'

acute pain during phlebotomy with a distraction intervention. *Applied Nursing Research, 10*(4), 168–173.

Cassileth, B. R., Lusk, E. J., Strouse, T. B., Miller, D. S., Brown, L. L., Cross, P. A., & Tenaglia, A. N. (1984). Psychosocial status in chronic illness: A comparative analysis of six diagnostic groups. *New England Journal of Medicine, 311*(8), 506–511.

Clark, J., & Lang, N. (1992). Nursing's next advance: An internal classification for nursing practice. *International Nursing Review, 39*(4), 109–111, 128.

Cook, T. D., & Campbell, D. T. (1979). *Quasi-experimentation: Design and analysis issues for field settings.* Chicago: Rand McNally.

Dansky, K. H., Dellasega, C., Shellenbarger, T., & Russo, P. C. (1996). After hospitalization: Home health care for elderly persons. *Clinical Nursing Research, 5*(2), 185–198.

Dellasega, C. (1988). Resource Utilization Checklist. Unpublished instrument.

Dunnihoo, D. R. (1990). *Fundamentals of gynecology and obstetrics.* Philadelphia: Lippincott.

Fetter, M. S., Fettham, S. L., D'Apolito, K., Chaze, B. A., Fink, A., Frink, B. B., Hougart, M. K., & Rushton, C. H. (1989). Randomized clinical trials: Issues for researchers. *Nursing Research, 38*(2), 117–120.

Fisher, R. A. (1935). *The design of experiments.* New York: Hafner.

Folstein, M., Folstein, S., & McHugh, P. (1978). Mini-mental state: A practical method for grading the cognitive state of patients for the clinician. *Journal of Psychiatric Research, 12*(3), 189–198.

Gardner, D. L. (1991). Fatigue in postpartum women. *Applied Nursing Research, 4*(2), 57–62.

Goldson, E. (1987). Non-nutritive sucking in the sick infant. *Journal of Perinatology, 7*(1), 30–34.

Goodwin, W. J., & Byers, P. (1993). Nutritional management of the head and neck cancer patient. *Medical Clinics of North America, 77*(3), 597–610.

Gruis, M. (1977). Beyond maternity: Postpartum concerns of mothers. *American Journal of Maternal Child Nursing, 2,* 182–283.

Harris, M. (1986). Oral-motor management of the high-risk neonate. *Physical and Occupational Therapy in Pediatrics, 6,* 231–253.

Harrison, M. J., & Hicks, J. A. (1983). Postpartum concerns of mothers and their sources of help. *Canadian Journal of Public Health, 74,* 325–328.

Kelly, K. C., Huber, D. G., Johnson, M., McCloskey, J. C., & Maas, M. (1994). The Medical Outcomes Study: A nursing perspective. *Journal of Professional Nursing, 10*(4), 209–216.

Kryger, M., Roth, T., & Dement, W. C. (1989). *Principles and practice of sleep medicine.* Philadelphia: Saunders.

Lillard, J., & McFann, C. L. (1990). A marital crisis: For better or worse…hospice involvement. *Hospice Journal—Physical, Psychosocial & Pastoral Care of the Dying, 6*(2), 95–109.

Medoff-Cooper, B., & Gennaro, S. (1996). The correlation of sucking behaviors and Bayley Scales of Infant Development at six months of age in VLBW infants. *Nursing Research, 45*(5), 291–297.

Milligan, R. A., Parks, P. L., & Lenz, E. R. (1990). An analysis of postpartum fatigue over the first 3 months of the postpartum period. In J. F. Wang, P. S. Simoni, & C. L. Nath (Eds.), *Proceedings of the West Virginia Nurses' Association research symposium* (pp. 245–251). White Sulphur Springs: West Virginia Nurses' Association Research Conference Group.

Minde, K., Whitelaw, A., Brown, J., & Fitzharding, P. (1983). Effect of neonatal complications in premature infants on early parent-infant interaction. *Developmental Medicine and Child Neurology, 25,* 763–777.

Moorcroft, W. (1989). *Sleep, dreaming, and sleep disorders: An introduction.* Lanham, MD: University Press of America.

Pearlin, L. I., Lieberman, M. A., Menaghan, E. G., & Mullan, J. T. (1981). The stress process. *Journal of Health and Social Behavior, 22*(4), 337–356.

Pugh, L. C., & Milligan, R. A. (1993). A framework for the study of childbearing fatigue. *Advanced Nursing Science, 15*(4), 60–70.

Radloff, L. S. (1977). The CES-D scale: A self-report depression scale for research in the general population. *Applied Psychological Measurement, 1,* 385–401.

Reese, J. L., Means, M. E., Hanrahan, K., Clearman, B., Colwill, M., & Dawson, C. (1996). Diarrhea associated with nasogastric feedings. *Oncology Nursing Forum, 23*(1), 59–68.

Ropka, M. E. (1996). Commentary [on Diarrhea associated with nasogastric feedings by Reese, Means, Hanrahan, Clearman, Colwill, & Dawson]. *Oncology Nursing Forum, 23*(1), 66–68.

Rosenberg, M. (1965). *Society and the adolescent self-image.* Princeton, NJ: Princeton University Press.

Russell, K. M., & Champion, V. L. (1996). Health beliefs and social influence in home safety practices of mothers with preschool children. *Image: Journal of Nursing Scholarship, 28*(1), 59–64.

Smith, M. P. (1989). Postnatal concerns of mothers: An update. *Midwifery, 5*(4), 182–188.

Spector, P. E. (1981). *Research designs.* Beverly Hills, CA: Sage.

Tolbert, S. R. (1986). *Concerns of mothers in the first month postpartum.* Unpublished master's thesis, University of British Columbia, Vancouver.

Troy, N. W., & Dalgas-Pelish, P. (1997). The natural evolution of postpartum fatigue among a group of primiparous women. *Clinical Nursing Research, 6*(2), 126–141.

Tyzenhouse, P. S. (1981). Technical notes: The nursing clinical trial. *Western Journal of Nursing Research, 3*(1), 102–109.

Waltz, C. F., & Bausell, R. B. (1981). *Nursing research: Design, statistics and computer analysis.* Philadelphia: Davis.

Willis, S. (1993). *Everyday problems test for cognitively challenged elderly.* University Park, PA: Pennsylvania State University.

Populations and Samples

Completing this chapter should enable you to:

1. *Describe sampling theory, including the following concepts: sample, population, subject, target population, elements of the population, sample criteria, sampling frame, sampling plan, accessible population, representativeness, statistics, precision, sampling error, and systematic bias.*
2. *Describe probability sampling methods.*
3. *Describe nonprobability sampling methods.*
4. *Differentiate probability from nonprobability sampling.*
5. *Examine elements that influence the decision on sample size.*
6. *Explain the purposes of power analysis.*
7. *Critique the sample section on quantitative nursing studies.*

Accessible population
Cluster sampling
Comparison group
Control group
Convenience sampling
Effect size
Elements
Generalization
Network sampling
Nonprobability sampling
Population
Power
Power analysis
Probability sampling
Purposive sampling

Quota sampling
Random sampling
Random variation
Representativeness
Sampling
Sampling criteria
Sampling frame
Sampling plan
Stratified random sampling
Systematic sampling
Systematic variation
Target population

*O*ne tends to enter the field of research with preconceived notions about samples and sampling, many of which are acquired through exposure to television advertisements, public opinion polls, market researchers in shopping centers, and newspaper reports of research findings. The television commercial boasts that four of five doctors recommend a particular product; the newscaster announces that John Jones is predicted to win the senate election by a margin of 3 to 1; the newspaper reports that scientists have now shown that treatment of early breast cancer with lumpectomy and radiation is as effective as mastectomy.

All of these examples use sampling techniques. However, some of the outcomes are more valid than others. The differences in validity are due in part to the sampling techniques used. Sampling is a key element of research methodology. Thus, in critiquing a study, you need to be able to identify the sampling method used in a published study and evaluate its adequacy. The sampling procedure is usually described in the methods section of a published paper. To judge its adequacy, you will need to understand some of the principles of sampling theory. This chapter discusses sampling theory and concepts, sampling plans, probability and nonprobability plans, and sample size.

Sampling Theory

Sampling involves selecting a group of people, events, behaviors, or other elements with which to conduct a study. A sampling plan defines the process of making the selections; the sample defines the selected group of people (or elements). Samples are expected to represent a population of people. The population might be all diabetics, all patients who have abdominal surgery, or all individuals who receive care from a nurse practitioner. However, in most cases, it would be impossible for a researcher to study an entire population. Sampling theory was developed to determine the most effective way to acquire a sample that would accurately reflect the population under study. Key concepts of sampling theory include elements, populations, sampling criteria, representativeness, sampling frames, and sampling plans. The following sections explain the meaning of these concepts. In later sections, these concepts are used to explain a variety of sampling techniques.

Elements and Populations

An individual unit of a population is called an *element.* An element can be a person, event, behavior, or any other single unit of a study. The element of the study could be the event of using iced or room-temperature injectate to measure cardiac output in a critical care unit. When elements are persons, they are referred to as "subjects." If a researcher studied the effect of preoperative teaching on length of hospital stay, the subjects of the study might be patients who were in the hospital for abdominal surgery. The sample represents a population. The *population,* sometimes referred to as the *target population,* is the entire set of individuals (or elements) who (that) met the sampling criteria (defined in the next section). Sampling criteria in the study of preoperative teaching would be patients admitted for abdominal surgery. An *accessible population* is the portion of the target population to which the researcher has reasonable access. The subjects for the study of preoperative teaching would be selected from the accessible population. The accessible population might be all patients admitted for abdominal surgery within a state, city, hospital, or nursing unit. For the preoperative teaching study, the researcher chose to limit the accessible population to a single hospital. The sample was obtained from the accessible population, and findings were generalized to the target population. *Generalization* involves extending the findings from the sample under study to the larger population. The generalization might tell you that the findings of the study can be applied to particular types of patients. With this information, you can decide whether it is appropriate for you to use these findings clinically in caring for specific patients.

Even though only subjects from a single hospital were studied, the researcher might generalize the findings to all patients admitted for abdominal surgery in the United States. In that case, the researcher is claiming that the study subjects are like all patients admitted for abdominal surgery throughout the United States. If the researcher defined the accessible population too narrowly, generalization to the broader target population might be difficult to defend. For example, if the accessible population included only white upper-middle-class individuals (common characteristics of patients in a private hospital), the researcher cannot justifiably generalize to nonwhite populations or to low-income populations (such as patients in a county hospital).

IN CRITIQUING a study, you need to identify the elements, accessible population, and target population and use your critical reasoning to evaluate the appropriateness of the generalization.

Sampling Criteria

Sampling criteria are the characteristics essential for inclusion in the target population. These criteria might include age limitations (over 18 years), ability to speak and read English at the sixth-grade level, and not having had previous surgery. The sample is selected from the accessible population that meets these sampling criteria. When the study is completed, the findings are generalized to the target population that meets these sampling criteria. The sampling criteria may be narrowly defined to make the sample as homogeneous (or similar) as possible or to control for extraneous variables. The criteria might be broadly defined to ensure a heterogeneous population with a broad range of values on the variables being studied. If the sampling criteria are narrow and restrictive, the researcher may have difficulty finding subjects who meet the criteria and may not be able to obtain a sufficiently large sample from the accessible population.

In discussing the generalization of findings in a published paper, researchers sometimes attempt to generalize beyond the sampling criteria. The researcher may contend that the sample was limited by the sampling criteria only for convenience in conducting the study but that the findings really apply to a larger population. For example, the sample may have been limited to subjects who speak and read English because the preoperative teaching would be performed in English and because one of the measurement instruments required that subjects be able to read English at the sixth-grade level. However, the researcher may believe that the findings can be generalized to non-English-speaking individuals.

IN CRITIQUING the study, you need to consider carefully the implications of using these findings with non-English-speaking populations. Perhaps these populations, because they come from another culture, might not have responded to the teaching in the same way as other populations. Perhaps the non-English-speaking groups have different knowledge about how to take care of themselves after surgery. Perhaps the knowledge provided in preoperative teaching would need to be expressed within the framework of the meanings their culture places on illness, surgery, and taking care of oneself after surgery. Thus, the preoperative teaching might have different effects on length of stay in populations of different cultures.

Generalizing to people unable to read English at the sixth-grade level might also be inappropriate. Poorly educated people would probably respond differently than other groups to the same preoperative teaching. They might not be able to read or comprehend written material given to them. They would probably be reluctant to ask questions when they did not understand. Many of them have difficulty organizing their ideas and would not be able to express them to another person. They might try to conceal their lack of understanding, making it difficult to clarify misconceptions. Thus, the preoperative teaching program developed for more educated populations is unlikely to alter the postoperative behavior or length of hospital stay of the poorly educated population.

The researcher may have limited the population to individuals who have had no previous surgery because they would have the least knowledge of the postoperative experience and how they might best care for themselves. To test differences among groups, the researcher chooses the most extreme groups so that the differences are as great as possible, and the statistical procedures are most likely to determine a difference. In this hypothetical study, one group would have no preoperative teaching (or only the small amount of teaching the hospital routinely provides). Thus, the researcher expects that their knowledge of how to take care of themselves after surgery would be limited and their length of stay longer. In the other group, the researcher could control the subjects' knowledge about how to take care of themselves after surgery by providing the information through preoperative teaching. The researcher hypothesizes that the subjects will use the knowledge to take care of themselves better after surgery and that that behavior will result in a shorter hospital stay.

However, the researcher might argue that the findings can be generalized to patients who have had previous surgery because although the effect of the preoperative teaching would be less than the effect on subjects in the study (they might already know some of the information taught), these patients would also be able to use the information to take care of themselves better after surgery and thus shorten their hospital stay. Thus, the researcher's claim that the findings can be generalized to patients who have had previous surgery may be justified.

IN CRITIQUING a study, use your critical reasoning to perform the following activities.

1. *Identify the sampling criteria.*
2. *Judge the appropriateness of the sampling criteria.*
3. *Determine if a homogeneous or heterogeneous sample was selected.*
4. *Evaluate the limitations of the study based on the sampling criteria. In interpreting the results, determine those cases in which the researcher generalized beyond the sampling criteria and evaluate the logic of that generalization.*

Beach, Smith, Luthringer, Utz, Ahrens, and Whitmire (1996) studied self-care limitations of persons after acute myocardial infarction, using Orem's model as their framework. They defined their sampling criteria as follows.

"The subjects in this study consisted of a convenience sample of 41 persons who had experienced their first AMI (acute myocardial infarction). The sample was drawn from an urban medical center and two private hospitals in northwest Ohio. Criteria for inclusion in the study were that the subject[s] [were] between the ages of 29 and 65, had experienced their first heart attack, and did not have open heart surgery during their initial hospitalization." (p. 25)

The researchers chose to include subjects from several hospital settings. This decision strengthens the study because it increases the probability of greater diversity in the sample. People cared for in an urban medical center may be different from those cared for in private hospitals. The sampling criteria seem appropriate to the study. By limiting the sample to subjects with no previous heart attacks, the researchers avoided patients who might have had previous experience with self-care after a heart attack. By restricting the sample to those who did not have open heart surgery, they avoided situations in which the self-care needs would be different. Limiting the study to subjects between the ages of 29 and 65 is curious. No rationale is given for this criterion.

The researchers did not attempt to generalize the findings of this descriptive study beyond the sample studied. Thus, they made no claim that their findings would apply to all patients experiencing their first heart attack. This is appropriate given the nature of their study. The study provides some initial insights that can be used to develop further research in this area.

Representativeness

Representativeness means that the sample, the accessible population, and the target population are alike in as many ways as possible. Representativeness needs to be evaluated in terms of the setting, characteristics of the subjects, and distribution of values on variables measured in the study. Individuals seeking care in a particular setting may be different from those who would seek care for the same problem in other settings or from those who choose to use self-care to manage their problems. The setting can influence representativeness in a variety of ways. Studies conducted in private hospitals usually exclude the poor. Other settings may exclude the elderly or the undereducated. Those who do not have access to care are usually excluded from studies. Subjects in research centers and the care they receive are different from patients and the care they receive in community hospitals, public hospitals, veterans' hospitals, or rural hospitals. People living in rural settings may respond differently to a health situation than those who live in urban settings. Obese individuals who chose to enter a program to lose weight may differ from those who did not enter such a program. Thus, gathering subjects across a variety of settings provides a sample more representative of the population than limiting the study to a single setting.

A sample needs to be representative in terms of characteristics such as age, gender, ethnicity, income, and education, which often influence study variables. It is especially important that the sample be representative in relation to the variables being examined in the study. For example, if the study examined attitudes toward AIDS, the sample should be representative of the distribution of attitudes toward AIDS that exists in the specified population. If a study involved blood pressures of patients in a surgical recovery room, one would expect the blood pressures of subjects to be representative of those usually noted in a surgical recovery unit.

Measurement values should also be representative. Measurement values in a study are expected to vary randomly among subjects. *Random variation* is the expected difference in values that occurs when different subjects from the same sample are examined. The difference is random because some values will be higher and others lower than the average (mean) population values. As sample size increases, random variation decreases, improving representativeness.

Systematic variation, or systematic bias—a serious concern in sampling—is a consequence of selecting subjects whose measurement values differ in some specific way from those of the population. This difference is usually expressed as a difference in the average (or mean) values between the sample and the population. Because the subjects have something in common, their values tend to be similar to those of others in the sample but different in some way from those of the population as a whole. These values do not vary randomly around the population mean. Most of the variation from the mean is in the same direction; it is systematic. For example, the sample mean may be higher than the mean of the target population. Increasing the sample size has no effect on systematic variation.

If all the subjects in a study examining some type of knowledge have an intelligence quotient (IQ) above 120, their scores will likely all be higher than the mean of a population that includes individuals with a wide variation in IQ. The IQs of the subjects have introduced a systematic bias. When a systematic bias occurs in an experimental study, it can lead the researcher to think that the treatment has made a difference, when in actuality the values would have been different even without the treatment.

The probability of systematic variation increases when the sampling process is not random. However, even in a random sample, systematic variation can occur as a consequence of potential subjects' declining participation. The greater the number who decline, the greater the possibility of a systematic bias. Unfortunately, researchers seldom report this number in the published study. Systematic variation may also occur in studies in which a number of subjects withdraw from the study before data collection is completed (sample mortality) or in which subjects withdraw from one group but not the other. In studies involving a treatment, subjects in the control group who will not receive the treatment may be more likely to withdraw from the study. Sample mortality should be reported in the published study.

IN CRITIQUING a published study, critically evaluate the representativeness of the sample. You might follow these guidelines.

1. *Compare the demographic characteristics of the sample with those of the target population. The researcher may provide information about the target population in the literature review. Otherwise, in making your judgment, you are limited to what you know about the target population.*
2. *Compare mean sample values of study variables with values of the target population determined from previous research.*
3. *Determine sample mortality. Does the author provide information on characteristics of subjects who left the study and why the subjects left? If the author does not directly report this information, you may be able to judge by comparing the number of subjects originally included in the study with the number used in reporting statistical results.*
4. *Evaluate the possibilities of systematic bias in the sample in terms of the setting, characteristics of the sample, and ranges of values on measured variables. Determine the number and characteristics of persons who declined to participate in the study. As the number of subjects who decline to participate increases, the probability of systematic bias increases. Subjects who decline may be different in important ways from those who agree to participate.*

Example Critique of Representativeness

Pellino (1997) conducted a study of the relationships between patient attitudes, subjective norms, perceived control, and analgesic use following elective orthopedic surgery. She described her sampling method and sample mortality as follows.

"Adults scheduled for elective orthopedic surgery were recruited from the outpatient practices of 32 orthopedic surgeons in two cities in the Midwest. Patients were excluded if they had a known history of drug or alcohol abuse. Two hundred and forty patients were approached and 172 patients agreed to participate (a 70% recruitment rate). Reasons for not participating included time constraints, the questionnaire was too long, and being overwhelmed by the prospect of having surgery. Complete data were available for 137 subjects who returned the postoperative questionnaire and had no missing data on critical variable(s). Subjects who used over two standard deviations more than the mean of the group for medication intake were dropped ($n = 2$).

The 69 women and 68 men who completed the study had an average age of 51.9 (SD = 16.1) years (range = 18–87 years). Subjects reported completing an average of 13.3 (SD = 2.6) years of education (range 6–23 years) and a middle economic status [M = 2.87; range = 1 (lower) to 5 (upper)]. A variety of orthopedic disorders (such as degenerative joint disease, scoliosis, and trauma) and procedures (such as total joint replacements, spinal fusions, and ligament reconstructions) were represented in the sample. The majority of patients ($n = 103$) had PCA [patient-controlled analgesia] ordered; intramuscular (IM), oral, or epidural analgesia was ordered as the primary pain medication for 34 patients." (p. 99)

In this study, the sampling criteria identified subjects as adults scheduled for elective orthopedic surgery. Exclusion criteria included a known history of drug or alcohol abuse. Given the focus of the study on analgesic use, this exclusion seems appropriate since persons with a history of drug or alcohol abuse could be expected to be different from others in their analgesic use, increasing the risk of bias in the sample. Selecting patients with a variety of diagnoses and procedures provides a heterogeneous sample that can be generalized to a larger population. Accessing subjects from the outpatient practices of 32 orthopedic surgeons decreases the bias that could occur from recruiting patients at a single surgical facility. However, this sampling strategy excludes patients financially unable to access this type of outpatient practice. Thus, the results cannot be generalized to low-income patients without further study. No ethnic description of subjects is provided. Since the literature provides evidence of cultural differences in attitudes, expression, and managment of pain, this seems a serious omission. Because of the lack of information provided about the sample, it is not possible to determine whether or not the findings can be generalized to various ethnic groups.

Random Sampling

From a sampling theory point of view, each individual in the population should have an opportunity to be selected for the sample. One method of providing this opportunity is referred to as *random sampling*. The purpose of random sampling is to increase the extent to which the sample is representative of the target population. However, random sampling must take place in an accessible population that is representative of the target population. It is rarely possible to obtain a purely random sample for clinical nursing studies because of informed consent requirements. Those who volunteer to participate in a study may differ in important ways from those not willing to participate. (Methods of achieving random samples are described later in the chapter.) The use of the term *control group* is limited to those studies using random sampling methods. If nonrandom methods are used for sample selection, the group not receiving a treatment is referred to as a *comparison group* because there is an increased possibility of preexisting differences in the experimental and comparison groups.

Sampling Frames

In order for each person in the accessible population to have an opportunity for selection in the sample, each person in the population must be identified. To accomplish this, a list of every member of the population must be acquired, using the sampling criteria to define membership. This list is referred to as the *sampling frame*. Subjects are then selected from the sampling frame using a sampling plan.

Sampling Plans

A *sampling plan* outlines strategies used to obtain a sample for a study. Like a design, a sampling plan is not specific to a study. The plan is designed to increase representativeness and decrease systematic bias. The sampling plan may use probability (random) or nonprobability (nonrandom) sampling methods.

IN CRITIQUING a study, you need to identify and describe the sampling plan the researcher used. Use your critical reasoning to answer the following questions

   1. *Did the researcher successfully implement the sampling plan?*
   2. *How effective was the sampling plan in achieving representativeness?*

continued

3. *In what ways is the sample not representative?*
4. *Were there possibilities for biases in the sample?*
5. *Were subjects selected from a sampling frame?*
6. *Was random sampling used?*
7. *Were control groups or comparison groups used in the study?*

Probability Sampling Methods

Probability sampling methods have been developed to increase the representativeness of the sample. In *probability sampling,* every member (element) of the population has a probability higher than zero of being selected for the sample. To achieve this probability, the sample is obtained randomly. All the subsets of the population, which may differ from each other but contribute to the parameters of the population, have a chance to be represented in the sample. There is less opportunity for systematic bias when subjects are selected randomly, although it is possible for a systematic bias to occur by chance. Without random sampling strategies, the researchers, who have a vested interest in the study, could tend (consciously or unconsciously) to select subjects whose conditions or behaviors are consistent with the study hypotheses. The researchers could decide that person X would be a better subject for the study than person Y. In addition, the researchers could exclude a subset of people from being selected as subjects because they do not agree with them, do not like them, or find them hard to deal with. Potential subjects could be excluded because they are too sick, not sick enough, coping too well, not coping adequately, uncooperative, or noncompliant. By using random sampling, the researcher leaves the selection to chance and thus increases the validity of the study. Four sampling designs have been developed to achieve probability sampling: simple random sampling, stratified random sampling, cluster sampling, and systematic sampling.

Simple Random Sampling

Simple random sampling is the most basic of the probability sampling plans. To achieve simple random sampling, elements are selected at random from the sampling frame. This can be accomplished in a variety of ways, limited only by the imagination of the researcher. If the sampling frame is small, names can be written on slips of paper, placed in a container, mixed well, and then drawn out one at a time until the desired sample size has been reached. The most common method of random selection is to use a table of random numbers. A section from a random numbers table is presented in Table 8-1. To use a table of random numbers, the researcher places a pencil or finger on the table with the eyes closed. That number is the starting place. Then, moving the pencil or finger up, down, right, or left, numbers are used in order until the desired

TABLE 8-1. Section from a Random Numbers Table									
06	84	10	22	56	72	25	70	69	43
07	63	10	34	66	39	54	02	33	85
03	19	63	93	72	52	13	30	44	40
77	32	69	58	25	15	55	38	19	62
20	01	94	54	66	88	43	91	34	28

sample size is obtained. If the pencil were initially placed on 58 in Table 8-1, which is the fourth column from the left and the fourth row down; if 5 subjects were to be selected from a population of 100; and if a decision were made to go across the columns to the right, the subject numbers would be 58, 25, 15, 55, and 38. This particular table is useful only when the population number is less than 100. However, tables and computer programs are available for selecting larger populations.

VandenBosch, Montoye, Satwicz, Durkee-Leonard, and Boylan-Lewis (1996) used a simple random sample in their study of nurse perception in identifying pressure ulcer risk. They describe their sample selection as follows.

> "The study took place in a 550-bed tertiary care community teaching hospital. Subjects were drawn from general care, intensive care, and a 40-bed inpatient rehabilitation unit. Hospitalized inpatients over 18 years of age with intact skin and no reddened areas over any bony prominence were asked to participate. Using a random numbers table and the daily list of admissions, subjects with an expected length of stay of at least 1 week were selected. Subjects were selected three times a week and were approached for informed consent within 48 hours of admission to the hospital." (p. 81)

It is not clear from the description provided how many subjects per day were selected. Was it a proportion of the daily list of admissions or a set number per day? Might this number have varied, depending on the number of data collectors available that day? Nonetheless, the method is effective in providing a random sample of subjects to address the purpose of the study.

Stratified Random Sampling

Stratified random sampling is used in situations in which the researcher knows some of the variables in the population that are critical to achieving representativeness. Variables commonly used for stratification include age, gender, ethnicity, socioeconomic status, diagnosis, geographic region, type of institution, type of care, and site of care. Stratification ensures that all levels of the identified variables will be adequately represented in the sample. With stratification, the researcher can use a smaller sample size and achieve the same degree of representativeness in relation to the stratified variable as a large sample acquired through simple random sampling. One disadvantage is that a large population must be available from which to select subjects.

If the researcher used stratification, categories (strata) of the variables selected for stratification would be defined in the published report. For example, using ethnicity for stratification, the researcher might have defined four strata: Caucasian, African American, Mexican American, and other. The population might have been 60% Caucasian, 20% African American, 15% Mexican American, and 5% other. The researcher might have selected a random sample for each stratum equivalent to the target population proportions of that stratum. Alternatively, equal numbers of subjects might have been randomly selected for each stratum. For example, if age was used to stratify a sample of 100 subjects, the researcher might have obtained 25 subjects under age 20, 25 subjects aged 20 to 39, 25 subjects aged 40 to 59, and 25 subjects over age 60.

O'Brien, Dalton, Konsler, and Carlson (1996) used stratified random sampling in their study, "The knowledge and attitudes of experienced oncology nurses regarding the management of cancer-related pain." The following text describes their sampling procedure.

"A sample of 1,400 RNs, stratified by educational levels and Area Health Education Center (AHEC) regions in which they work, were selected randomly to participate in the survey. The North Carolina Board of Nursing supplied the nurses' names; the selection process drew an equal number of nurses from each educational background (associate degree, diploma, baccalaureate, graduate) in each of the nine AHEC regions of the state." (p. 517)

Cluster Sampling

In *cluster sampling,* a sampling frame is developed that includes a list of all the states, cities, institutions, or organizations with which elements of the identified population would be linked. A randomized sample of these states, cities, institutions, or organizations would then be used in the study. In some cases, this randomized selection continues through several stages and is then referred to as "multistage sampling." For example, the researcher might first randomly select states, then randomly select cities within the sampled states. Then hospitals within the randomly selected cities might be randomly selected. Within the hospitals, nursing units might be randomly selected. At this level, all the patients on the nursing unit who fit the criteria for the study might be included or patients could be randomly selected.

Cluster sampling is used in two situations. The first is one in which the researcher considers it necessary to obtain a geographically dispersed sample but realizes that a simple random sample would be prohibitive in terms of travel time and cost. The second situation is one in which the individual elements making up the population are not known, thus preventing the development of a sampling frame. For example, there is no list of all open-heart surgery patients in the United States. In such a case, it is often possible to obtain lists of institutions or organizations with which the elements of interest are associated and randomly select institutions from which subjects will be acquired.

Golding (1996) used multistage probability sampling in her study, "Sexual assault history and limitations in physical functioning in two general population samples." The following text describes her sampling technique.

"Respondents were selected using multistage area probability sampling from household residents 18 years of age and older at each site. The Los Angeles sample was selected to represent adults in two mental health catchment areas in Los Angeles County, one of which was 83% Latino and the other 21% Latino. The Latino residents were largely of Mexican cultural or ethnic origin. . . . The North Carolina sample was selected to represent adults in two mental health catchment areas in North Carolina, one consisting of Durham County, which is primarily urban, and the other four contiguous rural counties." (p. 34)

The author used pooled data obtained from two sites of a five-site, National Institute of Mental Health (NIMH)-initiated program. Information provided about the sampling method is sparse. The researcher does not provide a rationale for the use of multistage sampling or reasons for choosing the selected sites. Although the author indicates that this is a probability sample, she does not indicate how the sites or subjects were randomly chosen. There is some indication that the original study may have intentionally chosen one Hispanic area, but no mention is made of a similar effort to include other minority groups. There also appeared to be an effort to include both urban and rural sites. There is insufficient information to judge the adequacy of the sampling plan.

Systematic Sampling

Systematic sampling can be conducted when an ordered list of all members of the population is available. The process involves selecting every *k*th individual on the list, using a starting point selected randomly. If the initial starting point is not random, the sample is not a probability sample. To use this design, the researcher must know the number of elements in the population and the size of the sample desired. The population size is divided by the desired sample size, giving *k*, the size of the gap between elements selected from the list. For example, if the population size was $N = 1,242$ and the desired sample size was $n = 50$, then $k = 24$. Every 24th person on the list would be included in the sample. This value is obtained by dividing 1,242 by 50. Some argue that this procedure does not truly give each element an opportunity to be included in the sample; it provides a random but not equal chance for inclusion.

Gross, Rocissano, and Roncoli (1989) used systematic sampling in their study, "Maternal confidence during toddlerhood: Comparing preterm and fullterm groups." They described their sampling procedure as follows.

"The fullterm population consisted of 4,000 mothers of toddlers born at a large northeastern metropolitan hospital between 1984 and 1986, who were fullterms delivered vaginally or by cesarian section, and products of single births with no known congenital anomalies. Systematic random sampling of hospital chart codes was used to identify a target population of 146 mothers to contact for participation. The preterm population consisted of 116 mothers of preterm infants born at the same hospital during the same time period, who had birthweights less than 2500 grams, were less than 36 weeks gestation at birth and who were products of a single birth with no known congenital anomalies." (p. 3)

All members of the preterm population were used in this study. The researchers wished to obtain an equivalent number of full-term mothers from a much larger population. Systematic sampling was effectively used to obtain that sample.

Nonprobability Sampling Methods

In *nonprobability sampling*, not every element of the population has an opportunity for selection in the sample. Although this approach increases the possibility of samples that are not representative, it has been commonly used in nursing studies. In an analysis of nursing studies published in six nursing journals from 1977 to 1986, only 9% used random sampling (Moody, Wilson, Smyth, Schwartz, Tittle, & Van Cott, 1988). Most of the studies examined were descriptive or correlational. Only 30% of the nursing studies reported during this period tested hypotheses (quasi-experimental or experimental). Thus, when you read published research, you will find few studies that have used random sampling methods. You must be able to discriminate among the various types of nonprobability sampling designs used in nursing studies. Each type addresses a different research need. The four nonprobability designs discussed here are convenience sampling, quota sampling, purposive sampling, and network sampling.

Convenience Sampling

Convenience sampling (also called "accidental sampling") is considered a poor approach because it provides little opportunity to control for biases; subjects are included in the study merely because they happened to be in the right place at the right time. A classroom of students, patients who attend a clinic on a specific day, subjects who attend a support group, patients currently admitted to a hospital with a specific diagnosis or nursing problem, and every fifth person who enters the emergency room are examples of types of frequently selected convenience samples. Available subjects are simply entered into the study until the desired sample size is reached. Multiple biases may exist in the sample, some of which may be subtle and unrecognized. However, serious biases are not always present in convenience samples.

Convenience samples are inexpensive, are accessible, and usually require less time to acquire than other types of samples. They provide means to conduct studies on topics that cannot be examined with probability sampling. However, this type of sampling should be used only when it is impossible to obtain a sample by other means.

Most quasi-experimental studies and clinical trials in both medicine and nursing use convenience sampling. As a component of the study design, subjects are randomly assigned to groups. This random assignment, which is not a sampling method, does not alter the high risk of biases resulting from convenience sampling. With these potential biases and the narrowly defined sampling criteria used to select subjects in most clinical trials, representativeness of the sample is a serious concern.

IN CRITIQUING a study using a convenience sample, you need to judge whether the researcher could have used other sampling methods to improve study validity given the circumstances of the study. From the description of the sample, identify biases and judge representativeness. If convenience sampling was used, the researcher should have identified and described known biases in the sample in the published report. Steps taken to increase the representativeness of the sample should also be explained.

Brandt, DePalma, Irwin, Shogan, and Lucke (1996) used convenience sampling in their study, "Comparison of central venous catheter [CVC] dressings in bone marrow transplant recipients." The following is a description of their sample selection.

"Researchers conducted the study on a seven-bed, high-efficiency particulate air-filtered BMT (bone marrow transplant) unit of a regional efficiency particulate air-filtered BMT unit of a regional oncology center. Following review and approval by the Institutional Review Board and the Nursing Research Committee, subjects ran-

continued

domly were assigned to one of the following CVC-dressing protocols: the standard care protocol with dry, sterile gauze dressing
(DSGD) changed every 24 hours or the experimental care protocol
with Opsite 3000 moisture vapor permeable dressing (MVPD)
changed weekly. Based on a cost comparison of the two dressing
protocols, researchers projected that the Opsite 3000 dressing
changed weekly would result in a weekly cost savings of $20 per
patient. This does not include the savings in nursing time required
to change the dressing weekly instead of daily. All other aspects of
CVC-related procedures occurred according to standard unit routine. The convenience sample consisted of 101 hospitalized, autolo-
gous BMT recipients with newly inserted long-term, silastic, triple-
lumen, tunneled Hickman® (Davol Inc., Cranston, RI) catheters.

Study participants had to be at least 18-years-old, alert, oriented,
and able to give written and verbal informed consent. They had to
have had a CVC inserted following hospital admission for autolo-
gous BMT. Subjects were excluded from the study if they had a preexisting bacteremia or fungemia within 14 days of study entry or if
the CVC placement was intended to be short-term. Patients received
the assigned CVC-care procedure until one of the following occurred: development of definitive catheter-related sepsis and subsequent CVC removal, removal of the CVC for any other reason (e.g.,
tunnel infection, mechanical or management complications), or
hospital discharge. At these end points, patients were considered
to have completed the study and were included in data analysis.
Exit-site infection or suspected CVC-related sepsis were considered
intervening variables; patients with these conditions were continued
on [the] study until one of the previously described off-study criteria
occurred." (p. 830)

"A total of 108 subjects were invited between January 1990 and April
1994 to participate in the study. Three patients chose not to participate because of a preference for gauze dressings or a history of skin
sensitivity to tape or transparent dressings. Four patients (two DSGD,
two MVPD) with histories of pre-BMT skin sensitivity (e.g., secondary
to drug rash, radiation skin reaction, abrasion) required an alternative dressing early after accrual and were taken off [the] study. The
final sample size was 101 subjects." (pp. 831–832)

This type of study is often referred to as a "randomized clinical trial"
and is often defined as experimental. In critiquing the sample, it is
important to examine the description of the sample and other information
provided about the subjects that might provide evidence of bias. In some
studies such as this, insufficient information is provided to judge the
presence of bias.

Quota Sampling

Quota sampling uses a convenience sampling technique with an added feature—a strategy to ensure the inclusion of subject types who are likely to be underrepresented in the convenience sample, such as females, minority groups, the aged, the poor, the rich, and the undereducated. The goal of quota sampling is to replicate the proportions of subgroups present in the population. The technique is similar to that used in stratified random sampling. Quota sampling requires that the researcher be able to identify subgroups in the target population important to achieving representativeness in the area being studied. In addition, the researcher must determine what proportion of the target population each identified subgroup represented. Quota sampling offers an improvement over convenience sampling and tends to decrease potential biases.

IN CRITIQUING a study using a quota sampling method, you need to use critical thinking to judge the adequacy of the subgroups selected in improving the representativeness of the sample. You might ask the following questions.

1. Were the subgroups selected appropriate for the study topic?
2. Were the proportions assigned to each subgroup reflective of the target population?

Topp, Estes, Dayhoff, and Suhrheinrich (1997) used quota sampling in their study, "Postural control and strength and mood among older adults." They described their sample selection as follows.

"Twenty-seven rural-dwelling older adults (22 women and 5 men; mean age 73.8 ± 6.4 years, range 64 to 87 years) were recruited for the present study as they completed a 4-month exercise clinical trial. Twelve subjects had completed 4 months of balance training, nine had completed the strength training, and six had attended a no-exercise control condition. Before participating in interventions subjects had undergone a history and physical to ensure they had no contraindications to participating in moderate intensity exercise. After completion of the 4-month interventions each subject was assessed for knee strength, ankle strength, and postural control. Subjects also completed a questionnaire that assessed their precursors to attention. The use of subjects who had completed different types of intervention programs was intended to assure variability in measures of strength and postural control among the sample." (pp. 12–13)

Purposive Sampling

Purposive sampling, sometimes referred to as "judgmental or theoretical sampling," involves the conscious selection by the researcher of certain subjects or elements to include in the study. Efforts might be made to include typical subjects or situations. Examples of good and poor care or good and bad patients might be used. The strategy has been criticized because there is no way to evaluate the precision of the researcher's judgment. How does one determine that the patient or element was typical, good, bad, effective, or ineffective? However, this sampling method may be a way to get some beginning ideas about an area not easily examined with other sampling techniques.

IN CRITIQUING a study using a purposive sampling method, identify the characteristics for which subjects were purposively selected. Use critical reasoning to answer the following questions.

1. What rationale did the researcher(s) give for selecting those characteristics?
2. Does the rationale seem logical to you?
3. Does (do) the researcher(s) provide information on how subjects were determined to have the characteristics selected?

Dildy (1996) used purposive sampling in a study of "Suffering in people with rheumatoid arthritis." Her description of sample selection is as follows.

> Purposive or theoretical sampling, a procedure involving selection of persons who represent the desired perspective, was used. Fourteen people (nine women and five men), diagnosed with rheumatoid arthritis and followed in local rheumatologists' offices, were selected for the study. The informants ranged in age from 39 to 76 years old (M = 59.5). All of the informants were White, seven informants were married, three were widowed, three were divorced, and one had never married. The amount of formal education completed ranged from 8 to 18 years. Two male and three female informants were still employed on a full-time basis. Individuals whose disease was in remission, as well as those in an active phase, were purposefully included to gain a broader perspective. The length of illness from time of diagnosis ranged from 6 months to 35 years (M = 16.75). (pp. 177–178)

Although the researcher indicated the use of purposive sampling as the method of obtaining the study sample, no information was given regarding the purpose for selecting particular subjects or what perspective was desired.

Network Sampling

Network sampling, sometimes referred to as "snowballing," holds promise for locating samples difficult or impossible to obtain in other ways. Network sampling takes advantage of social networks and the fact that friends tend to have characteristics in common. When the researcher has found a few subjects with the necessary criteria, he or she asks their assistance in getting in touch with others with similar characteristics. This strategy is particularly useful for finding subjects in socially devalued populations such as alcoholics, child abusers, sex offenders, drug addicts, and criminals. These individuals are seldom willing to make themselves known. Other groups, such as widows, grieving siblings, or those successful at lifestyle changes, can be located using this strategy. These individuals are outside the existing health care system and are difficult to find. Biases are built into this sampling process because the subjects are not independent of each other.

IN CRITIQUING a study using a network sampling method, you might follow these guidelines.

1. Identify the chain of networks used to obtain the sample.

2. Evaluate the possibility of biases in the study findings based on the sampling procedure.

3. Identify other sampling procedures the researcher could have used to obtain a similar sample.

Armstrong (1991) used network sampling to obtain subjects for her study, "Career-oriented women with tattoos." She describes her sampling procedure as follows.

> "Subjects were contacted after word-of-mouth inquiry at exercise clubs, physical examination centers, doctors' offices and nursing organizations in the state. . . . Next, participants were sought from a wide geographic region by placing advertisements in alternative newspapers in nine cities: Washington, DC, Philadelphia, New Orleans, Atlanta, Chicago, Portland, Madison, WI, San Francisco and San Diego. Respondents ($N = 155$) voluntarily phoned or wrote to the investigator (47 percent), or were referred by other respondents (38 percent). Others were sought by word-of-mouth (24 percent)." (p. 217)

In this study, at least 62% of the sample was obtained with network sampling. No obvious biases are present in the sample. This sampling method would tend to exclude individuals who were reticent about their tattoo (such as concealing it from others). These individuals could not be referred by others, who would probably not know about their tattoo. This portion of the population of tattooed professional women would not be represented in this sample.

Sample Size

One of the most troublesome questions that arise during the critique of a study is whether the sample size was adequate. If the study was designed to make comparisons and significance was found, the sample size was adequate. Questions about the adequacy of the sample size occur only when no significance was found. Thus, in critiquing a study in which no significance was found in at least one of the hypotheses or research questions, you need to evaluate the adequacy of the sample size. The question is, is there in fact no difference or relationship, or is there really a difference or relationship that was not found because of inadequacies in the research methods?

Currently, the adequacy of the sample size is evaluated using a *power analysis*. *Power* is the capacity of the study to detect differences or relationships that actually exist in the population. Expressed another way, it is the capacity to correctly reject a null hypothesis. The minimum acceptable level of power for a study is .80 (Cohen, 1988). This power level results in a 20% chance of a Type II error, in which the study fails to detect existing effects (differences or relationships).

The researcher should perform a power analysis to evaluate the adequacy of the sample size for all nonsignificant findings. The results of this analysis should be reported in the published study. Nurse researchers have only recently begun using power analysis to evaluate sample size. Polit and Sherman (1990) evaluated the sample size of 62 studies published in 1989 in *Nursing Research* and *Research in Nursing & Health.* They found that most of the studies examined had inadequate sample sizes for making comparisons between groups. The studies needed an average of 218 subjects per group to have a power level of .80. Therefore, in most of these studies, the risk of a Type II error was extremely high. In only one of the studies was a power analysis performed to determine the adequacy of the sample size.

Other factors that influence the adequacy of sample size (because they affect power) include effect size, type of study, number of variables, sensitivity of the measurement tools, and data analysis techniques. In critiquing the adequacy of the sample size, you need to consider the influence of all of these factors.

Effect Size

The effect is the presence of the phenomenon examined in a study. *Effect size* is the extent to which the null hypothesis is false. In a study in which two populations are compared, the null hypothesis states that the difference between the two populations is zero. However, if the null hypothesis were false, there would be an effect. If the null hypothesis is false, it is false to some degree; this is the effect size (Cohen, 1988). The statistical test tells you that there is a difference between groups. The effect size tells you how much difference there is between groups.

When the effect size is large (e.g., considerable difference between groups), detecting it is easy and requires only a small sample; when the effect size is small (e.g., only a small difference between groups), detecting it is more difficult and requires larger samples. Broadly, a small effect size would be about .2, a medium effect size .5, and a large effect size .8 (Cohen, 1988). Effect size is smaller with a small sample, and thus effects are more difficult to detect. Increasing the sample size also increases the effect size, making it more likely that the effect will be detected.

In the nursing studies examined by Polit and Sherman (1990), 52.7% of the effect sizes computed were small. These researchers found that in nursing studies, for small effects, average power was under .30. Thus, there was less than a 30% probability that acceptance of the null hypothesis was correct. In most cases, this was due to an insufficient sample size. Even when the effect size was moderate, the average power in the nursing studies examined was only .70. Only when the effect size was large did nursing studies reach an acceptable level of power, and 11% of these studies were underpowered. Only 15% of the studies had sufficient power for all of their analyses.

Type of Study

Case studies tend to have very small samples. Comparisons between groups are not performed, and problems related to sampling error and generalization have little relevance for these studies. A small sample size may be more useful in examining the situation in depth from various perspectives. Descriptive studies (particularly those using survey questionnaires) and correlational studies often require very large samples. In these studies, multiple variables may be examined, and extraneous variables are likely to affect subject response(s) to the variables under study. Statistical comparisons are often made on multiple subgroups in the sample, requiring that an adequate sample be available for each subgroup being analyzed. Quasi-experimental and experimental studies use smaller samples more often than do descriptive and correlational studies. As control in the study increases, the sample size can decrease and still approximate the population. Instruments in these studies tend to be more refined, thus increasing precision. Designs that use blocking or stratification usually increase the total sample size required. Designs that use matched pairs of subjects have increased power and thus require a smaller sample (Winer, 1962).

Number of Variables

As the number of variables under study increases, the sample size needed may increase. Including variables such as age, gender, ethnicity, and education in the data analyses can increase the sample size needed to detect differences between groups. Using them only to describe the sample does not cause a problem in terms of power. A number of the studies analyzed by Polit and Sherman (1990) had sufficient sample size for the primary analyses but failed to plan for analyses involving subgroups, such as analyzing the data by age category or ethnic group. The inclusion of multiple dependent variables also increases the sample size needed.

Measurement Sensitivity

Well-developed instruments measure phenomena with precision. A thermometer, for example, measures body temperature precisely. Tools measuring psychosocial variables tend to be less precise. However, a tool with strong reliability and validity tends to measure more precisely than a tool that is less well developed. Variance tends to be higher in a less well-developed tool than in one that is well developed. For example, if anxiety were being measured and the actual anxiety score of several subjects was 80, measures ranging from 70 to 90 might be obtained with a less well-developed tool. There is much more variation from the true score than from the use of a well-developed tool, which would tend to show a score closer to the actual score of 80 for each subject. As variance in instrument scores increases, the sample size needed to obtain significance increases. Measurement sensitivity is discussed further in Chapter 9.

Data Analysis Techniques

Data analysis techniques vary in their ability to detect differences in the data. Statisticians refer to this as the "power of the statistical analysis." There is also an interaction between the measurement sensitivity and the power of the data analysis technique. The power of the analysis technique increases as precision in measurement increases. Larger samples are needed when the power of the planned statistical analysis is weak.

For some statistical procedures, such as the *t*-test and ANOVA, equal group sizes will increase power because the effect size is maximized. The more unbalanced the group sizes, the smaller the effect size. Therefore, in unbalanced groups, the total sample size must be larger (Kraemer & Theimann, 1987). Chi-square is the weakest of the statistical tests and requires very large sample sizes to achieve acceptable levels of power. As the number of categories increases, the sample size increases. Also, if there are small numbers in some of the categories, the sample size must be increased.

Critiquing the Adequacy of the Sample

IN CRITIQUING the sample, use critical reasoning to perform the following activities.

1. Describe the sample.
2. List the sampling criteria.

3. *Identify the sample size; list the sample sizes for each group.*
4. *Indicate whether any power analyses were reported.*
5. *Discuss the characteristics of the sample.*
6. *Determine sample mortality.*
7. *Describe the method used to obtain the sample.*
8. *Evaluate the representativeness of the sample.*
9. *Explore the possibility of Type II error.*
10. *Identify potential biases in the sample.*
11. *If groups were used, determine whether the groups are equivalent.*
12. *Determine whether the researcher(s) defined the target population to which the findings are generalized.*

SUMMARY

Sampling involves selecting a group of people, events, behaviors, or other elements with which to conduct a study. Sampling defines the process of making the selections; sample defines the selected group of elements. Sampling theory was developed to determine the most effective way of acquiring a sample that would accurately reflect the population under study. Important concepts in sampling theory include population, elements of the population, sampling criteria, representativeness, randomization, sampling frame, and sampling plan.

A sampling plan is developed to increase representativeness, decrease systematic bias, and decrease sampling error. The two main types of sampling plans are probability and nonprobability. Probability sampling plans have been developed to ensure some degree of precision in estimating the population values. Thus, probability samples reduce sampling error. To obtain a probability sample, the researcher must know every element in the population. A sampling frame must be developed and the sample randomly selected from the sampling frame. Five sampling designs have been developed to achieve probability sampling: simple random sampling, stratified random sampling, cluster sampling, systematic sampling, and random assignment.

In nonprobability sampling, not every element of the population has an opportunity for selection in the sample. There is no sampling frame. There are several types of nonprobability sampling designs, each addressing a different research need. The four nonprobability designs discussed in this chapter are convenience sampling, quota sampling, purposive sampling, and network sampling.

A major concern in critiquing the sampling procedure is evaluating the adequacy of the sample size. Factors that must be considered in making decisions about sample size include the type of study, number of variables, sensitivity of the measurement tools, data analysis techniques, and expected effect size.

REFERENCES

Armstrong, M. L. (1991). Career-oriented women with tattoos. *Image: Journal of Nursing Scholarship, 23*(4), 215–220.

Beach, E. K., Smith, A., Luthringer, L., Utz, S. K., Ahrens, S., & Whitmire, V. (1996). Self-care limitations of persons after acute myocardial infarction. *Applied Nursing Research, 9*(1), 24–28.

Brandt, B., DePalma, J., Irwin, M., Shogan, J., & Lucke, J. F. (1996). Comparison of central venous catheter dressings in bone marrow transplant recipients. *Oncology Nursing Forum, 23*(5), 829–836.

Cohen, J. (1988). *Statistical power analysis for the behavioral sciences* (2nd ed.). New York: Academic Press.

Dildy, S. P. (1996). Suffering in people with rheumatoid arthritis. *Applied Nursing Research, 9*(4), 177–183.

Golding, J. M. (1996). Sexual assault history and limitations in physical functioning in two general population samples. *Research in Nursing & Health, 19*(1), 33–44.

Gross, D., Rocissano, L., & Roncoli, M. (1989). Maternal confidence during toddlerhood: Comparing preterm and fullterm groups. *Research in Nursing & Health, 12*(1), 1–9.

Kraemer, H. C., & Theimann, S. (1987). *How many subjects? Statistical power analysis in research.* Newbury Park, CA: Sage.

Moody, L. E., Wilson, M. E., Smyth, K., Schwartz, R., Tittle, M., & Van Cott, M. L. (1988). Analysis of a decade of nursing practice research: 1977–1986. *Nursing Research, 37*(6), 374–379.

O'Brien, S., Dalton, J. A., Konsler, G., & Carlson, J. (1996). The knowledge and attitudes of experienced oncology nurses regarding the management of cancer-related pain. *Oncology Nursing Forum, 23*(3), 515–521.

Pellino, T. A. (1987). Relationships between patient attitudes, subjective norms, perceived control, and analgesic use following elective orthopedic surgery. *Research in Nursing & Health, 20*(2), 97–105.

Polit, D. F., & Sherman, R. E. (1990). Statistical power in nursing research. *Nursing Research, 39*(6), 365–369.

Topp, R., Estes, P. K., Dayhoff, N., & Suhrheinrich, J. (1997). Postural control and strength and mood among older adults. *Applied Nursing Research, 19*(1), 11–18.

VandenBosch, T., Montoye, C., Satwicz, M., Durkee-Leonard, K., & Boylan-Lewis, B. (1996). Predictive validity of the Braden Scale and nurse perception in identifying pressure ulcer risk. *Applied Nursing Research, 9*(2), 80–86.

Winer, B. J. (1962). *Statistical principles in experimental design.* New York: McGraw-Hill.

Measurement and Data Collection in Research

Completing this chapter should enable you to:

1. Discuss measurement theory and the relevant concepts (directness of measurement, measurement error, levels of measurement, reliability, and validity).
2. Examine the types of measurement error.
3. Compare and contrast the four levels of measurement (nominal, ordinal, interval, and ratio) and provide an example of each.
4. Describe the three aspects of reliability (stability, equivalence, and homogeneity) and specify how the reliability of a measurement technique is determined.
5. Discuss the types of measurement validity and specify how the validity of a measurement technique is determined.
6. Describe the reliability and validity of physiologic measures.
7. Examine the common measurement approaches used in nursing research: physiologic measures, observations, interviews, questionnaires, and scales.
8. Examine the methods section of a written report.
9. Critique the measurement section in a research article.
10. Critique the data collection section in a research article.

Data collection	Random error
Direct measure	Rating scale
Equivalence	Ratio-scale measurement
Homogeneity	Reliability
Indirect measure	Scale
Interrater reliability	Semantic differential scale
Interval-scale measurement	Serendipity
Interview	Split-half reliability
Levels of measurement	Stability
Likert scale	Structured interview
Measurement error	Systematic error
Nominal-scale measurement	Test-retest reliability
Observational measurement	True score
Ordinal-scale measurement	Unstructured interview
Physiologic measurement	Validity
Questionnaire	Visual analogue scale

*T*he purpose of measurement is to produce trustworthy data that can be used in statistical analyses. In critiquing a published study, you must judge the trustworthiness of the measurement methods used in the study. To produce trustworthy measures, rules have been established to ensure that values or categories will be assigned consistently from one subject (or event) to another and, eventually, if the measurement strategy is found to be meaningful, from one study to another. The rules of measurement established for research are similar to those used in nursing practice. For example, when pouring a liquid medication, the rule is that the measuring container must be placed at eye level. This ensures accuracy and consistency in the dose of medication. When measuring abdominal girth to detect changes in ascites, the skin on the abdomen is marked to be sure that the measure is always taken the same distance below the umbilicus. Using this method, any change in measurement can be attributed to a change in ascites rather than to an inadvertent change in the measurement site. Understanding the logic of measurement is important for critiquing the adequacy of measurement methods in a nursing study. This chapter includes a discussion of some of the concepts of measurement theory, measurement strategies in nursing, and the process of data collection.

Concepts of Measurement Theory

Measurement theory guides the development and use of measurement methods. The following section discusses some of the basic concepts of measurement theory, including directness of measurement, measurement error, levels of measurement, reliability, and validity.

Directness of Measurement

To measure, the researcher must first clarify the object, characteristic, or element to be measured. In some cases, identification of the measurement object and measurement strategies is quite simple and straightforward, as when the researcher measures concrete factors such as a person's height or wrist circumference. These are referred to as *direct measures.* Direct measures of concrete elements such as height, weight, temperature, time, space, movement, heart rate, and respiration are commonly used in nursing. Technology is available to measure many bodily functions and biological and chemical characteristics. The focus of measurement in these instances is on the precision of measurement. Nurses are also experienced in gathering direct measures of attribute or demographic variables such as age, gender, ethnic origin, diagnosis, marital status, income, and education.

However, in many cases in nursing research, the characteristic the researcher needs to measure is an abstract idea such as stress, caring, coping, anxiety, compliance, or pain. When abstract concepts are measured, *indirect measures,* indicators or attributes of the concept, are used to represent the abstraction. For example, indicators of coping might be the frequency or accuracy of problem identification, the speed or effectiveness of problem resolution, level of optimism, and self-actualization behaviors. Rarely, if ever, can a single measurement strategy completely measure all the aspects of an abstract concept.

IN CRITIQUING a study, you need to determine what variables were measured and what methods were used to measure each variable. Determine whether the measure is direct or indirect.

Measurement Error

The ideal, perfect measure is referred to as the "true measure." However, error is inherent in any measurement strategy. *Measurement error* is the difference between the *true* score and what in reality is measured. The amount of difference varies from one measurement to the next. Thus, there may be considerable error in one measurement and very little in the next. Measurement error exists in both direct and indirect measures and can be random or systematic. With direct measures, one can actually see the object being measured and the measurement that is taken. Direct measures, which are generally expected to be highly accurate, are subject to error. For example, the weight scale may not be accurate, the precisely calibrated thermometer may decrease in precision with use, or the tape measure may not be held at exactly the same tightness. With indirect measures, one can see neither the thing being measured nor the measure that is taken. For example, in measuring hope, one can physically see neither hope nor the measurement scale that gives us numerical values from mathematical calculations. There is an even greater chance of error in using indirect measures. Efforts to measure concepts such as hope usually result in measuring only part of the concept. Sometimes measures may identify an aspect of the concept but may also include other elements that are not part of the concept. For example, an instrument designed to measure anxiety might also measure aspects of fear.

Two types of error are of concern in measurement: random error and systematic error. The difference between random and systematic error is the direction of the error. In *random error*, the difference between the actual value obtained through measurement and the ideal true value is without pattern or direction (random). In one measure, the actual value may be lower than the true value, whereas in the next measure, the actual value may be higher than the true value. A number of situations can occur during the measurement process that can result in random error. For example, there may be variations in the administration of the measurement procedure; subjects completing a paper-and-pencil scale may accidentally mark the wrong column; or the wrong key may be punched while data are being entered into the computer. Our purpose in measuring is to estimate the true value, usually by combining a number of values and calculating an average. Thus, an average such as the mean is an estimate of the true value. As random errors increase, that estimation is less precise. We know this because there is much variation in the measurement values from the average we have calculated, and the variation is scattered in a number of directions.

Measurement error that is not random is referred to as systematic error. In *systematic error*, the variation in measurement values from the calculated average is primarily in the same direction. For example, most of the variation may be higher or lower than the average we calculated. Systematic error occurs because something else is being measured in addition to the concept. A weight scale that weighed subjects at 2 pounds more than their true weights would result in systematic error. All of the weights would be high and, as a result, the mean would be higher than it should be. Some systematic error occurs in almost any measure. Because of its importance in a study, researchers spend considerable time and effort refining their measurement instruments in order to minimize systematic error.

IN CRITIQUING a published study, you will not be able to judge the extent of measurement error directly. However, you may find clues to the amount of error in the published report. For example, if the researcher has described the method of measurement in great detail, providing evidence of accuracy and consistency of measurement, the probability of error will be reduced. If weight scales are recalibrated periodically during data collection, error will be reduced. Measurement will be more precise if the researcher has used a well-developed paper-and-pencil scale than if a newly developed scale was used, and less measurement error will occur.

Accuracy of measurement is of concern clinically and in the conduct of research. Craft and Moss (1996) discuss error in the assessment of infant emesis volume.

> "Liquid amounts are particularly difficult to verify because of the instability of the configuration from event to event. When visualized, the variety in edges, colors, and direction of the liquid in each occurrence makes a template for comparison difficult.
>
> Liquid volumes in the form of emesis are often estimated in nurseries and pediatric units at hospitals. The smaller the patient, the more crucial is accurate fluid output assessment. Infants demand the accurate estimation of fluid loss, and measures to increase accuracy in visual processing are needed. The emesis of infants is particularly difficult to estimate because the infant cannot verbalize the presence of nausea, which would help nurses anticipate vomiting. Therefore, nurses are often unable to preweight bibs, spit cloths, or bed linen, or to catch the fluid in a container for objective measurement." (p. 3)

continued

"The non-experimental study was conducted using 109 subjects who had a large range of experience in assessing infant emesis volume. Practicing pediatric nurses were invited to participate in the study by displaying posters on pediatric and neonatal areas in a large university hospital. Nursing students from the university also were invited to participate.

Because the purpose of this study was to determine the accuracy of assessing infant emesis volume, a realistic situation was provided, using displays of actual formula volumes on receiving blankets that were all folded to one eighth of their original size. Subjects were asked to write down the correct volume perceived and to state whether they had picked up the blanket to evaluate the weight of the display.

Twenty receiving blankets were used as displays. The amounts of formula to be poured on the blankets was randomly selected by writing amounts on slips of paper . . . the subjects were read the following scenario: 'You have just fed Timmy 50 ML of formula before he vomits. You are to determine how much he has vomited.' Subjects began at display 1 and walked to display 20, writing down their volume estimations.

Absolute accuracy was defined as subject choosing the exact number of milliliters corresponding to what was measured and poured on the display. . . . The investigators were concerned about the small number of displays that were assessed accurately. This small number necessitated a change from analyzing accuracy to analyzing relative error. Relative error was determined by the range of milliliter chosen on either side of the exact amount. . . . The findings showed that novice subjects, or students, overestimated an average of 1% of the correct volume, whereas more experienced subjects underestimated an average of 16% of the volume. Subjects who stated they were unsure of what method they used underestimated an average of 60%, and subjects who said they used 'experience' as a method underestimated an average of 50% of the correct volume.

Thus, the amount of error in judging amounts of emesis is high, and is problematic both clinically and in nursing studies. Experience alone does not increase accuracy although teaching a method for estimating volume is related to accuracy in judgments about volume." (p. 4)

Levels of Measurement

The traditional *levels of measurement* were developed by Stevens in 1946. Stevens organized the rules for assigning numbers to objects so that a hierarchy in measurement was established. The levels of measurement from low to high are nominal, ordinal, interval, and ratio.

Nominal-Scale Measurement

Nominal-scale measurement is the lowest of the four measurement categories. It is used when data can be organized into categories of a defined property, but the categories cannot be compared. For example, you might categorize people by diagnosis. However, you cannot say that the category kidney stone is higher than the category peptic ulcer or that ovarian cyst is closer to kidney stone than to peptic ulcer. The categories differ in quality but not quantity. Therefore, one cannot say that subject A possesses more of the property being categorized than does subject B. (Rule: The categories must be unorderable.) Categories must be established in such a way that a datum will fit into only one of the categories. (Rule: The categories must be exclusive.) All the data must fit into the established categories. (Rule: The categories must be exhaustive.) Data such as gender, ethnicity, marital status, and diagnoses are examples of nominal data.

Ordinal-Scale Measurement

With *ordinal-scale measurement,* data that can be measured at the ordinal level can be assigned to categories that can be ranked. To rank data, one category is judged to be (or is ranked) higher or lower, better or worse, than another category. Rules govern how one ranks data. As with nominal data, the categories must be exclusive and exhaustive. With ordinal data, the quantity can also be identified. For example, if you were measuring intensity of pain, you could identify differing levels of pain. You would develop categories that ranked these differing levels of pain, such as excruciating, severe, moderate, mild, and no pain. However, using these categories, as in all ordinal measures, there is no certainty that the intervals between the ranked categories are equal. A greater difference might exist between mild and moderate pain than between intense and severe pain. Therefore, ordinal data are considered to have unequal intervals.

Many scales used in nursing research are ordinal levels of measurement. For example, one could rank degrees of coping, levels of mobility, ability to provide self-care, or daily amount of exercise on an ordinal scale. Using daily exercise, the scale could be 0 = no exercise, 1 = moderate exercise with no sweating, 2 = exercise to the point of sweating, 3 = strenuous exercise with sweating for at least 30 minutes a day, and 4 = strenuous exercise with sweating for at least 1 hour per day. The measurement is ordinal because we cannot claim that equal distances exist between the rankings we have developed. There may be a greater difference between our ranking of 1 and our ranking of 2 than there is between our ranking of 2 and our ranking of 3.

Interval-Scale Measurement

Interval-scale measurement uses interval scales, which have equal numerical distances between intervals of the scale. These scales follow the rules of mutually exclusive categories, exhaustive categories, and rank ordering and are assumed to be a continuum of values. Thus, the magnitude of the attribute can be much more precisely defined. However, it is not possible to provide the absolute amount of the attribute because of the absence of a zero point on the interval scale. Temperature is the most commonly used example of an interval scale. A difference between a temperature of 70° and one of 80° is the same as the difference between a temperature of 30° and one of 40°. Changes in temperature can be precisely measured. However, it is not possible to say that a temperature of 0° means the absence of temperature.

Ratio-Scale Measurement

Ratio-scale measurement is the highest form of measurement and meets all the rules of other forms of measurement: mutually exclusive categories, exhaustive categories, rank ordering, equal spacing between intervals, and a continuum of values. In addition, ratio-level measures have absolute zero points. Weight, length, and volume are commonly used examples of ratio scales. All three have absolute zero points at which a value of zero indicates the absence of the property being measured; zero weight means the absence of weight. In addition, because of the absolute zero point, one can justifiably say that object A weighs twice as much as object B or that container A holds three times as much as container B.

IN CRITIQUING a published study, you need to determine the level of each measurement used in the study. In some studies, the researcher will indicate the level of measurement used. In others, you will need to determine the level of measurement from the description of the measurement method used.

Johnson (1996), in a study of "Social support and physical health in the rural elderly," described her approach to measuring health status as follows.

"Perceived health status of the subjects was determined by asking them to choose one statement indicating their current state of physical health. Choices ranged from 1, indicating that 'I think my present health is very good' to 5, indicating 'I think my present health is very poor.' The use of a single question asking subjects to rate their own health is the most frequently used method to determine the assessment of one's health. Subjectively rated health status correlates highly with physicians' evaluations of health (Weinberger, Hiner, & Tierney, 1987)." (p. 63)

This measure has the characteristics of an ordinal scale.

Reliability

Reliability is concerned with how consistently the measurement technique measures the concept of interest. For example, if one were using a scale to obtain the weight of subjects, one would expect the scale to indicate the same weight if the subject stepped on and off the scale several times. A scale that did not show the same weight each time would be unreliable.

Reliability testing is considered a measure of the amount of random error in the measurement technique. It is concerned with such characteristics as dependability, consistency, accuracy, and comparability. Because all measurement techniques contain some random error, reliability exists in degrees and is usually expressed as a form of correlation coefficient, with 1.00 indicating perfect reliability and .00 indicating no reliability. A reliability of .80 is considered the lowest acceptable coefficient for a well-developed measurement tool. For a newly developed instrument, a reliability of .70 is considered acceptable (Burns & Grove, 1997). Estimates of reliability are specific to the sample being tested. Thus, high reported reliability values on an established instrument do not guarantee that reliability will be satisfactory in another sample or with a different population. Therefore, reliability testing needs to be performed on each instrument used in a study before other statistical analyses are performed. These values should be included in published reports of the study. Reliability testing focuses on three aspects of reliability: stability, equivalence, and homogeneity.

Stability

Stability is concerned with the consistency of repeated measures. This is usually referred to as *test-retest reliability*. This measure of reliability is generally used with physical measures, technological measures, and paper-and-pencil scales. Use of the technique requires an assumption that the factor to be measured remains the same at the two testing times and that any change in the value or score is a consequence of random error. A high correlation coefficient between the test and the retest indicates high reliability.

In Redeker, Mason, Wykpisz, and Glica's (1996) study of sleep patterns in women after coronary artery bypass surgery, a method was needed to measure sleep. The Mini-Motionlogger (Ambulatory Monitoring, Inc., Ardsley, NY) was used for this purpose. The authors describe how this instrument measures sleep as follows:

"This battery-operated actigraph is an electronic accelerometer that senses motion in three dimensions with a ceramic bimorph beam that generates a charge when subjected to the force of acceleration and deceleration; it counts the number of movements over a prepro-

continued

grammed period of time (epoch) and stores the data. Depending on the epoch length, the Mini-Motionlogger can collect data for several weeks without a battery change." (p. 116)

Test-retest reliability was reported on the Mini-Motionlogger as follows: "Reliability of the actigraph is supported by reproducing virtually identical measurements of the repeated swing of a pendulum in the laboratory" (p. 117).

Equivalence

Equivalence focuses on comparing measurements made by two or more observers measuring the same event and is referred to as *interrater reliability*. Interrater reliability values need to be reported in any study in which observational data are collected or judgments are made by two or more data gatherers. Two or more raters independently observe and record the same event using the data collection procedure developed for the study, or the same rater observes and records an event on two occasions. Every data collector used in the study needs to be tested for interrater reliability. There is no absolute value below which interrater reliability is unacceptable. However, any value below .80 should generate serious concern about the reliability of the data. A value of .90 is more desirable. The numerical reliability value needs to be reported in published studies.

Johnson and Miller (1996), in a study examining various methods of measuring healing in leg ulcers, reported interrater and intrarater reliability of the measures tested. The measures and findings related to reliability were described in the published study as follows.

"Stereophotogrammetry is a technique that obtains measurements of an object from [its] photographic images (Avery, 1977). . . . Planimetry is the measurement of surface area. A freehand tracing of the outline of the ulcer is digitized, and the surface area of the ulcer is calculated with the aid of a computer . . . the Kundin Wound Gauge (Pacific Technologies & Development Corp, San Mateo, CA) consists of four cross-arms and a vertical arm that can be placed over and into the wound. Four reference points are assessed and provide the radii for the calculation of surface area. The vertical insert allows for volume calculation. . . . The Johnson (1984) criterion-referenced scale assesses wound characteristics. The criteria used were exudate, necrosis, and granulation, with each ranging in score from 0 (none) to 3 (heavy). Both exudate and necrosis are negative values and are subtracted from the wound score. Totaling the three criteria provides the wound characteristic score. . . . A semantic differential scale named the Healing Scale was designed by the authors to assess the perception of the nurse over 7 days as to how well the ulcer was healing. The key adjectives were derived from previous subjective methods using a similar scale with intervals ranging from 1 (rapidly deteriorating) to 7 (rapidly healing)." (pp. 205–206)

"Subjective methods performed poorly in this study. The perception of healing (Healing Scale) and changes in wound characteristics (Johnson Scale) did not correlate to objective measures of healing (sterophotogrammetry measurement of rate of healing). Interrater reliability was not shown in these scales, but intrarater reliability was supported. If scales are to be used clinically, they should show interrater reliability because the likelihood of the same nurse rating the patient is minimal in many clinical settings. Planimetry showed satisfactory intrarater and interrater reliability and concurrent validity." (p. 207)

Homogeneity

Tests of instrument *homogeneity* are used primarily with paper-and-pencil tests and address the correlation of various items within the instrument. The original approach to determining homogeneity was *split-half reliability*. This strategy was a way of assessing test-retest reliability without administering the test twice. Instead, the instrument items were split in half, and a correlational procedure was performed between the two halves. The Spearman-Brown correlation formula has generally been used for this procedure (Burns & Grove, 1997).

More recently, testing the homogeneity of all the items in the instrument has been considered a better approach to determining reliability. This procedure examines the extent to which all items in the instrument consistently measure the construct. It is a test of internal consistency. The statistical procedure used for this process is Cronbach's alpha coefficient. If the coefficient value is 1.00, each item in the instrument is consistently measuring the same thing. When this occurs, one might question the need for more than one item. A slightly lower coefficient (.8 to .9) indicates an instrument that will reflect more richly the fine discriminations in levels of the construct.

In a study examining positioning to minimize fatigue in breastfeeding women, Milligan, Flenniken, and Pugh (1996) used a fatigue scale tested for reliability using Cronbach's alpha.

"Fatigue symptoms were measured using the Modified Fatigue Symptoms Checklist (MFSC), a list of 30 symptoms of fatigue, with established reliability and validity (Milligan, Parks, & Lenz, 1990).

continued

In past work using this instrument with 259 postpartum women, Milligan, Parks, and Lenz (1990) reported the internal consistency (Kuder-Richardson formula) to be .85 at 6 weeks postpartum. . . . The MFSC measures fatigue as a subjectively experienced phenomenon involving discomfort and decreased efficiency during the first 3 months postpartum. The instrument is scored by totaling the number of symptoms the postpartum subject has checked. Scores range from zero (no fatigue symptoms) to 30 symptoms (maximum fatigue)." (p. 69)

IN CRITIQUING a study, you need to determine the method used to evaluate reliability and identify the reliability value obtained. Using this information, you need to judge the adequacy of reliability for each measurement method used in the study. In some studies, the author does not report the reliability. In others, the author states that the reliability has been reported to be acceptable in previous studies. If no reliability values are provided for these previous studies, you have little information on which to judge previous reliability and none on which to judge reliability in the study being reported. This does not mean that the reliability is poor; it simply means that you do not have sufficient information on which to base a judgment of the adequacy of measurement reliability in the study.

Validity

The *validity* (sometimes referred to as "construct validity") of an instrument is a determination of the extent to which the instrument actually reflects the abstract construct (or concept) being examined (Berk, 1990; Rew, Stuppy, & Becker, 1988). Validity, like reliability, is not an all-or-nothing phenomenon but rather a matter of degree. No instrument is completely valid. Thus, one determines the degree of validity of a measure rather than whether validity exists. Validity will vary from one sample to another and from one situation to another; therefore, validity testing actually validates the use of an instrument for a specific group or purpose rather than being directed to the instrument itself. An instrument may be very valid in one situation but not valid in another.

Several sources that provide evidence of validity are described below: content, contrasting groups, convergence, divergence, discriminant analysis, prediction of future events, predicting concurrent events, and successive verification of validity (information obtained from repeated use of the same method of measurement).

Content-Related Validity. This is the extent to which the method of measurement includes all the major elements relevant to the concept being measured. In reporting content-related validity, the researcher may cite sources from the literature, seek feedback from individuals who might be subjects in a study using the measurement, or seek feedback from individuals who are considered experts in measuring the concept. These experts may complete a form referred to as the Content Validity Index (CVI), which evaluates the validity of the method of measurement. In this case, the researcher will report a numerical value indicating the level of content-related validity.

Evidence of Validity from Constrasting Groups or Known Groups. This evidence can be obtained by identifying groups who are expected to have contrasting scores on the instrument. The researcher selects samples from at least two such groups. For example, the researcher might measure hope in newly married individuals and in hospitalized suicidal individuals. If the groups' responses are significantly different in the expected directions, the researcher reports it as evidence of the validity of the instrument.

Evidence of Validity from Examining Convergence. This evidence is obtained by comparing the instrument with other instruments that measure the same concept. This type of comparison is particularly important for newly developed instruments. To evaluate convergent validity, the researcher administers all of the selected instruments concurrently to a sample of subjects. Then statistical analyses are performed to determine how closely related the scores are. The statistical result would be a value (r) ranging from 0 to $+1$. If the convergent measures are closely related, the validity of each instrument is strengthened.

Evidence of Validity from Examining Divergence. This evidence can be obtained if the researcher can locate instruments that measure a concept opposite to the concept measured by the newly developed instrument. For example, if the newly developed instrument was a measure of hope, the researcher would search for an instrument that measured hopelessness. The researcher would then administer the two instruments to a single sample of subjects. Statistical analyses (usually correlation) would be performed to determine the extent to which measures from the two instruments were opposite each other (negatively correlated). The statistical result would be a correlational value (r) ranging from -1 to 0. If the divergent measure was negatively correlated with other measures, validity for each of the instruments would be strengthened.

Evidence of Validity from Discriminant Analysis. This evidence can be obtained if instruments have been developed to measure concepts closely related to the concept measured by the newly developed instrument. For example, two instruments might measure the closely related concepts of coping and adaptation. The researcher would administer the two instruments to a single sample and then perform statistical analyses to test the extent to which both instruments can discriminate finely between these concepts.

Evidence of Validity from Prediction of Future Events. This evidence can be obtained by testing the ability of the instrument to predict future performance or attitudes based on instrument scores. For example, nurse researchers might determine the ability of a scale that measures health-related behaviors to predict the future health status of individuals.

Evidence of Validity from Predicting Concurrent Events. This evidence can be tested by examining the ability to predict the current value of one measure based on the value obtained on the measure of another concept. For example, one might be able to predict the self-esteem score of an individual who had a high score on an instrument that measured coping.

Successive Verification of Validity. This verification is obtained through repeated use of the instrument. Each time a researcher uses the instrument, more knowledge is gained about its validity. When a researcher uses the instrument, information on validity is reported from previous studies. In addition, researchers may report further information on validity obtained in their study. Thus, with each successive study, the validity of the instrument is further verified.

IN CRITIQUING a study, you need to judge the validity of the measures that were used. However, you cannot consider validity apart from reliability. If a measurement method does not have acceptable reliability, its validity becomes a moot issue. Unfortunately, not all published studies include information on the validity and reliability of instruments. Selby-Harrington, Mehta, Jutsum, Riportella-Muller, and Quade (1994) found that 47% of a random sample of 55 nursing studies published in 1989 had no evidence of validity for any data collection instruments, 36% had no evidence of reliability, and 29% had no evidence of either validity or reliability. Content validity was addressed in only 27% of the studies.

IN CRITIQUING the validity of an instrument used in a published study, you might follow these guidelines.

1. *Check for information on reliability.*
2. *Look for reports of the validity of the instrument in previous studies. Unfortunately, in some cases, the researcher will simply state that previous research has found validity of the measurement method to be acceptable. This statement does not provide the information you need to judge validity. Thus, in critiquing validity in this case, you would simply state that you had insufficient information on which to judge validity other than the author's statement that the validity was acceptable.*
3. *Look for reports of pilot studies performed by the researcher to examine the validity of the instrument.*
4. *Examine the discussion of findings near the end of the report. The researcher may have used data from the present study to examine instrument validity.*

Wineman, Schwetz, Goodkin, and Rudick (1996) report reliability and validity information on an instrument used to measure hope in their study, "Relationships among illness uncertainty, stress, coping and emotional well-being at entry into a clinical drug trial."

> "Hopefulness was defined as . . . anticipation for a continued good state, an improved state, or a release from a perceived entrapment (Miller & Powers, 1988, p. 6). It was measured using the Miller Hope Scale, which is composed of 48 items measured using a five-point Likert-type format. Summary scores were obtained by adding [the] subject's responses on this scale. The higher the score, the more hopeful the subject felt. The estimate of internal consistency in the present study was .96. A published report of reliability and validity is based on a 40-item version. Estimates of internal consistency (Cronbach's alpha = .93) and test-retest reliability (r = .812) were adequate; discriminant and convergent validity were supported (Miller & Powers, 1988)." (pp. 55–56)

Reliability and Validity of Physiologic Measures

Reliability and validity of physiologic and biochemical measures tend not to be reported in published studies. The assumption, not always correct, is made that routine physiologic measures are valid and reliable. The most common physiologic measures used in nursing studies are blood pressure, heart rate, weight, and temperature. These measures are often obtained from the patient's record, with no consideration of their accuracy. Researchers using physiologic measures need to provide evidence of the validity of their measures; Gift and Soeken (1988) identify five terms that are critical to evaluation of physiologic measures: accuracy, selectivity, precision, sensitivity, and error.

Accuracy. Accuracy is comparable to validity in that evidence of content-related validity addresses the extent to which the instrument measured the concept defined in the study. Thus, it is an evaluation of the adequacy of the operational definition. For example, arterial blood gases may be a more accurate measure of oxygen saturation than is pulse oxymetry.

Selectivity. "Selectivity, an element of accuracy, is the ability to identify correctly the signal under study and to distinguish it from other signals" (Gift & Soeken, 1988, p. 129). For example, electrocardiographic readings allow one to distinguish electrical signals coming from the myocardium from similar signals coming from skeletal muscles. Content validity of biochemical measures can be determined by contacting experts in the laboratory procedure and asking them to judge the appropriateness of the measure for the concept being measured.

Precision. Precision is the degree of consistency or reproducibility of measurements using physiologic instruments. Precision is comparable to reliability. The reliability of most physiologic instruments is determined by the manufacturer and is part of quality control testing. Recalibration of mechanical equipment is used in many physiologic studies to maintain precision. Because of fluctuations in most physiologic measures, test-retest reliability is inappropriate.

Sensitivity. "Sensitivity of physiologic measures is related to the amount of change of a parameter that can be measured precisely" (Gift & Soeken, 1988, p. 130). If changes are expected to be very small, the instrument must be highly sensitive in order to detect the changes. For example, a bathroom scale is not sufficiently sensitive to detect very small changes in weight. The stability of the instrument is also related to sensitivity. Stability may be judged in terms of the ability of the system to resume a steady state after a disturbance in input. For example, in a weight scale, does the scale return to zero quickly after a weight is removed (return to a steady state) or does an unsteady state affect the measurement of the next item placed on it? For electrical systems, this is referred to as "freedom from drift" (Gift & Soeken, 1988).

Error. Error has a number of sources in physiologic measures. Environmental factors such as temperature, barometric pressure, and static electricity can alter measures. Variations in operation of equipment can occur as a result of different users, changes in supplies, and/or changes in procedures. Machine error may be related to calibration or to the stability of the machine. Signals transmitted from the machine can result in misinterpretation (Gift & Soeken, 1988).

Biological variability in biochemical measures can occur because of factors such as age, gender, body size, diurnal rhythms, and seasonal cycles. Patient intake of food and/or drugs, exercise, and emotional stress can also cause variations. Materials, equipment, procedures, and personnel used to perform measures can cause errors. Errors can also occur in the recording of measurement values.

IN CRITIQUING a study, you need to judge the adequacy of accuracy, selectivity, precision, and sensitivity of any physiologic measures used in the study. Keep in mind, however, that initial attempts to measure a physiologic element important to nursing practice are likely to be less valid than those that have been refined in several studies. Much work is needed to clarify specific elements of physiologic assessment in nursing practice; the use of these in research requires even more rigor.

Medoff-Cooper and Gennaro (1996) used the Kron Nutritive Sucking Apparatus in a study correlating sucking behaviors and development in infants. They described the instrument as follows.

"The hardware of the Kron Nutritive Sucking Apparatus continuously measures negative pressure generated by the infant during sucking. The sucking apparatus incorporates a calibrated capillary tube for metering flow of nutrient into an ordinary nipple by embedding it in silicone rubber. A second tube embedded in the silicone measures the intraoral pressure and is connected to a Cobe pressure transducer. The volume per suck (consumption) is proportional to the pressure-time integral, or area under the pressure-time curve of the suck. Flow is calibrated such that a sustained 100 mmHg pressure yields a constant flow of 10 ml/min. All materials are nontoxic and easily sterilized. The pressure signal was fed online to an IBM-compatible computer, which displays the pattern of sucks throughout the session and creates a sucking record for off-line analysis. Customized software generates a range of session summary parameters, including number of sucks, number of bursts, sucks per burst, interburst width (time between bursts), suck width (length of time for an individual suck), intersuck interval, and mean maximum sucking pressures, intersuck width (time between sucks), and mean maximum pressure. In addition, the burst/pause organization and changes in sucking patterns over time within the session were characterized. The session was divided into five parts (epochs), with a mean duration equal to 58 seconds. An array of sucking parameters was generated for each quintile, including number of sucks per epoch (on average, 58 seconds), number of bursts, mean duration of sucking within a burst, percentage of time bursting, and suck frequency within burst." (p. 293)

A CRITIQUE of Medcoff-Cooper and Gennaro's study follows.

Accuracy. *Accuracy, the extent to which the instrument measures sucking, appears to be high. The measure provides detailed information on an array of sucking parameters.*
Selectivity. *The instrument is highly selective in distinguishing measures of sucking from other signals.*
Precision. *The authors report that flow is calibrated such that a sustained 100 mmHg pressure yields a constant flow of 10 ml/min. Thus, it would be feasible to test that calibration. However, no information is provided on testing the precision of that calibration.*
Sensitivity. *The description of the instrument gives the impression of a very sensitive instrument. However, specific information on the amount of change that can be measured is not provided.*

Measurement Strategies in Nursing

Nursing studies examine a wide variety of phenomena and thus require the availability of an extensive array of measurement tools. Many nursing phenomena have not been examined because no one has thought of a way to measure them. This has implications for clinical practice as well as for research. This section describes some of the most common measurement approaches used in nursing research, including physiologic measurement, observational measurement, interviews, questionnaires, and scales.

Physiologic Measurement

Physiologic nursing research has lagged behind studies of psychosocial dimensions of nursing practice because of measurement problems. Some of the first physiologic nursing studies examined basic care activities such as mouth care; decubitus care; the effect of preoperative teaching on postoperative recovery; and infection control related to urinary bladder catheterization, intravenous therapy, and tracheotomy care. Even at this fairly simple level, developing valid ways to measure the variables of interest was difficult and required considerable time and expense. For example, how does one measure changes in a decubitus ulcer? What criteria can be used to determine the effectiveness of a mouth-care regimen? Creativity and attention to detail are needed to develop effective *physiologic measurement* strategies.

Increased need for means to measure the outcomes of nursing care has also generated more nursing studies that include physiologic measures. The outcome of interest may be the outcome of all nursing care received for a particular care episode or the outcome of a particular nursing intervention. An important focus of physiologic measurement is finding means to quantify changes that occur as a consequence of nursing practice. This upsurge of interest in outcome measures has broadened the base of physiologic research beyond nurse physiologists to include nurse clinicians. The number of nursing studies including physiologic measures has increased dramatically in recent years. The detailed description of physiologic measures in a research report should include the exact procedure followed and specific descriptions of equipment used in measurement, as can be seen from some of the following examples.

There are a variety of approaches to obtaining physiologic measures. Some are relatively easy and are an extension of the measurement methods used in nursing practice, such as obtaining weight and blood pressure. Others are not difficult but require imaginative approaches to measuring phenomena that are traditionally observed in clinical practice but not measured. Some physiologic measures are obtained using self-report or paper-and-pencil scales.

Jarrett, Cain, Heitkemper, and Levy (1996) used self-report to obtain information on stool frequency and stool consistency for their study. "Subjects were asked to record the number and consistency of each stool on a scale . . . that included pictorial and written descriptions of stool consistency, e.g., none (0), hard (1), dry to watery (9) (Heitkemper & Jarrett, 1992)" (p. 47).

Data on physiologic parameters are sometimes obtained using observational data collection methods.

Algase, Kupferschmid, Beel-Bates, and Beattie (1997) measured wandering behavior of cognitively impaired elders using observational methods. Their description of the observational method follows.

"Ambulation cycles were measured using time-study techniques. Observers recorded time of onset and cessation for each ambulation episode on the Datamyte 1010 (Allen-Bradley, Minnetonka, MN). The Datamyte 1010 is a portable terminal with programmable clock, solid-state memory, and storage capacity to 64K characters in computer-readable format. Each locomoting phase was also coded for impetus (self- or other-directed starts) and pattern (direct, lapping, pacing, or random).

Data were downloaded directly to a microprocessor for analysis. Cycle period was computed as the time elapsed from the onset of one ambulation episode to the onset of the next. Locomoting phase duration was the time elapsed from the onset of an episode of locomotion to its cessation; nonlocomoting phase was the time elapsed from the cessation of an episode of locomotion to the onset of the next episode. Percent-of-cycle-locomoting was the locomoting phase divided by the cycle period ($\times$ 100). All ambulation episodes were observed, but only those coded as self-initiated were analyzed. Of those, lapping, pacing, and random patterns were considered wandering, while the direct pattern was not." (p. 174)

Measurement of physiologic variables can be either direct or indirect. Direct measures are more valid. Norman, Gadaleta, and Griffin (1991) used both direct and indirect measures of blood pressure in their study. The measurement of arterial pressure waveforms through an arterial catheter provides a direct measure of blood pressure, whereas use of a stethoscope and sphygmomanometer provides an indirect measure.

Kotzer (1990) describes a creative method of indirectly measuring physiologic parameters of the preverbal infant.

"Heart rate, respirations and mobility are monitored through passive-motion sensors embedded in a mattress that fits into the infant's bassinet. The data are fed directly into a computer where the physiologic record is analyzed and categorized into quiet sleep, active sleep, transitions, indeterminant, awake, and crying." (p. 50)

Sometimes, physiologic measures are obtained from laboratory or x-ray results. If so, the same detailed description of the process of obtaining the values to be included in the study is expected.

Carson (1996) used a lipid profile measure in her study of the impact of relaxation on the lipid profile. She describes the process of conducting a lipid profile as follows.

"Blood samples were obtained for total cholesterol, HDL, LDL, and triglycerides after a 14-hour fast.... Lipid specimens were processed through the local medical center laboratory. This laboratory reports an intra-laboratory coefficient of variation (CV) of 1.3% (personal communication, F. Lembo, November 1995) as determined through participation in the VA-CDC [Veterans Administration–Centers for Disease Control] national Cholesterol Standardization and Certification Program. Laboratory procedures for testing precision and bias meet the general recommendations of the NCEP [National Cholesterol Education Program] Laboratory Standardization Panel (Laboratory Standardization Panel, 1990). Total cholesterol, HDL, and triglycerides were measured directly. Reagents and methodology conformed to descriptions by Catechem Inc. (Bridgeport, CT). High-density lipoproteins were obtained after precipitation of low-density and very low-density lipoproteins from the serum with phosphotungstate reagent. Lipid specimens were processed on a centrifugal analyzer. LDL concentrations were estimated with the Friedewald formula (Friedewald, Levy, & Fredrickson, 1972). This calculation provides a reliable standard for indirect measurement of LDL (McNamara, Cohn, Wilson, & Schaefer, 1990)." (p. 272)

IN CRITIQUING physiologic measures, you might ask the following questions.

1. Is the method of measurement clearly described?
2. Is the method of measurement direct or indirect?
3. How accurate, precise, selective, and sensitive is the measure?

Observational Measurement

Although *observational measurement* is most commonly used in qualitative research, it is used to some extent in all types of studies. Unstructured observations involve spontaneously observing and recording what is seen with minimum planning. Although unstructured observations give the observer freedom, there is a risk of loss of objectivity and a possibility that the observer may not remember all the details of the observed event. In structured observational measurement, the researcher carefully defines what is to be observed and how the observations are to be made, recorded, and coded. In most cases, a category system is developed for organizing and sorting the behaviors or events being observed. Checklists are often used to indicate whether a behavior occurred or did not occur. Rating scales allow the observer to rate the behavior or event. This provides more information for analysis than dichotomous data, which indicate only that the behavior either occurred or did not occur.

Observation tends to be more subjective than other types of measurement and thus is often considered less credible. However, in many cases, this approach is the only way to obtain important data for nursing's body of knowledge. As with any means of measurement, consistency is very important; thus, data on interrater reliability are essential.

Becker, Engelhardt, Steinmann, and Kane (1997) used observational methods to record mother-infant interaction during feeding behaviors and teaching behaviors of mothers of infants with mental delay. They describe the method of measurement as follows.

"Mother-infant interaction was rated in two contexts, feeding and teaching, using the Nursing Child Assessment Feeding and Teaching Scales (Barnard, 1980; Sumner & Spietz, 1994). The feeding scale consists of 50 mother and 26 infant behaviors, marked present or absent. The teaching scale consists of 50 mother and 23 infant items. Each scale has four mother subscales: sensitivity to infant cues (16 items feeding, 11 items teaching), response to distress (11, 11), social-emotional growth fostering (social-emotional support) (11, 14), and cognitive growth fostering (cognitive support) (17, 9); and two infant subscales: clarity of cues (15, 10) and responsiveness to parent (responsivity) (11, 13). Cronbach's alpha for the feeding and teaching total scales, respectively, are reported as .83 for each mother score, and .73 and .78 for the infant scores. . . . Concurrent validity for the NCAST [Nursing Child Assessment Satellite Training] scales is reported in terms of significant correlations with the HOME assessment of the caretaking environment (Bradley, Caldwell, & Elardo, 1977), and predictive validity in terms of significant correlations with the Bayley Scales of Infant Development (Sumner &

continued

Spietz, 1994). Interrater reliability was established prior to the study and checked at approximately 3-month intervals following the NCAST protocol. Reliability ranged from 85% to 100% absolute agreement for the feeding total scale and 85% to 96% for the teaching total scale." (p. 43)

IN CRITIQUING observational measures, you might ask the following questions.

1. Is what is to be observed clearly identified and defined?
2. Is interrater reliability described?
3. Are the techniques for recording observations described?

Interviews

An *interview* involves verbal communication between the researcher and the subject during which information is provided to the researcher. Although this measurement strategy is most commonly used in qualitative and descriptive studies, it can also be used in other types of studies. A variety of approaches can be used to conduct an interview, ranging from a totally *unstructured interview,* in which the content is completely controlled by the subject, to a *structured interview,* in which the content is similar to a questionnaire, with the possible responses to questions carefully designed by the researcher.

Unstructured interviews may be initiated by asking a broad question, such as "Describe for me your experience with . . ." After the interview has begun, the role of the interviewer is to encourage the subject to continue talking, using techniques such as nodding the head or making sounds that indicate interest. In some cases, the subject may be encouraged to elaborate further on a particular dimension of the topic of discussion.

Structured interviews involve strategies that provide increasing amounts of control by the researcher over the content of the interview. Questions the interviewer asks are designed by the researcher before the initiation of data collection, and the order of the questions is specified. In some cases, the interviewer is allowed to explain further the meaning of the question or to modify the way in which the question is asked so that the subject can understand it better. In more structured interviews, the interviewer is required to ask the question precisely as it has been designed.

Because nurses frequently use interviewing techniques in nursing assessment, the dynamics of interviewing are familiar; however, using the technique for measurement in research requires greater sophistication. Interviewing is a flexible technique that allows the researcher to explore meaning in greater depth than can be obtained with other techniques. Interpersonal skills can be used to facilitate cooperation and elicit more information. There is a higher response rate to interviews than to questionnaires, leading to a more representative sample. Interviewing allows collection of data from subjects who are unable or unlikely to complete questionnaires, such as those who are very ill or whose ability to read, write, and express themselves is marginal.

Interviews are a form of self-report, and it must be assumed that the information provided is accurate. Because of time and costs, sample size is usually limited. Subject bias is always a threat to the validity of the findings, as is inconsistency in data collection from one subject to another.

Hatton (1997) conducted interviews to gather data about "Managing health problems among homeless women with children in a transitional shelter." She describes the data gathering as follows.

"[T]he investigator conducted 30 indepth, semi-structured interviews with a convenience sample of women living in transitional housing. The sample was 13 Latina, 11 White, and 6 African American women. The typical respondent was age 20 to 30. The investigator interviewed each woman at least once, and, in most cases, obtained additional data from later informal conversations. Questions during the interviews included: How is your health? What makes you say you are healthy or unhealthy? Do you have any current concerns about particular diseases? What will you do about these? Have you ever had a sickness that lasted for a long time? When was the last time you went to a health care provider—such as a nurse or doctor? Each question was explored in further detail with the investigator asking how respondents perceived various symptoms, how their severity was managed, and how they decided on various treatments.

An interpreter assisted during the interviews with Spanish-speaking women ($n = 10$). The researcher familiarized the interpreter, who had considerable experience translating, with the overall purpose of the study. After each interview, the researcher and interpreter held debriefing sessions to review what each woman said and to discuss its meaning.

Interviews lasted from 30 minutes to 2 hours depending on the client's desire to talk with the researcher and the woman's busy schedule that included responsibilities for child rearing. All but two of the respondents had children. The two women without children were pregnant. At the beginning of the study, the investigator audiotaped the interviews and transcribed them verbatim ($n = 7$). As the study proceeded, however, women commented that they did not want their interviews audiotaped because they discussed problems they considered shameful. As Vredevoe, Shuler, and Woo (1992) have noted, disclosure can be a methodological problem when doing research among the homeless. Thus, during the latter part of the study, the investigator did not audiotape the interviews but took extensive notes that were later transcribed ($n = 23$)." (p. 34)

IN CRITIQUING measures obtained through an interview, you might ask the following questions.

1. Do the interview questions address concerns expressed in the research problem?
2. Are the interview questions relevant for the research purpose and objectives, questions, or hypotheses?
3. Does the design of the questions tend to bias subjects' responses?
4. Does the sequence of questions tend to bias subjects' responses?

Questionnaires

A *questionnaire* is a printed self-report form designed to elicit information that can be obtained through written or verbal responses of the subject. The information obtained from questionnaires is similar to that obtained by an interview, but the questions tend to have less depth. The subject is unable to elaborate on responses or ask for clarification of questions, and the data collector cannot use probing strategies. However, questions are presented in a consistent manner, and there is less opportunity for bias than in the interview. Questionnaires tend to be used in descriptive studies designed to gather a broad spectrum of information from subjects, such as facts about the subject or about persons known by the subject; facts about events or situations known by the subject; or beliefs, attitudes, opinions, levels of knowledge, or intentions of the subject. Like interviews, questionnaires can have varying degrees of structure. Some questionnaires ask open-ended questions, which require written responses from the subject. Others ask closed-ended questions, which have options selected by the researcher. A recent modification is the use of computers to gather questionnaire data (Saris, 1991).

Stotts, Henderson, and Burns (1988) used a questionnaire to examine smoking patterns of nurses in the state of Texas. Items from that questionnaire are shown in Figure 9-1.

Although questionnaires can be distributed to very large samples, either directly or through the mail, the response rate to questionnaires is generally lower than that of other forms of self-report, particularly if the questionnaires are mailed. If the response rate is lower than 50%, the representativeness of the sample is seriously in question. The response rate for mailed questionnaires is usually small (25% to 30%), so the researcher is frequently unable to obtain a representative sample, even with random sampling methods. Respondents commonly fail to mark responses to all the questions, especially on long questionnaires. This can threaten the validity of the instrument.

1. Do you currently smoke cigarettes?
   a. no
   b. yes

2. How old were you when you started smoking?
   a. under 15   e. 18 years   h. 21 years
   b. 15 years   f. 19 years   i. 22 years
   c. 16 years   g. 20 years   j. over 22 years
   d. 17 years

3. Before entering your basic (GENERIC) nursing education program, on the average, about how many cigarettes a day did you smoke?
   a. didn't smoke at all   d. 15–24 cigarettes/day
   b. didn't smoke every day   e. 25–39 cigarettes/day
   c. less than 15 cigarettes/day   f. 40 or more cigarettes/day

4. During your basic nursing (GENERIC) education program, on the average, about how many cigarettes a day did you smoke?
   a. didn't smoke at all   d. 15–24 cigarettes/day
   b. didn't smoke every day   e. 25–39 cigarettes/day
   c. less than 15 cigarettes/day   f. 40 or more cigarettes/day

5. How many organized programs have you attended to help you quit smoking?
   a. none   d. three   g. six
   b. one   e. four   h. seven
   c. two   f. five   i. more than seven

6. What is the longest single period you have stopped smoking?
   a. have never stopped   e. more than 1 month but less than 1
   b. less than a day   year
   c. less than a week   f. more than 1 year but less than 3
   d. less than a month   years
                             g. 3 years or more

7. Aside from what you think you actually could do, which would you most like to do?
   a. quit smoking   d. not sure at this time
   b. cut down   e. smoke as much as now
   c. cut down just a little

FIGURE 9-1
Example of items from a smoking questionnaire.

IN CRITIQUING a published study using a questionnaire, you need to evaluate the adequacy of the questionnaire to measure the concepts important to the study (content-related validity evidence). In most studies, only a brief description of the questionnaire is provided. The questionnaire itself will not be available for you to examine. Compare the questionnaire contents described with the conceptual definitions they are intended to reflect. Search for information on content-related validity. If the CVI was used, report the value obtained.

In most questionnaires, researchers analyze individual items rather than sum the items and obtain a total score for use in data analysis. Responses to items are usually measured at the nominal or ordinal level. Because individual items may address a variety of topics associated with the research area, attempting to determine reliability using tests of homogeneity may not be logical.

Chang and Hill (1996) used a questionnaire in their study of "HIV/AIDS related knowledge, attitudes, and preventive behavior of pregnant Korean women." They describe the questionnaire used in the study as follows.

"Data were collected in 1993 using self-administered questionnaires given to a convenience sample of 409 pregnant women attending prenatal clinics at six diverse health care facilities in Seoul, Korea: 70 of the 479 women approached (15%) chose not to participate. The questionnaire consisted of 18 demographic items, 22 AIDS-related knowledge items, 19 attitude items, and 7 preventive behavior items. Knowledge items measured risk factors, transmission modes, and general basic information. Responses to knowledge items were True, False, and Don't Know. Correct answers were scored as 1 and incorrect answers were scored as 0. Attitude and preventive behavior items were measured by a five-point scale (a score of 4 indicated strongly agree: 0 indicated strongly disagree). Cronbach's alphas of the attitude and preventive behavior scales were .83 and .77 respectively. . . .

The questionnaire was first prepared in English and content validity was assessed by five senior American AIDS researchers. It was translated into Korean by the first author of this article and validated by another Korean nurse researcher and a Korean doctoral student in health education. The Korean version of the questionnaire was then reviewed for face validity by one Korean language scholar, two nurse researchers, and three clinical nurses. Minor wording changes were made to increase idiomatic expression but no changes were made in format or item content." (p. 322)

Scales

The *scale,* a form of self-report, is a more precise means of measuring phenomena than the questionnaire. Most scales measure psychosocial variables. However, scaling techniques can be used to obtain self-reports on physiologic variables such as pain, nausea, or functional capacity. The various items on most scales are summed to obtain a single score. These are referred to as "summated scales." Less random and systematic error exists when the total score of a scale is used. The various items in a scale increase the dimensions of the concept that are reflected in the instrument. The types of scales described below include rating scales, the Likert scale, the semantic differential, and the visual analogue scale.

Rating Scales

Rating scales are the crudest form of measure using scaling techniques. A *rating scale* lists an ordered series of categories of a variable and is assumed to be based on an underlying continuum. A numerical value is assigned to each category. The fineness of the distinctions among categories varies with the scale. Rating scales are commonly used by the general public. In conversations, one can hear statements such as, On a scale of one to ten, I would rank that . . . This type of scale is often used in observational measurement to guide data collection. Burns (1974) used the rating scale in Figure 9-2 to examine differences in nurse-patient communication of cancer patients and other medical-surgical patients.

Motzer and Stewart (1996) used a rating scale to measure social support in their study of "Sense of coherence as a predictor of quality of life in persons with coronary heart disease surviving cardiac arrest." Their description of the rating scale is as follows.

"Perceived social support (SUPPORT) was measured by the Burck-hardt Perceived Support Score (1985), modified to enhance content validity by adding an item about financial help to the other three areas of assistance (physical help, social time, and advice or prob-lem-solving help) that one could expect to receive from each of six support persons if one wanted or needed the support. This 24-item measure reflected degree of perceived social support on a 0 = none to 3 = a lot scale." (p. 292)

IN CRITIQUING a rating scale, you might ask the following questions.

1. *Is the instrument clearly described?*
2. *Are the techniques that were used to administer and score the scale provided?*
3. *Are validity and reliability information on the scale from previous studies described?*
4. *Are validity and reliability information on the scale from the present sample described?*
5. *If the scale was developed for the study, was the instrument development process described?*

1. Nurses come into my room
   a. rarely
   b. sometimes
   c. whenever I call them
   d. frequently just to speak or check me
2. I would <u>like</u> nurses to come into my room
   a. rarely
   b. sometimes
   c. whenever I call them
   d. frequently just to speak or check me
3. When a nurse enters my room, she usually
   a. talks very little
   b. tries to talk about things I do not wish to discuss
   c. talks only about casual things
   d. is willing to listen or discuss what concerns me
4. When a nurse enters my room, I would <u>prefer</u> that she
   a. talk very little
   b. talk only when necessary
   c. talk only about casual things
   d. be willing to listen or discuss what concerns me
5. When a nurse talks with me she usually seems
   a. not interested
   b. in a hurry
   c. polite but distant
   d. caring for me as a person
6. When a nurse talks with me, I would <u>prefer</u> that she be
   a. not interested
   b. in a hurry
   c. polite but distant
   d. caring for me as a person
7. When a nurse talks with me she usually
   a. stands in the doorway
   b. stands at the foot of the bed
   c. stands at the side of the bed
   d. sits beside the bed
8. When a nurse talks with me I would <u>prefer</u> that she
   a. stand in the doorway
   b. stand at the foot of the bed
   c. stand at the side of the bed
   d. sit beside the bed
9. When a nurse talks with me, she is
   a. strictly business
   b. casual
   c. friendly but does not talk about feelings
   d. open to talking about things I worry or think about
10. When a nurse talks with me, I would <u>prefer</u> that she keep the conversation
   a. strictly business
   b. casual
   c. friendly but not talking about feelings
   d. open to talk about things I worry or think about

FIGURE 9-2
A rating scale used to measure the nature of nurse-patient communications.

11. Nurses talk with me about things important to me
   a. rarely
   b. sometimes
   c. frequently
   d. as often as I need to talk
12. I would <u>like</u> for the nurse to talk with me about things important to me
   a. rarely
   b. sometimes
   c. frequently
   d. as often as I need to talk
13. The nurse looks me in the eye when she talks with me
   a. rarely
   b. sometimes
   c. frequently
   d. very frequently
14. I would <u>prefer</u> that the nurse look me in the eye when she talks with me
   a. rarely
   b. sometimes
   c. frequently
   d. very frequently
15. When a nurse talks to me, she touches me
   a. rarely
   b. sometimes
   c. frequently
   d. very frequently
16. When a nurse talks with me, I would <u>prefer</u> that she touch me
   a. rarely
   b. occasionally
   c. frequently
   d. very frequently
17. My feelings about nurses talking to me are
   a. They should do their work well and otherwise leave me alone.
   b. They may talk if they need to; it does not bother me.
   c. I enjoy talking with the nurses.
   d. When the nurse lets me talk with her about things important to me, I feel that she cares for me as a person.

On question 18, please mark as many answers as you wish.
18. I would like to feel free to talk with the nurse about my
   a. illness
   b. future
   c. financial problems
   d. feelings about myself
   e. feelings about my family
   f. life up to this time

FIGURE 9-2 Continued

	Strongly Disagree	Disagree	Uncertain	Agree	Strongly Agree
People with cancer almost always die					
Chemotherapy is very effective in treating cancer					
We are close to finding a cure for cancer					
I would work next to a person with cancer					
I could develop cancer					
Nurses take good care of patients with cancer					

FIGURE 9-3
Example of items that could be included in a Likert scale.

Likert Scale

The *Likert scale,* which was designed to determine the opinion on or attitude toward a subject, contains a number of declarative statements with a scale after each statement. The Likert scale is the most commonly used scaling technique. The original version of the scale consisted of five categories. However, sometimes seven options are given, sometimes only four. Values are placed on each response, with a value of 1 on the most negative response and a value of 5 on the most positive response (Nunnally, 1978). Response choices on a Likert scale most commonly address agreement, evaluation, or frequency. Agreement responses may include options such as strongly agree, agree, uncertain, disagree, and strongly disagree. Evaluation responses ask the respondent for an evaluative rating along a good/bad dimension, such as positive to negative or excellent to terrible. Frequency responses may include options such as rarely, seldom, sometimes, occasionally, and usually. The values from each item are summed to provide a total score. Figure 9-3 illustrates the form used for this type of scale.

LoBiondo-Wood, Williams, Wood, and Shaw (1997) used a Likert -type scale to measure quality of life in their study of the impact of liver transplantation on quality of life. Their description of the instrument follows.

> "The Quality of Life Index-Liver Transplant Version (QLI-LT), which measures subjectively perceived quality of life, was used to measure quality of life (Ferrans & Powers, 1985). This instrument is derived from Campbell's framework of quality of life (1976, 1981). The 72-item, 6-point Likert-type instrument has two sections: (1) satisfaction with various life domains, and (2) importance of life domains. The QLI-LT yields an overall index of quality of life (QLI total) and four subscale scores reflecting the domains of (a) health and functioning (HF), (b) socioeconomic (SE), (c) psychological/spiritual (PS), and (d) family (F). The QLI-LT yields an adjusted score that reflects an individual's satisfaction with, and the importance of, each domain and an overall quality of life score. Alpha reliability coefficients for the QLI-LT range from .73 to .93 (Ferrans, 1990; Ferrans & Powers, 1985; Hicks, Larson, & Ferrans, 1992). The potential scores range is 0 to 30 for the subscales and total scale." (p. 29)

IN CRITIQUING a Likert scale, you might ask the following questions.

1. *Is the instrument clearly described?*
2. *Are the techniques to complete and score the scale provided?*
3. *Are validity and reliability information on the scale from previous studies described?*
4. *Are reliability and validity information on the scale from the present sample described?*
5. *If the scale was developed for the study, was the instrument development process described?*

Semantic Differentials

The *semantic differential* measures attitudes or beliefs. A semantic differential scale consists of two opposite adjectives with a 7-point scale between them. The subject is to select one point on the scale that best describes his or her view of the concept being examined. Values of 1 to 7 are assigned to each space, with 1 being the most negative response and 7 the most positive. The placement of negative responses to the left or right of the scale should be randomly varied to avoid global responses (in which the subject places checks in the same column of each scale). The values for the scales are summed to

CANCER

Certain Death |⎯⎯⎯⎯⎯⎯⎯| Being Cured

Punishment |⎯⎯⎯⎯⎯⎯⎯| No Punishment

Painless |⎯⎯⎯⎯⎯⎯⎯| Severe Constant Untreatable Pain

Abandoned |⎯⎯⎯⎯⎯⎯⎯| Cared For

FIGURE 9-4
Example of items from the Burns Cancer Beliefs Scales.

obtain one score for each subject. Burns (1981, 1983) developed a semantic differential to measure beliefs about cancer that uses descriptive phrases. Figure 9-4 includes descriptive phrases from this 23-item scale.

IN CRITIQUING a semantic differential, you might ask the following questions.

1. *Is the instrument clearly described?*
2. *Are the techniques to administer and score the scale provided?*
3. *Are the validity and reliability information on the scale from previous studies described?*
4. *Are validity and reliability information on the scale from the present sample described?*
5. *If the scale was developed for the study, was the instrument development process described?*

Visual Analogue Scales

The *visual analogue scale* is a line 100 mm long with right angle stops at either end. The line may be horizontal or vertical. Bipolar anchors are placed beyond either end of the line. These end anchors should include the entire range of sensations possible in the phenomenon being measured (e.g., all and none, best and worst, no pain and pain as bad as it could possibly be).

The subject is asked to place a mark through the line to indicate the intensity of the stimulus. A ruler is then used to measure the distance between the left end of the line and the subject's mark. This measure is the value of the stimulus. The visual analogue scale has been used to measure pain, mood, anxiety, alertness, craving for cigarettes, quality of sleep, attitudes toward environmental conditions, functional abilities, and severity of clinical symptoms (Wewers & Lowe, 1990). An example of a visual analogue scale is shown in Figure 9-5.

Strategies commonly used to evaluate the reliability of scales are not useful for visual analogue scales. Because these scales are used to measure phenomena that are erratic over time, test-retest reliability is inappropriate, and because

Visual Analogue Scale

No pain |——| Pain as bad as it
                                                                                                                      can possibly be

FIGURE 9-5
Example of a visual analogue scale.

the scale consists of a single item, other methods of determining reliability cannot be used.

IN CRITIQUING a visual analogue scale, you might ask the following questions.

1. *Is the instrument clearly described?*
2. *Are the techniques to administer and score the scale provided?*
3. *Is the validity information on the scale from previous studies described?*
4. *Is validity information on the scale from the present sample described?*
5. *If the scale was developed for the study, was the instrument development process described?*

Defining an Experimental Intervention

In quasi-experimental and experimental studies, an intervention is developed that is expected to result in differences in posttest measures of the treatment and control or comparison groups. This intervention may be physiologic, psychosocial, educational, or a combination of these. The details of the intervention should have been carefully planned and a rationale given for providing the intervention in a particular way. The researcher should describe the intervention in detail in the published study. Labels for interventions, such as "preoperative teaching," limit the reader's ability to understand the exact nature of the intervention. We may be easily led astray since each of us has our own expectations of what should occur during preoperative teaching. Nursing is currently developing classifications of nursing interventions. These classifications should be useful to the researcher in clarifying the intervention provided (Egan, Snyder, & Burns, 1992). The intervention should maximize the differences between the groups. Thus, it should be the best intervention that can be provided in the circumstances of the study, an intervention that should make a difference in the experimental group.

Although control and comparison groups traditionally received no intervention, this circumstance is not possible in many nursing studies. For example, it would be unethical not to provide preoperative teaching to a patient. In addition, in many studies, it is possible that just spending time with a patient or having a patient participate in activities that he or she considers beneficial may itself cause an effect. Therefore, the study often includes a control or comparison group intervention. This intervention is commonly the usual treatment the patient would receive if a study were not being conducted. The researcher should describe the intervention the control or comparison group receives in detail so that the study can be more adequately critiqued. Because the quality of this usual treatment is likely to vary considerably among subjects, variance in the control or comparison group is likely to be high, and the risk of a Type II error is greater than when the control or comparison group receives no treatment.

Johnson, Fieler, Wlasowicz, Mitchell, and Jones (1997) studied the effects of nursing care guided by self-regulation theory on coping with radiation therapy. They describe their nursing intervention as follows.

"The control-group patients received the routine nursing care that was usual practice at the institution. The aspect of care relevant to the study was patient information. The only specific standards for patient teaching were that it had to take place and be documented. What was taught, when it was taught, and amount of detail included varied among nurses. In general, nurses would 'catch' a patient during the first week of treatment, and they would meet for 10 to 15 minutes in any space that was available. The nurses would provide a brief overview of the procedures involved in RT [radiation therapy] and inform the patients about possible side effects. Some of the nurses would talk about self-care management of the side effects, and others would tell the patient 'Let me know when you have [the side effect], and I will give you more information.' Patient teaching sheets that contained general information about RT and self-care activities for specific side effects were available. Nurses usually gave the sheets to patients during the first week of treatment.

The theory-based nursing care consisted of interventions delivered at four points in time: (a) before the simulation (treatment planning) procedure, (b) the first week of treatment, (c) the last week of treatment, and (d) one month posttreatment. Nurses made 30-minute appointments with patients to deliver the interventions. At the beginning of each appointment nurses told patients the topics that would be covered and that the information would help them to handle the experience of receiving RT because they would know what to expect. At the end of each intervention session, patients were told the time of the next appointment and the topics that would be covered. . . . The expected experiences were described by the nurses in concrete, objective terms without reference to subjective features such as severity and amount of distress that might be experienced." (p. 1043)

The Process of Data Collection

Data collection is the process of acquiring subjects and collecting the data needed for the study. The actual steps of collecting the data are specific to each study and are dependent on the research design and measurement techniques. During the data collection period, the researcher focuses on obtaining subjects, training data collectors, collecting data in a consistent way, maintaining research controls, protecting the integrity (or validity) of the study, and solving problems that threaten to disrupt the study.

The researcher should describe the data collection process in the published study. The strategies used to approach potential subjects who meet the sampling criteria need to be clear. The number and characteristics of subjects who decline to participate in the study should be reported. The approach used to perform measurements, the timing, and the setting of measurements need to be described. The result should be a step-by-step description of exactly how, where, and in what sequence the data were collected.

In many studies, data collection forms are used to gather data. These forms may be used to record data from the patient record or to ask the subject for information such as demographic data. The form itself is not a measurement tool. In many cases, each item on these forms is a separate measurement. Thus, the researcher should report the source of information and describe the method and level of measurement of each item on the form. An example of a data collection form is shown in Figure 9-6.

Data Collection Tasks

In both quantitative and qualitative research, the investigator performs five tasks during the data collection process. These tasks are interrelated and occur concurrently rather than in sequence. The tasks include selecting subjects, collecting data in a consistent way, maintaining research controls as indicated in the study design, protecting the integrity (or validity) of the study, and solving problems that threaten to disrupt the study.

DATA COLLECTION FORM

Subject Identification Number _____   Date _____

A. Age _____   B. Gender: 1. Male   2. Female

C. Weight _____ pounds   D. Height _____ inches

E. Surgical diagnosis _____

F. Surgery Date _____ and Time _____

G. Narcotics Ordered after Surgery _____

_____

H. Narcotic Administration:
   Date   Time   Type of Narcotic   Dose
   1.
   2.
   3.
   4.
   5.

I. Patient Instructed on Pain Scale: Date _____ Time _____
   Comments:

J. Type of Treatment: 1. TENS   2. Placebo-TENS   3. No-treatment Control

K. Treatment Implemented: Date _____   Time _____
   Comments:

L. Dressing Change: Date _____   Time _____
   Hours since Surgery _____

M. Score on Visual Analogue Pain Scale _____

   Date _____   Time _____

Data Collector's Name: _____ Comments:

FIGURE 9-6
Hypothetical data collection form for Hargreaves and Lander's (1989) study, The use of trans-electrical nerve stimulation (TENS) for management of postoperative pain.

Recruiting Subjects

Subjects may be recruited only at the initiation of data collection or throughout the data collection period. The design of the study determines the method of selecting subjects. Recruiting the number of subjects originally planned is critical because data analysis and interpretation of findings depend on an adequate sample size. Factors related to subject recruitment and selection need to be continually examined to determine possible biases in the sample obtained.

Recruiting subjects for research is becoming more difficult for a variety of reasons, including the following: (1) an increasing number of nurses are conducting research, (2) clinical agencies are placing constraints on the time staff nurses can be released from patient care for research activities, (3) patients are being protected from participating in too many investigations, and (4) access to patients is being limited so that agency personnel can use these patients for their own research (Cronenwett, 1986). Thus, in the future, nurse researchers will need to be creative and persistent in recruiting adequate numbers of subjects. In recruiting subjects, researchers have found that direct contact with potential subjects is the most effective method, telephone contact is less effective, and mail contact is least effective. Direct contact in small groups is usually more effective for subject recruitment than is contact in large groups (Crosby, Ventura, Finnick, Lohr, & Feldman, 1991). The researcher must determine the most effective recruitment approach based on the purpose of the study, the type and number of subjects required, and the design of the study.

Maintaining Consistency

The key to accurate data collection in any study is consistency. Consistency involves maintaining the data collection pattern for each collection event as it was developed in the research plan. A good plan will facilitate consistency and maintain the validity of the study. However, developing a consistent plan is easier than implementing it. Deviations, though minor, need to be noted and evaluated for their impact on the interpretation of the findings. When data collectors are used in a study, they need to be trained to note deviations during the data collection process.

Maintaining Controls

Research controls were built into the plan to minimize the influence of intervening forces on study findings. Maintenance of these controls is essential; these controls are not natural in a field setting, and letting them slip is easy. In some cases, the controls slip without the researcher's realizing it. In addition to maintaining the controls identified in the plan, the researcher needs to watch continually for previously unidentified extraneous variables that might have an impact on the data being collected. These variables are often specific to a study and tend to become apparent during the data collection period. The extraneous variables identified during data collection must be considered during data analysis and interpretation. These variables also need to be noted in the research report to allow future researchers to control them.

Protecting Study Integrity

Maintaining consistency and controls during subject selection and data collection protects the integrity or validity of the study. In addition, the integrity of the study needs to be considered in a broad context. To accomplish this, you must shift from examining the elements of data collection to viewing the process of data collection as a whole. Changes in one small component of data collection can modify other elements and thus alter the entire process in ways that threaten the validity of the outcomes.

Harrison, Wells, Fisher, and Prince (1996) conducted a study to evaluate evidence of the effectiveness of practice guidelines for the prediction and prevention of pressure ulcers. They used a Demographic and Clinical Profile Form to capture information about age, sex, length of hospital stay, admission, diagnosis, pressure relief devices being used, and type of nursing unit. The Prevalence Grid was used to identify 20 specific assessment sites to assess skin integrity. If ulcers were present, a staging classification system was used to define ulcers from Stage I to Stage IV. The Braden Scale was used to assess the risk of pressure ulcers. The authors described their data collection procedure as follows.

"A survey team of 23 registered nurses conducted a head-to-toe skin assessment and administered the Braden Scale to consenting subjects. The surveyors were prepared through an education workshop that included an orientation to the study purpose and procedures, the use of data collection instruments, and a theoretical and practical 'hands-on' component to stage ulcers and conduct risk assessment. The training films developed by Bergstrom and Braden were included in the workshop format. Reliability was assessed on a range of known cases where team members went to clinical areas, staged ulcers, and then had these assessments checked by a clinical expert (enterostomal therapist).

On prevalence day, the surveyors were divided into four data collection teams plus a validation team. Each had a team leader who was not directly involved in data collection to attend to administrative tasks, such as tracking admissions and discharges, and deploying surveyors. The team members were assigned to clinically familiar areas (e.g., critical care nurses to critical care areas) but not to their home units where they would know the patients. The enterostomal therapist was on call at all times if the surveyors required a second opinion on an assessment of ulcer stage.

The validation team, comprised of two registered nurse surveyors, reassessed a randomly selected subsample of 10% of the prevalence population to assess reliability. Correlation of the survey team and validation team on total Braden scores was calculated using Pearson's product moment correlation. Correlation of the survey team and validation team assessments was $r - .87$.

The degree of association indicates a strong relationship between assessments.

The surveyors conducted a full skin examination and administered the Braden Scale for risk assessment on prevalence day. The risk assessment was completed using the chart, plan of care, clinical assessment, and consultation with the patient's assigned nurse to complete the data collection. The Braden Scale was administered in this manner because it closely emulates the way in which clinical staff would use such a scale if implemented institutionwide.

To determine the Braden Scale's accuracy in the setting, the same data (full skin assessment and administration of the Braden Scale) was collected in a 20 week follow-up on a Monday-Wednesday-Friday schedule by a subsample of the surveyors. They had no information of the subjects' prior risk scores, and with the number of surveyors, computer calculation of total scores, and the large number of patients in the study, the likelihood of bias by remembering an assessment was minimal.

To evaluate the Braden Scale and the risk cut-off scores, the sensitivity (i.e., percentage of all subjects who developed a pressure ulcer and were so predicted by the scale), specificity (i.e., percentage of all subjects who did not develop pressure ulcers and were so predicted by the scale), positive predictive value (i.e., percentage of subjects who were predicted to be at risk and did develop a pressure ulcer), and the negative predictive value (i.e., percentage of subjects who were predicted to be at low risk and did not develop a pressure ulcer) were calculated. The calculations are well described by Bergstrom, Demuth, and Braden (1987)." (pp. 12–13)

Problem Solving

Problems can be perceived either as a frustration or as a challenge. The fact that the problem occurred is not as important as the success of problem resolution. Therefore, the final and perhaps most important task of the data collection period may be problem resolution. Little has been written about the problems encountered by nurse researchers. The research reports often read as though everything went smoothly. The implication is that if you are a good researcher, you will have no problems, which is not true. Research journals generally do not provide sufficient space to allow description of the problems encountered, and this gives a false impression to the inexperienced researcher. A more realistic picture can be obtained through personal discussions with researchers about the data collection process.

IN CRITIQUING the data collection process of a published study, you might follow these guidelines.

1. Describe and evaluate the way subjects were obtained.
2. Describe and evaluate the data collection procedures.
3. Search the descriptions of the data collection process for possible threats to validity.
4. Describe and evaluate the training of data collectors.
5. Identify and evaluate the use of data collection forms.

Serendipity

Serendipity is the accidental discovery of something useful or valuable. During the data collection phase of studies, researchers often become aware of elements or relationships not previously identified. Therefore, in some published studies, the researcher has gathered data, made observations, or recorded events not originally planned. These aspects may be closely related to the study being conducted or have little connection with it. They come from the increased awareness of close observation. Because the researcher is focused on close observation, other elements in the situation can come into clearer focus and take on new meaning. Serendipitous findings are important to the development of new insights in nursing. They can lead to new areas of research that generate new knowledge.

SUMMARY

The purpose of measurement is to produce trustworthy evidence that can be used in evaluating the outcomes of research. The rules of measurement ensure that the assignment of values or categories is performed consistently from one subject (or event) to another and, eventually, if the measurement strategy is found to be meaningful, from one study to another. Measurement begins by clarifying the object, characteristic, or element to be measured. Direct measurement is the measurement of concrete factors such as height or wrist circumference. Indirect measurement is used to measure abstract concepts such as stress, caring, coping, anxiety, compliance, and pain. Measurement error is the difference between what exists in reality and what is measured.

The levels of measurement from low to high are nominal, ordinal, interval, and ratio. Nominal-scale measurement is used when data can be organized into categories of a defined property, but the categories cannot be compared. Data that can be measured at the ordinal-scale level can be assigned to categories of an attribute that can be ranked. In addition to following the rules of mutually exclusive categories, exhaustive categories, and rank ordering, interval scales have equal numerical distance between intervals of the scale. Ratio-level measures are the highest form of measure and meet all the rules of other forms of measures, and they have absolute zero points.

Reliability in measurement is concerned with how consistently the measurement technique measures the concept of interest. Reliability testing is considered a measure of the amount of random error in the measurement technique. Reliability testing focuses on three aspects of reliability: stability, equivalence, and homogeneity. The validity of an instrument is a determination of the extent to which the instrument actually reflects the abstract concept being examined. Validity, like reliability, is not an all-or-nothing phenomenon but rather a matter of degree. No instrument is completely valid. Validity is considered a single broad method of measurement evaluation referred to as construct validity. Validity testing validates the use of an instrument for a specific group or purpose rather than being directed to the instrument itself. An instrument may be very valid in one situation but not valid in another. There are a number of sources for obtaining evidence of the validity of an instrument. Reliability and validity of physiologic and biochemical measures tend not to be reported in published studies. It is erroneously assumed that routine physiologic measures are valid and reliable. Evaluation of physiologic measures requires a different perspective than does evaluation of behavioral measures.

Nursing studies require the availability of an extensive array of measurement tools. Common measurement approaches used in nursing research include physiologic measures, observation, interviews, questionnaires, and scales. Many questions in nursing research require the measurement of physiologic dimensions. Measurements of physiologic variables can be either direct or indirect. Many physiologic measures require the use of specialized equipment; some require laboratory analysis. In publishing the results of a physiologic study, the measurement technique needs to be described in great detail.

Observational measurement may be unstructured or structured. In structured observational studies, category systems must be developed. Checklists or rating scales are developed from the category systems and are used to guide data collection. Interviews involve verbal communication between the researcher and the subject, during which information is provided to the researcher. A questionnaire is a printed self-report form designed to elicit information that can be obtained through written responses of the subject. Scales, a form of self-report, are a more precise means of measuring phenomena than questionnaires. A rating scale lists an ordered series of categories of a variable; the scale is assumed to be based on an underlying continuum. The Likert scale is designed to determine the opinion or attitude of a subject and contains a number of declarative statements with a scale after each statement. A semantic differential scale consists of two opposite adjectives with a 7-point scale between them. The visual analogue scale is a line 100 mm long with right angle stops at either end. Adjectives expressing the opposite extremes of psychosocial or behavioral responses (such as pain, mood, or anxiety) are placed beyond either end of the line.

In quasi-experimental and experimental studies, an intervention is developed that is expected to result in differences in posttest measures of the treatment and control groups. The researcher should describe the intervention in detail in the published study. Although control groups traditionally received no intervention, many nursing studies include a control group intervention. This intervention is commonly the usual treatment the patient would receive if a study were not being conducted.

The researcher performs five tasks during the process of data collection: (1) obtaining subjects, (2) collecting data in a consistent way, (3) maintaining research controls, (4) protecting the integrity (or validity) of the study, and (5) solving problems that threaten to disrupt the study. It is important to critique the description of the data collection process for threats to validity. During data collection, the researcher may make an accidental discovery of valuable information unrelated to the planned study; this is referred to as serendipity.

REFERENCES

Algase, D. L., Kupferschmid, B., Beel-Bates, C. A., & Beattie, E. R. (1997). Estimates of stability of daily wandering behavior among cognitively impaired long-term care residents. *Nursing Research, 46*(3), 172–178.

Avery, T. E. (1977). *Interpretation of aerial photographs* (3rd ed.). Broken Arrow, OK: Burgess.

Barnard, K. (1980). *Nursing child assessment training/ learning resource manual.* Seattle: NCAST Project.

Becker, P. T., Engelhardt, K. F., Steinmann, M. F., & Kane, J. (1997). Infant age, context, and family system influences on the interactive behavior of mothers of infants with mental delay. *Research in Nursing & Health, 20*(1), 39–50.

Bergstrom, N., Demuth, P. J., & Braden, B. J. (1987). A clinical trial of the Braden Scale for predicting pressure sore risk. *Nursing Clinics of North America, 22*(2), 417–428.

Berk, R. A. (1990). Importance of expert judgment in content-related validity evidence. *Western Journal of Nursing Research, 12*(5), 659–671.

Bradley, R., Caldwell, B. M., & Elardo, R. (1977). Home environment, social status, and mental test performance. *Journal of Educational Psychology, 69*, 697–701.

Burckhardt, C. S. (1985). The impact of arthritis on quality of life. *Nursing Research, 34*(1), 11–16.

Burns, N. (1974). *Nurse-patient communication with the advanced cancer patient.* Unpublished master's thesis, Texas Woman's University, Dallas.

Burns, N. (1981). *Evaluation of a supportive-expressive group for families of cancer patients.* Unpublished doctoral dissertation, Texas Woman's University, Denton.

Burns, N. (1983). Development of the Burns cancer beliefs scale. *Proceedings of the American Cancer Society Third West Coast Cancer Nursing Research Conference Proceedings*, 308–329.

Burns, N., & Grove, S. K. (1997). *The practice of nursing research: Conduct, critique, and utilization* (3rd ed.). Philadelphia: Saunders.

Campbell, A. (1976). Subjective measures of well being. *American Psychologist, 31*, 117–124.

Campbell, A. (1981). *The sense of well being in America.* New York: McGraw-Hill.

Carson, M. A. (1996). The impact of a relaxation technique on the lipid profile. *Nursing Research, 45*(5), 271–276.

Chang, S. B., & Hill, M. N. (1996). HIV/AIDS related knowledge, attitudes, and preventive behavior of pregnant Korean women. *Image: Journal of Nursing Scholarship, 28*(4), 321–324.

Craft, M. J., & Moss, J. (1996). Accuracy of infant emesis volume assessment. *Applied Nursing Research, 9*(1), 2–8.

Cronenwett, L. (1986). Research reflections: Access to research subjects. *Journal of Nursing Administration, 16*(1), 8–9.

Crosby, F., Ventura, M. R., Finnick, M., Lohr, G., & Feldman, M. J. (1991). Enhancing subject recruitment for nursing research. *Clinical Nurse Specialist, 5*(1), 25–30.

Egan, E. C., Snyder, M., & Burns, K. R. (1992). Intervention studies in nursing: Is the effect due to the independent variable? *Nursing Outlook, 40*(4), 187–190.

Ferrans, C. E. (1990). Development of a Quality of Life Index for cancer patients. *Oncology Nursing Forum, 17*(3 Suppl), 15–19.

Ferrans, C. E., & Powers, M. (1985). Quality of Life Index: Development of psychometric properties. *Advances in Nursing Science, 8*(1), 15–24.

Friedewald, W. T., Levy, R. I., & Fredrickson, D. S. (1972). Estimation of the concentration of low-density lipoprotein cholesterol in plasma without use of the preparative ultracentrifuge. *Clinical Chemistry, 18*, 499–502.

Gift, A. G., & Soeken, K. L. (1988). Assessment of physiologic instruments. *Heart & Lung, 17*(2), 128–133.

Harrison, M. B., Wells, G., Fisher, A., & Prince, M. (1996). Practice guidelines for the prediction and prevention of pressure ulcers: Evaluating the evidence. *Applied Nursing Research, 9*(1), 9–17.

Hargreaves, A., & Lander, J. (1989). Use of transcutaneous electrical nerve stimulation for postoperative pain. *Nursing Research, 38*(3), 159–161.

Hatton, D. C. (1997). Managing health problems among homeless women with children in a transitional shelter. *Image: Journal of Nursing Scholarship, 29*(1), 33–37.

Heitkemper, M. M., & Jarrett, M. (1992). Pattern of gastrointestinal and somatic symptoms across the menstrual cycle. *Gastroenterology, 102*, 505–513.

Hicks, F. D., Larson, J. L., & Ferrans, C. E. (1992). Quality of life after liver transplant. *Research in Nursing & Health, 15*(2), 111–119.

Jarrett, M., Cain, K. C., Heitkemper, M., & Levy, R. L. (1996). Relationship between gastrointestinal and dysmenorrheic symptoms at menses. *Research in Nursing & Health, 19*(1), 45–51.

Johnson, A. (1984, November 28). Towards rapid tissue healing. *Nursing Times, 80*(48), 39–43.

Johnson, J. E. (1996). Social support and physical health in the rural elderly. *Applied Nursing Research, 9*(2), 61–66.

Johnson, J. E., Fieler, V. K., Wlasowicz, G. S., Mitchell, M. L., & Jones, L. S. (1997). The effects of nursing care guided by self-regulation theory on coping with radiation therapy. *Oncology Nursing Forum, 24*(6), 1041–1050.

Johnson, M., & Miller, R. (1996). Measuring healing in leg ulcers: Practice considerations. *Applied Nursing Research, 9*(4), 204–208.

Kotzer, A. M. (1990). Creative strategies for pediatric nursing research: Data collection. *Journal of Pediatric Nursing, 5*(1), 50–53.

Laboratory Standardization Panel of the National Cholesterol Education Program. (1990). *Recommendations for improving cholesterol measurement: Executive summary* (NIH Pub. No. 90-2964A). Bethesda, MD: National Institutes of Health.

LoBiondo-Wood, G., Williams, L., Wood, R. P., & Shaw, B. W. (1997). Impact of liver transplantation on quality of life: A longitudinal perspective. *Applied Nursing Research, 10*(1), 27–32.

McNamara, J. R., Cohn, J. S., Wilson, P. W. F., & Schaefer, E. J. (1990). Calculated values for low-density lipoprotein cholesterol in the assessment of lipid abnormalities and coronary disease risk. *Clinical Chemistry, 36*, 36–42.

Medoff-Cooper, B., & Gennaro, S. (1996). The correlation of sucking behaviors and Bayley Scales of Infant Development at six months of age in VLBW infants. *Nursing Research, 45*(5), 291–296.

Miller, J. F., & Powers, M. J. (1988). Development of an instrument to measure hope. *Nursing Research, 37*(1), 6–10.

Milligan, R. A., Flenniken, P. M., & Pugh, L. C. (1996). Positioning intervention to minimize fatigue in breastfeeding women. *Applied Nursing Research, 9*(2), 67–70.

Milligan, R. A., Parks, P., & Lenz, E. (1990). An analysis of postpartum fatigue over the first three months of the postpartum period. In J. Wang, P. Simoni, & C. Nath (Eds.), *Vision of excellence: The decade of the nineties* (pp. 245–251). Charleston: West Virginia Nurses' Association Research Conference Group.

Motzer, S. U., & Stewart, B. J. (1996). Sense of coherence as a predictor of quality of life in persons with coronary heart disease surviving cardiac arrest. *Research in Nursing & Health, 19*(4), 287–298.

Norman, E., Gadaleta, D., & Griffin, C. C. (1991). An evaluation of three blood pressure methods in a stabilized acute trauma population. *Nursing Research, 40*(2), 86–89.

Nunnally, J. C. (1978). *Psychometric theory* (2nd ed.). New York: McGraw-Hill.

Redeker, N. S., Mason, D. J., Wykpisz, E., & Glica, B. (1996). Sleep patterns in women after coronary artery bypass surgery. *Applied Nursing Research, 9*(3), 115–122.

Rew, L., Stuppy, D., & Becker, H. (1988). Construct validity in instrument development: A vital link between nursing practice, research, and theory. *Advances in Nursing Science, 10*(4), 10–22.

Saris, W. E. (1991). *Computer-assisted interviewing*. Newbury Park, CA: Sage.

Selby-Harrington, M. L., Mehta, S. M., Jutsum, V., Riportella-Muller, R., & Quade, D. (1994). Reporting of instrument validity and reliability in selected clinical nursing journals, 1989. *Journal of Professional Nursing, 10*(1), 47–56.

Stevens, S. S. (1946). On the theory of scales of measurement. *Science, 103*(2684), 677–680.

Stotts, C., Henderson, A., & Burns, N. (1988). *Health exemplar? Nurses, nursing students and smoking behavior*. XIII World Conference on Health Education Proceedings, Houston, TX, August 28–September 2.

Sumner, G., & Spietz, A. (1994). *Caregiver/parent-child interaction teaching and feeding manuals*. Seattle: NCAST Publications, University of Washington.

Vredevoe, D. L., Shuler, P., & Woo, M. (1992). The homeless population. *Western Journal of Nursing Research, 14*(6), 731–740.

Weinberger, M., Hiner, S. L., & Tierney, W. M. (1987). In support of hassles as a measure of stress in predicting health outcomes. *Journal of Behavioral Medicine, 10*(1), 19–31.

Wewers, M. E., & Lowe, N. K. (1990). A critical review of visual analogue scales in the measurement of clinical phenomena. *Research in Nursing & Health, 13*(4), 227–236.

Wineman, N. M., Schwetz, K. M., Goodkin, D. E., & Rudick, R. A. (1996). Relationships among illness uncertainty, stress, coping, and emotional well-being at entry into a clinical drug trial. *Applied Nursing Research, 9*(2), 53–60.

Understanding Statistics in Research

Completing this chapter should enable you to:

1. *Identify the purposes of statistical analysis.*
2. *Describe the process of data analysis: (a) preparation of the data for analysis; (b) description of the sample; (c) testing the reliability of the measurement methods; (d) exploratory analysis of the data; (e) confirmatory analyses guided by objectives, questions, or hypotheses; and (f) post-hoc analyses.*
3. *Differentiate probability theory from decision theory.*
4. *Describe the process of inferring from a sample to a population.*
5. *Discuss the distribution of the normal curve.*
6. *Compare and contrast Type I error and Type II error.*
7. *Differentiate a one-tailed test of significance from a two-tailed test.*
8. *Discuss the clinical versus the statistical significance of findings.*
9. *Differentiate the ungrouped frequency distribution from the grouped frequency distribution.*
10. *Describe the three measures of central tendency (mean, median, and mode).*
11. *Discuss the purpose of measures of dispersion.*
12. *Discuss the purposes and interpretation of results of chi-square analysis, t-test, analysis of variance, Pearson's correlation, and regression analysis.*
13. *Critique the use of chi-square analysis, t-test, analysis of variance, Pearson's correlation, and regression analysis in published studies.*
14. *Describe the five types of results obtained from quasi-experimental and experimental studies that are interpreted within a decision theory framework: (a) significant and predicted results, (b) nonsignificant results, (c) significant and unpredicted results, (d) mixed results, and (e) unexpected results.*
15. *Differentiate the results, findings, and conclusions in a study.*
16. *Examine findings for statistical significance and practical significance in a study.*
17. *Identify the following elements of a research report: findings, conclusions, significance of findings, generalization of findings, implications, and suggestions for further study.*
18. *Given a study, critique the findings, conclusions, generalizations, implications, and suggestions for further study.*

Analysis of covariance (ANCOVA)
Analysis of variance (ANOVA)
Bivariate correlation
Chi-square test of independence
Clinical significance
Conclusions
Confirmatory analysis
Decision theory
Degrees of freedom (df)

Dependent groups
Descriptive statistics
Effect size
Empirical generalizations
Exploratory analysis
Factor analysis
Findings
Frequency distribution
Generalization

Grouped frequency distribution
Implications
Independent groups
Inference
Level of significance
Mean
Measures of central tendency
Measures of dispersion
Median
Mode
Nonsignificant results
Normal curve
One-tailed test of significance
Outliers
Pearson's product-moment correlation

Post-hoc analyses
Power
Power analysis
Probability theory
Regression analysis
Significant results
Standard deviation
Standardized scores
Statistical significance
t-Test
Two-tailed test of significance
Type I error
Type II error
Ungrouped frequency distribution
Z-score

*N*urses probably have more anxiety about knowledge of statistics and data analysis than they do about any other aspect of the research process, whether they need the knowledge to critique published studies or to conduct research. We hope this chapter will dispel some of that anxiety. The statistical information in this chapter is provided from the perspective of reading, understanding, and critiquing published studies rather than from that of selecting statistical procedures or performing statistical analyses. To critique a quantitative study, you need to be able to (1) identify the statistical procedures used; (2) judge whether these procedures were appropriate to the hypotheses, questions, or objectives of the study and to the data available for analysis; (3) comprehend the discussion of data analysis results; (4) judge whether the author's interpretation of the results is appropriate; and (5) evaluate the clinical significance of the findings.

The chapter begins with a discussion of some of the more pragmatic aspects of quantitative data analyses: the purposes of statistical analyses and the process of performing data analyses. The reasoning behind statistics is explained, and some of the more common statistical procedures used to describe and test hypotheses are introduced. The chapter concludes with strategies for judging statistical suitability and evaluating the interpretation of statistical outcomes.

The Process of Data Analysis

Statistical procedures are used to examine the numerical data gathered in a study. In critiquing a study, it may be helpful to understand the process the researcher uses to perform data analyses. There are several stages in quantitative data analyses: (1) preparation of the data for analysis; (2) description of the sample; (3) testing the reliability of measurement methods; (4) exploratory analysis of the data; (5) confirmatory analyses guided by the hypotheses, questions, or objectives; and (6) post-hoc analyses. Although not all of these stages are equally reflected in the final published report of the study, they all contribute to the insights that can be gained from analysis of the data.

Preparation of the Data for Analysis

Except in very small studies, computers are almost universally used for data analyses. The first step of the process is entering the data into the computer. The researcher uses a systematic plan for data entry designed to reduce errors during the entry phase. After entry, the data are "cleaned." This process is time intensive and tedious but essential to ensuring the accuracy of the data. If the size of the data file allows, every datum on the printout is cross-checked with the original datum for accuracy. Otherwise, data points are randomly checked for accuracy. All identified errors are corrected. Missing data points are identified. If the information can be obtained, the missing data are entered into the data file. If data are missing on a large number of subjects in relation to specific variables, the researcher will have to determine whether there are sufficient data to perform analyses using those variables. In some cases, subjects must be excluded from an analysis because of missing data considered essential to that analysis.

IN CRITIQUING a study, search for information on the amount of missing data and clues to the accuracy of the data.

Description of the Sample

Next, the researcher obtains as complete a picture of the sample as possible. First, frequencies of descriptive variables related to the sample are obtained. Estimates of central tendency (such as the mean) and dispersion (such as the standard deviation) of variables relevant to the sample are calculated. Variables relevant to describing the sample might include age, education level, health status, gender, and ethnicity. If the study is composed of more than one sample, the researcher might compare the various groups in relation to these variables. For example, it might be important to know whether the age distribution of the various groups was similar. If the groups being compared are not equivalent in ways important to the study, the researcher needs to make a decision regarding the justification of continuing the analysis.

IN CRITIQUING a study, you need to judge the representativeness of the sample and the equivalence of groups that are compared in the statistical analyses.

Testing the Reliability of Measurement

Next, the researcher will examine the reliability of the measurement methods used in the study. Reliability of observational or physiologic measures may have been determined during the data collection phase but will be noted again at this point. If paper-and-pencil scales were used in data collection, alpha coefficients will be performed. If the coefficient is unacceptably low (below .70), the researcher must make a decision regarding the justification of performing an analysis using data from the instrument.

IN CRITIQUING a study, search for information on the reliability of measures used to gather data for the analyses.

Exploratory Analysis

The next step, *exploratory analysis,* is to examine all of the data descriptively. This step will be discussed in more detail later in the section "Using Statistics to Describe." The researcher must become as familiar as possible with the nature of the data obtained on variables that will be used to test hypotheses, research questions, or objectives. Data on each variable are examined using measures of central tendency and dispersion to determine the nature of variation in the data and to identify *outliers*—subjects with extreme values that seem unlike the rest of the sample. The most valuable insights from a study often come from careful examination of outliers (Tukey, 1977). In many studies, relationships among variables and differences between groups are explored using statistical procedures that are also used in confirmatory studies. However, when these procedures are used for exploratory purposes, the results are not generalized to a larger population, but rather are used to give a better understanding of the sample being examined.

IN CRITIQUING a study, examine the values obtained on variables. Do they appear to be representative of values you would expect to find in the population under study? Is the full range of values for each variable represented in the data? What is the nature of outliers in the sample? Is it likely that data from outliers affected the analysis results? Are analyses used for exploratory or confirmatory purposes?

Confirmatory Analyses

Confirmatory analysis is performed to confirm expectations regarding the data that are expressed as hypotheses, questions, or objectives. This step will be discussed in more detail later in the section "Statistics Used to Test Hypotheses." When confirmatory analyses are performed, the findings are generalized from the sample to appropriate populations. Statistical procedures designed for the purpose of making inferences (inferential statistical procedures) are used. To justify generalization of the results of confirmatory analyses, a rigorous research methodology is needed—including a strong research design, reliable and valid measurement methods, and a large sample size.

IN CRITIQUING a study, identify the confirmatory analyses performed. Is the research methodology sufficiently rigorous to warrant using confirmatory analyses?

Post-Hoc Analyses

Some statistical analyses, such as chi-square analyses and analyses of variance (ANOVA), are used to test for differences among groups in studies including more than two groups. These statistical procedures indicate significant differences among groups but do not specify which groups are different. For example, a study might examine the proportion of the sample who smoked in four occupational groups to determine differences in smoking behavior among the groups. Chi-square analysis or ANOVA might indicate that there were significant differences among the groups, but the researcher would not be able to determine which groups were different. In these studies, when significant differences are found, *post-hoc analyses* using statistical procedures specific to this purpose are performed after the initial statistical analyses to identify the specific groups that are different.

IN CRITIQUING a study, you need to identify the specific post-hoc analyses that are used. These should be indicated in the research report.

The Reasoning Behind Statistics

One reason that nurses tend to avoid statistics is that many were taught only the mathematical procedures of calculating statistical equations, with little or no explanation of the logic behind those procedures or the meaning of the results. Computation is a mechanical process usually performed by a computer, and information about the calculation procedure is not necessary to begin understanding statistical results. We will approach data analysis from the perspective of enhancing the reader's understanding of the meaning underlying statistical analysis. This understanding can then be used to critique data analyses or results sections of research reports.

The ensuing discussion presents a brief explanation of some of the concepts commonly used in statistical theory. The concepts presented include probability theory, decision theory, hypothesis testing, level of significance, inference, generalization, the normal curve, tailedness, Type I and Type II errors, power, and degrees of freedom. For a more extensive discussion of these topics, see Burns and Grove (1997).

Probability Theory

Probability theory, which is deductive, is used to explain the extent of a relationship, the probability of an event's occurring in a given situation, or the probability of accurately predicting an event. The researcher might be interested in the probability that a particular outcome will result from a nursing action. For example, the researcher might want to know the probability that urinary catheterization during hospitalization will lead to a bladder infection after discharge from the hospital. The researcher might want to know the probability that subjects in the experimental group are actually members of the same larger population from which the control group subjects were taken. Probability is expressed as a lowercase letter p, with values expressed as percentages or as a decimal value ranging from 0 to 1. If the exact probability is known, for example, to be .23, this would be expressed as $p = .23$. This means that there is a 23% probability that a particular outcome (such as a bladder infection) will occur. Probability values could be expressed as less than a specific probability value such as .05, expressed as $p < .05$. (The symbol $<$ means "less than.") The researcher could state in a research report the finding that the probability that the experimental group subjects were members of the same larger population as the control group subjects was less than or equal to 5% ($\leq .05$). Probability values are often given in reporting the results of statistical analyses. Thus, in critiquing studies, it is useful to be able to recognize these symbols and understand what they mean.

Decision Theory, Hypothesis Testing, and Level of Significance

Decision theory, which is inductive, assumes that all of the groups in a study (such as experimental and control groups) used to test a particular hypothesis are components of the same population in relation to the variables under study. This expectation (or assumption) is traditionally expressed as a null hypothesis stating that there is no difference between (or among) the groups in a study in terms of the variables included in the hypothesis. It is up to the researcher to provide evidence that, in reality, there is a difference between the groups. For example, the researcher might hypothesize that there is no difference in the frequency of urinary tract infections after discharge from the hospital in patients who were catheterized during hospitalization and those who were not. To test the assumption of no difference, a cutoff point is selected prior to data collection. The cutoff point, referred to as alpha (α), or the *level of significance*, is the probability level at which the results of statistical analysis are judged to indicate a statistically significant difference between the groups. The level of significance selected for most nursing studies is .05. This means that if the level of significance found as a result of the statistical analyses is $\leq$ .05, the experimental and control groups are considered to be significantly different (members of different populations). In some studies, the more rigorous level of significance of .01 may be chosen. This may be indicated in some studies, particularly on tables and figures, as $\alpha = .01$.

Decision theory requires that the cutoff point selected for a study be absolute. Absolute means that even if the value obtained is only a fraction above the cutoff point, the samples are considered to be from the same population and *no* meaning can be attributed to the differences. Thus, it is inappropriate when using decision theory to state that the findings *approached* significance at the .051 level if the alpha level was set at .05. Using decision theory rules, this finding indicates that the groups tested are not significantly different, and the null hypothesis is not rejected. On the other hand, once the level of significance has been set at .05 by the researcher, if the analysis reveals a significant difference of .001, this result is not considered more significant than the .05 originally proposed (Slakter, Wu, & Suzaki-Slakter, 1991). The level of significance is dichotomous; it is either significant or not significant; there are no degrees of significance. However, some individuals, not realizing that their reasoning has shifted from decision theory to probability theory, indicate in their research report that the .001 result makes the findings more significant than if they had obtained only a .05 level of significance. The researcher might state that the findings are "highly" significant, which is unacceptable from the perspective of decision theory.

From the perspective of probability theory, there is considerable difference in the risk of a Type II error between a probability of .05 and .001. If $p = .001$, the probability that the two groups are components of the same population is 1 in 1,000 compared with $p = .05$, which indicates that the probability of the groups belonging to the same population is 5 in 100. In other words if $p = .05$, 5 times out of 100, groups with statistical values such as those found in the statistical analyses are actually members of the same population, and the conclusion that the groups are different is erroneous.

In computer analysis, the probability value obtained from each data analysis (e.g., $p = .03$ or $p = .07$) is frequently provided on the printout and is often reported by the researcher in the published study, as is the level of significance set prior to the analysis. The probability (p) value will tell you the risk of a Type II error. The alpha (α) value will tell you whether the probability value for a particular analysis met the cutoff point for deciding whether there is a significant difference between or among groups.

IN CRITIQUING a study, you need to identify the level of significance and determine whether the findings show significant differences. You need to judge the risk of a Type II error. (Type I and Type II errors are defined and discussed later in the chapter.)

Inference and Generalization

An *inference* is a conclusion or judgment based on evidence. Statistical inferences are made cautiously and with great care. The decision theory rules related to interpreting the results of statistical procedures increase the probability that inferences are accurate. A *generalization* is the application of information to a general situation that has been acquired from a specific instance. One must infer in order to make a generalization; both require the use of inductive reasoning. Inductively, one infers from a specific case to a general truth, from a part to the whole, from the concrete to the abstract, and from the known to the unknown. In research, one infers from the study findings obtained from a specific sample to a more general population, using information obtained through statistical analyses. Thus, the researcher might conclude in a research report that a significant difference in the number of urinary tract infections was found between a sample of patients who had been catheterized during hospitalization and a sample who had not, and that this difference could be expected in all patients who had been cared for in hospitals. The findings are generalized from the sample studied to all previously hospitalized patients. Statisticians and researchers can never prove things using inferential reasoning; they can never be certain that their inferences and generalizations are correct. For example, the researcher's generalization of the incidence of urinary tract infection may not be carefully thought out; the findings may be generalized to too broad a population. It is possible that in the more general population, there is no difference in the incidence of urinary tract infection based on whether the patient was catheterized.

IN CRITIQUING a study, you must judge whether generalizations made by the researcher are justified based on the study results.

The Normal Curve

The theoretical *normal curve* is an expression of statistical theory (Fig. 10-1). It is a theoretical frequency distribution of all *possible* values in a population;

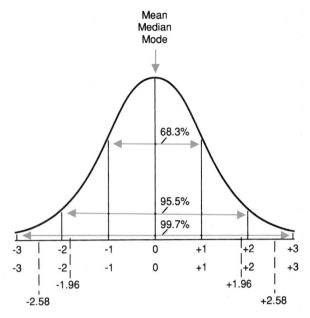

FIGURE 10-1
The normal curve.

however, no *real* distribution exactly fits the normal curve. The idea of the normal curve was developed by an 18-year-old mathematician, Johann Gauss, in 1795. He found that data from variables measured repeatedly in many samples from the same population (such as the mean of each sample) can be combined into one large sample. From this large sample, one can develop a more accurate representation of the pattern of the curve in that population than is possible with only one sample. Surprisingly, in most cases, the curve is similar, regardless of the specific variables examined or the population studied.

Levels of significance and probability levels are based on the logic of the normal curve. This normal curve in Figure 10-1 shows the distribution of values for a single population. Notice that 95.5% of the values are within 2 standard deviations of the mean, ranging from −2 to +2 standard deviations. (Standard deviations are defined and discussed in the section "Using Statistics to Describe.") Thus, there is approximately a 95% probability that a given measured value (e.g., the mean of a group) would fall within 2 standard deviations of the population mean, and there is a 5% probability that the value would fall in the tails of the normal curve (the extreme ends of the normal curve—below −2 standard deviations [2.5%] or above +2 standard deviations [2.5%]). If groups being compared were from the same population (not significantly different), you would expect the value (e.g., the mean) of each group to fall within the 95% range of values on the normal curve. If the groups were from (significantly) different populations, you would expect one of the group values to be outside the 95% range of values. A statistical analysis performed to determine differences between or among groups, using a level of significance set at .05, would test that expectation. If the statistical test indicates a significant difference (the value of one group does not fall within the 95% range of values), the groups are considered to belong to different populations. However, in 5% of the statistical tests, the value of one of the groups can be expected to fall outside the 95% range of values but still belong to the same population (a Type I error).

Tailedness

Nondirectional hypotheses usually assume that an extreme score (obtained because the group with the extreme score did not belong to the same population) can occur in either tail of the normal curve (Fig. 10-2). If the hypothesis is nondirectional, the analysis is referred to as a *two-tailed test of significance*. In a *one-tailed test of significance*, the hypothesis is directional, and extreme statistical values that occur on a single tail of the curve are of interest. The hypothesis states that the extreme score is higher or lower than that of 95% of the population, indicating that the sample with the extreme score is not a member of the same population. In this case, all 5% of statistical values that are considered significant will be in one tail. Extreme statistical values occurring on the other tail of the curve are not considered significantly different. In Figure

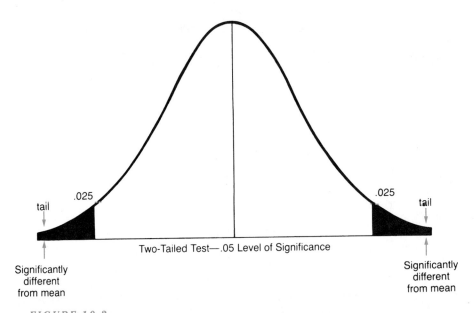

FIGURE 10-2

The two-tailed test of significance.

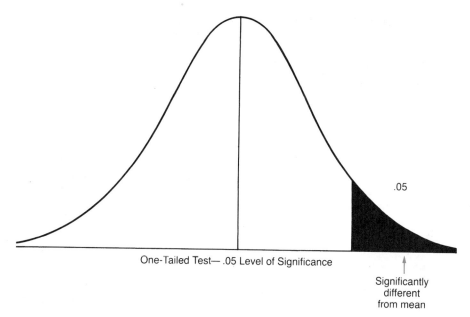

One-Tailed Test— .05 Level of Significance

.05

Significantly
different
from mean

FIGURE 10-3
The one-tailed test of significance.

10-3, which is a one-tailed figure, the portion of the curve in which statistical values will be considered significant is the right tail. Developing a one-tailed hypothesis requires that the researcher have sufficient knowledge of the variables to predict whether the difference will be in the tail above the mean or in the tail below the mean. One-tailed statistical tests are uniformly more powerful than two-tailed tests, decreasing the possibility of a Type II error.

IN CRITIQUING a study, determine whether there are one-tailed or two-tailed hypotheses. If the researcher states a one-tailed hypothesis, judge whether there is sufficient knowledge on which to base a one-tailed statistical test.

Type I and Type II Errors

According to decision theory, two types of error can occur in making decisions about the meaning of a value obtained from a statistical test: Type I and Type II. A *Type I error* occurs when the null hypothesis is rejected when it is true (e.g., when the results indicate that there is a significant difference when, in reality, there is not). The risk of a Type I error is indicated by the level of significance. There is a greater risk of a Type I error with a .05 level of significance

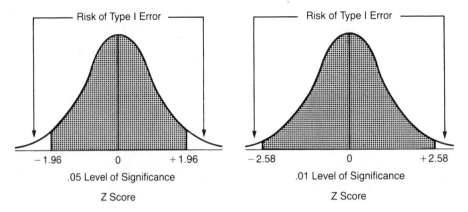

FIGURE 10-4
Risk of Type I error.

than with a .01 level of significance. As the level of significance becomes more extreme, the risk of a Type I error decreases, as illustrated in Figure 10-4.

A *Type II error* occurs when the null hypothesis is regarded as true when in fact it is false. For example, the statistical analyses might indicate that there were not significant differences between groups when, in reality, the groups were different. There is a greater risk of a Type II error with a .01 than with a .05 level of significance. However, Type II errors are often a consequence of flaws in the research methods. In nursing research, many studies are conducted with small samples and with instruments that are not precise measures of the variables under study. In many nursing situations, multiple variables interact to lead to differences within populations. However, when one is examining only a few of the interacting variables, small differences can be overlooked, leading to a false conclusion that there are no differences between the samples. Thus, the risk of a Type II error is high in many nursing studies.

IN CRITIQUING a study, evaluate the risk of a Type I or Type II error.

Power—Controlling the Risk of a Type II Error

Power is the probability that a statistical test will detect a significant difference that exists. The risk of a Type II error can be determined using *power analysis.* Cohen (1988) has identified four parameters of a power analysis: the level of significance, sample size, power, and effect size. If three of the four are known, the fourth can be calculated using power analysis formulas. The minimum acceptable power level is .80. The level of significance and sample size are determined by the researcher. *Effect size* is "the degree to which the phenomenon is present in the population, or the degree to which the null hypothesis is false" (Cohen, 1988, pp. 9–10). For example, if one were measuring changes in anxiety level in a group of preoperative patients, measured first when the patients were at home and then just prior to surgery, effect size would be large if a great change in anxiety occurred in the group across the two time periods. If one were examining the effect of a preoperative teaching program on amount of anxiety, the effect size would be the difference in the posttest level of anxiety in the experimental group compared with that in the control group. If only a small change in the level of anxiety was expected, the effect size would be small. In most nursing studies, only small effect sizes can be expected; larger samples are required to detect differences. The power level should be reported in studies that fail to reject the null hypothesis (or have nonsignificant findings). If the power level is below .80, you should question the validity of nonsignificant findings.

IN CRITIQUING a study, look for reports of the effect size and the power level.

Degrees of Freedom

The concept of *degrees of freedom* (*df*) is important in calculating statistical procedures and in interpreting the results using statistical tables. However, it is difficult to explain because of the complex mathematics involved. Degrees of freedom involve the freedom of a score's value to vary given the other existing scores' values and the established sum of these scores. Degrees of freedom are often indicated in reporting statistical results.

Using Statistics to Describe

Data analysis begins with *descriptive statistics* (also called "summary statistics") in any study in which the data are numerical. For some descriptive studies, descriptive statistics are the only approach to analysis of the data. For other studies, descriptive statistics are used primarily as a means to describe the characteristics of the sample from which the data were collected and to describe values obtained from the measurement of variables. Descriptive statistics presented include frequency distributions, measures of central tendency, measures of dispersion, and standardized scores.

Frequency Distributions

Frequency distribution is usually the first strategy used to organize the data for examination. There are two types of frequency distribution: ungrouped and grouped.

Ungrouped Frequency Distribution

Most studies have some categorical data that are presented in the form of an *ungrouped frequency distribution,* in which a table is developed to display all numerical values obtained on a particular variable, with each datum shown. This approach is generally used on discrete rather than continuous data. Examples of data commonly organized in this manner include gender, ethnicity, marital status, diagnostic category of study subjects, and values obtained from the measurement of variables. In Table 10-1, LoBiondo-Wood, Williams, Wood, and Shaw (1997) present the ungrouped frequency of subject characteristics in their study of the impact of liver transplantation on quality of life.

Grouped Frequency Distribution

Grouped frequency distributions are used when continuous variables, such as age, are being examined. Many measures taken during data collection are continuous, including temperature, vital lung capacity, weight, scale scores, and time. Any method of grouping results in loss of information. For example, if age is grouped, a breakdown of under 65 and over 65 provides considerably less information about the data than groupings of 10-year spans. As with levels of measurement, rules have been established to guide classification systems. There should be at least 6 but not more than 20 groups. The classes established must be exhaustive; each datum must fit into one of the identified classes. The classes must be exclusive; each datum must fit into only one. A common mistake occurs when the ranges contain overlaps that would allow a datum to fit into more than one class. For example, the researcher might have classified age ranges as 20 to 30, 30 to 40, 40 to 50, and so on. In this case, subjects aged 30, 40, and so on could have been classified into more than one class. The range of each class must be equivalent; with age, for example, if 10 years is the range, each class must include 10 years of ages. This rule is violated in some cases to allow the first and last categories to be open-ended and worded to include all scores above or below a specified point. In Table 10-1, "Income" is a grouped frequency.

Percentage Distributions

Percentage distributions indicate the percentage of the sample whose scores fall into a specific group, as well as the number of scores in that group. Percentage distributions are particularly useful in comparing the present data with findings

TABLE 10-1. Subject Characteristics		
Variable	*n*	*Percentage*
Gender		
Male	19	46.3
Female	22	53.7
Marital status		
Single	4	9.8
Married	32	78.0
Divorced	4	9.8
Widowed	1	2.4
Education		
High school	18	43.9
Attended/completed college	12	29.3
Attended/completed graduate school	10	24.4
Income—Family		
Below 20,000	14	34.4
20,001–30,000	6	14.6
30,001–40,000	7	17.1
40,001–50,000	5	12.2
50,001–60,000	3	7.3
Above 60,000	3	7.3
Diagnosis		
Cirrhosis	24	58.5
Primary biliary cirrhosis	8	19.5
Primary sclerosing cholangitis	7	17.1
Secondary biliary cirrhosis	1	2.4
Malignancy	1	2.4
Occupation		
Unemployed	20	48.8
Laborer	6	14.6
Semiskilled	2	4.9
Skilled	1	2.4
Clerical	2	4.9
Semiprofessional	2	4.9
Minor/lesser professional	6	14.6
Professional	3	7.3

From LoBiondo-Wood, G., Williams, L., Wood, R. P., & Shaw, B. W. (1997). Impact of liver transplantation on quality of life: A longitudinal perspective. *Applied Nursing Research, 10*(1), 29, with permission.

from other studies that have varying sample sizes. The percentage distribution is provided for each variable in Table 10-1. A cumulative distribution is a type of percentage distribution in which the percentages and frequencies of scores are summed as one moves from the top of the table to the bottom. Thus, the bottom category would have a cumulative frequency equivalent to the sample size and a cumulative percentage of 100 (Table 10-2). Frequency distributions are also displayed using tables or graphs (e.g., pie charts, bar charts, histograms, and frequency polygons). Graphic displays of the grouped frequency distribution of data from Table 10-2 are presented in Figure 10-5.

| | | | Cumulative | Cumulative |
Score	Frequency	Percent	Frequency (f)	Percent
1	4	8	4	8
3	6	12	10	20
4	8	16	18	36
5	14	28	32	64
7	8	16	40	80
8	6	12	46	92
9	4	8	N = 50	100

TABLE 10-2. Example of a Cumulative Frequency Table

Measures of Central Tendency

A *measure of central tendency* is frequently referred to as an "average"—a lay term not commonly used in statistics because it is vague. The measures of central tendency are the most concise statement of the nature of the data; the three that are commonly used in statistical analyses are the mode, median, and mean. In the normal curve, these are equal (see Fig. 10-1); however, there are usually differences in these three values in data obtained from real samples.

Mode

The *mode* is the numerical value or score that occurs with greatest frequency; it does not necessarily indicate the center of the data set. The mode can be determined by examination of an ungrouped frequency distribution of the data. In Table 10-2, the mode is the score of 5, which occurred 14 times in the data set. The mode can be used to describe the typical subject or to identify the most frequently occurring value on a scale item. The mode is the appropriate measure of central tendency for nominal data. A data set can have more than one mode. If two modes exist, the data set is referred to as "bimodal," as illustrated in Figure 10-6. More than two modes would be multimodal.

Median

The *median* is the score at the exact center of the ungrouped frequency distribution—the 50th percentile. The median is obtained by rank ordering the scores. If the number of scores is uneven, exactly 50% of the scores are above the median and 50% are below it. If the number of scores is even, the median is the average of the two middle scores; thus, the median may not be an actual score in the data set. The median is not affected by extreme scores in the data (outliers), as is the mean. The median is the most appropriate measure of central tendency for ordinal data. The median for the data in Table 10-2 is 5.

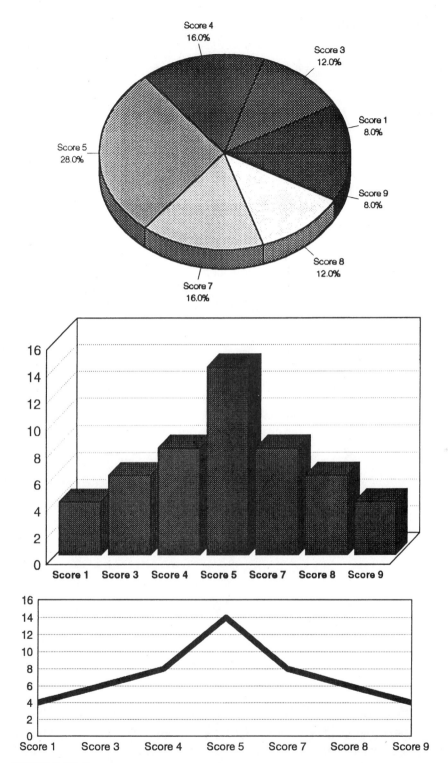

FIGURE 10-5
Commonly used graphic displays of frequencies distribution.

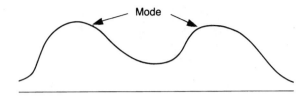

FIGURE 10-6
Bimodal distribution.

Mean

The most commonly used measure of central tendency is the mean. The *mean* is the sum of the scores divided by the number of scores being summed. Thus, like the median, the mean may not be a member of the data set. The mean is the appropriate measure of central tendency for interval and ratio level data. The mean for the data in Table 10-2 is 5.28.

Measures of Dispersion

Measures of dispersion, or variability, are measures of individual differences of the members of the sample. They give some indication of how scores in a sample are dispersed around the mean. These measures provide information about the data that is not available from measures of central tendency. They indicate how different the scores are—the extent to which individual scores deviate from one another. If the individual scores are similar, measures of variability are small, and the sample is relatively homogeneous, or similar, in terms of those scores. A heterogeneous sample has a wide variation in scores. The measures of dispersion most commonly used are range, variance, and standard deviation. Standardized scores may be used to express measures of dispersion. Scatterplots are frequently used to illustrate the dispersion in the data.

Range

The simplest measure of dispersion is the *range*, which is obtained by subtracting the lowest score from the highest score. The range for the scores in Table 10-2 is calculated as follows: 9   1 = 8. The range is a difference score, which uses only the two extreme scores for the comparison. It is a very crude measure and is sensitive to outliers.

Variance

The *variance* is calculated using a mathematical equation. The numerical value obtained from the calculation is dependent upon the measurement scale used; it has no absolute value and can be compared only with data obtained using similar measures. Generally, however, the larger the variance, the larger the dispersion of scores. The variance for the data in Table 10-2 is 4.94.

Standard Deviation

The *standard deviation* is the square root of the variance. Just as the mean is the average score, the standard deviation is the average difference (deviation) score. The standard deviation provides a measure of the average deviation of a score from the mean in that particular sample. It indicates the degree of error that would be made if the mean alone were used to interpret the data. In the normal curve, 68% of the scores will be within 1 standard deviation above or below the mean, 95% will be within 2 standard deviations above or below the mean, and 99% will be within 3 standard deviations above or below the mean (see Fig. 10-1).

The standard deviation for the data in Table 10-2 is 2.22. Because we know that the mean is 5.28, we can determine that the score of a subject 1 standard deviation below the mean would be $5.28 - 2.22$ (3.06). The score of a subject 1 standard deviation above the mean would be $5.28 + 2.22$ (7.50). Thus, we know that approximately 68% of the sample (and perhaps the population from which it was derived) can be expected to have scores in the range of 3.06 to 7.50. Extending this calculation further, the score of a subject 2 standard deviations above the mean would be $5.28 + 2.22 + 2.22$ (9.72). Using this strategy, the entire distribution of scores can be estimated. The score of a single individual can be compared with the scores of the total sample. Standard deviation is an important measure, both for understanding dispersion within a distribution and for interpreting the relationship of a particular score to the distribution.

Standardized Scores

Because of differences in the characteristics of various distributions, comparing a score in one distribution with a score in another is difficult. Let's say, for example, that you wanted to compare test scores from two classroom examinations. The highest possible score in one test was 100 and in the other 70; the scores would be difficult to compare. To facilitate this comparison, a mechanism was developed to transform raw scores into *standardized scores.* Numbers that make sense only within the framework of measurements used within a specific study are transformed into numbers (standardized scores) that have a more general meaning. Transformation into standardized scores allows an easy conceptual grasp of the meaning of the score. A common standardized score is called a *Z-score.* It expresses deviations from the mean (difference scores) in terms of standard deviation units (see Fig. 10-1). A score that falls above the mean will have a positive Z-score, whereas a score that falls below the mean will have a negative Z-score. The mean expressed as a Z-score is zero. The standard deviation is equal to the Z-score. Thus, a Z-score of 2 indicates that the score from which it was obtained is 2 standard deviations above the mean. A Z-score of -0.5 indicates that the score was 0.5 standard deviations below the mean.

Scatterplots

A *scatterplot* has two scales: horizontal and vertical. Each scale is referred to as an "axis." The vertical scale is called the "Y axis"; the horizontal scale is the "X axis." A scatterplot can be used to illustrate the dispersion of scores on a variable. In this case, the X axis would represent the possible values of the variable. The Y axis would represent the number of times each value of the variable occurred in the sample. Scatterplots can also be used to illustrate the relationship of scores on one variable with scores on another. In this case, each axis would represent one variable. For example, if a graph was developed to illustrate the relationship between days of hospitalization and decubitus ulcer stage, the horizontal axis might represent days and the vertical axis decubitus ulcer stage. For each unit or subject, there is a value for X and a value for Y. The point at which the values of X and Y for a single subject intersect is plotted on the graph (Fig. 10-7). When the values for each subject in the sample have been plotted, the degree of relationship between the variables is revealed (Fig. 10-8).

In a published study, descriptive statistics are often reported in the text of the results section, usually in describing the sample and values obtained on

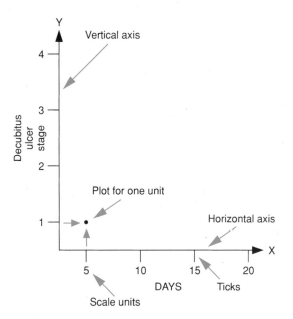

FIGURE 10-7
Structure of a plot.

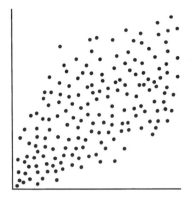

FIGURE 10-8
Example of a scatterplot.

study variables. However, in some studies, descriptive statistics may be summarized in a table. Froman and Owen (1997), in two related studies conducted to examine the validity of the AIDS Attitude Scale, used a table to report descriptive statistics. The sample of the first study included 21 baccalaureate-prepared practicing nurses who worked in a variety of clinical settings. The sample of the second study compared pediatric and adult care nurses practicing in intensive care units and general care settings. The results of descriptive analysis of these data are presented in Table 10-3.

TABLE 10-3. Means and SDs by Patient Age and Setting, Validity Study 2

| | Setting of Care | | | |
| | General Care | | ICU | |
Patient Age	M	SD	M	SD
Pediatric[a]				
Avoidance	2.09	0.60	1.99	0.75
Empathy	5.51	0.67	5.64	0.43
Adult[b]				
Avoidance	1.75	0.58	2.37	0.82
Empathy	5.67	0.41	5.09	0.74

[a]General care, $n = 16$; ICU, $n = 12$.
[b]General care, $n = 16$; ICU, $n = 20$.
From Froman, R. D., & Owen, S. V. (1997). Further validation of the AIDS Attitude Scale. *Research in Nursing & Health, 20*(2), 166. ©1997. Reprinted with permission of John Wiley and Sons, Inc.

Statistics Used to Test Hypotheses

In this section, some of the statistical procedures frequently used to test hypotheses or address research objectives or questions are briefly explained. The purpose of each procedure and the interpretation of the results are discussed. For a more detailed presentation of statistical procedures, see Burns and Grove (1997).

Chi-Square Test of Independence

The *chi-square test of independence* determines whether two variables are independent or related; it can be used with nominal or ordinal data. The procedure examines the frequencies of observed data and compares them with the frequencies that could be expected to occur if the data categories were actually independent of each other. The procedure is not very powerful; thus, the risk of a Type II error is high, and large samples are needed to reduce this risk. Therefore, most studies using this procedure place little importance on results in which no differences are found. Researchers frequently perform multiple chi-square tests in a sample. However, results are generally presented only for significant chi-square analyses.

Interpretation of Results

The result of the mathematical calculation is a chi-square statistic, which is compared with the chi-square values in a statistical table. If the value of the statistic is equal to or greater than the value identified in the chi-square statistical table, the researcher can conclude that there are significant differences between the two variables. The exact location of specific differences among categories of variables cannot be determined from this analysis. Post-hoc analyses can be used to determine in exactly which categories the differences lie. In some published studies, the researchers discuss the results as if they knew where the differences lie without having performed post-hoc analyses. Readers must view these reports with skepticism.

In a published study, chi-square results may be reported as text in the results section. Alexy, Nichols, Heverly, and Garzon (1997), in a study examining rural/urban differences in prenatal outcomes in the Public Health Service, compared the rural and urban groups using chi square analysis. A .05 level of significance was set for the study. Of particular interest was differences in the proportion of cesarean deliveries and vaginal deliveries. The authors report their findings as follows.

> "Method of delivery was significantly different between the rural and urban groups. In the rural group, 90 (24.9%) infants were delivered by cesarean section compared with 65 (15.7%) cesarean deliveries in the urban group, χ^2 ($df = 1$, $N = 776$) = 10.37, $p < .001$." (p. 65)

Often, the first reaction to a sentence such as this by those unfamiliar with reading statistical results is panic. The next reaction might be to avoid looking at the sentence and skip to the next one. Maybe it will make more sense. However, a sentence such as this provides a great deal of information in a small amount of space. Rather than trying to take in the entire sentence in one glance, examine the component parts first. In the component, "χ^2 $(df = 1, N = 776)$ $= 10.37, p <.001$)," the author is using chi-square analysis to compare the rural and urban groups. The author provides the information within the parentheses on degrees of freedom $(df = 1)$ and sample size $(N = 776)$ to enable the reader to validate the accuracy of the results using a statistical chi-square table. The numerical value after the parentheses, 10.37, is the chi-square value obtained from calculating the chi-square equation (probably using a computer). This value has no inherent meaning other than to determine significance on a statistical table. As noted earlier, the symbol p is the abbreviation for probability; the symbol $<$ means "less than." The groups were significantly different because p $<.001$ is below the cutoff point of .05. The phrase also indicates that the probability is less than .001 (.1%) that these groups come from the same population.

Chi-square results are sometimes provided within a table. Alexy and colleagues (1997) used a table as well as textual discussion to report chi-square results from their study. Table 10-4 indicates the results of chi-square analyses examining rural/urban differences among a number of variables examined in the study. The following text discusses the results presented in Table 10-4.

"Poor diet and low prepregnancy weight/inadequate weight gain were more prevalent in the rural group. The urban group had a higher incidence of previous abortion, cigarette use, drug use, maternal complications, and neonatal complications." (p. 65)

TABLE 10-4. Comparison of Prenatal/Perinatal Factors in Rural and Urban Samples

Variable	Rural (N = 364) n (%)	Urban (N = 415) n (%)	χ^2	df	p
Previous abortion	90 (24.9%)	181 (46.0%)	47.53	6	<.001
Cigarette use	54 (15.0%)	161 (38.8%)	54.45	1	<.001
Poor diet (by history)	317 (87.1%)	43 (10.4%)	459.26	1	<.001
Low prepregnancy wt./inadequate wt. gain	191 (52.5%)	85 (20.5%)	86.75	1	<.001
Neonatal complications	50 (13.9%)	161 (38.8%)	60.03	1	<.001
Maternal complications	90 (25.0%)	265 (63.9%)	117.24	1	<.001
History of emotional/physical abuse	2 (0.5%)	14 (3.4%)	7.69	1	.01
Drug use	3 (0.8%)	13 (3.1%)	5.04	1	.03

From Alexy, B., Nichols, B., Heverly, M. A., & Garzon, L. (1997). Prenatal factors and birth outcomes in the Public Health Service: A rural/urban comparison. *Research in Nursing & Health, 20*(1), 65. ©1997. Reprinted by permission of John Wiley and Sons, Inc.

t-*Tests*

One of the most common analyses used to test for significant differences between statistical measures of two samples is the t-*test*. A variety of *t*-tests have been developed for various types of samples. Frequently researchers misuse the *t*-test by using multiple *t*-tests to examine differences in various aspects of data collected in a study. When this is done, there is an escalation of significance that results in a greatly increased risk of a Type I error. Bonferroni's procedure, which controls for the escalation of significance, may be used when various *t*-tests must be performed on different aspects of the same data.

Interpretation of Results

The result of the mathematical calculation is a t statistic. This statistic is compared with the *t* values in a statistical table. The table is used to identify the critical value of *t*. If the computed statistic is equal to or greater than the critical value, the groups are significantly different.

Alexy and colleagues (1997) used a *t*-test to compare prenatal and demographic factors in rural and urban samples. They reported the results of the *t*-test in the text as follows.

"There were no between-group differences in alcohol use, hypertension, elevated glucose levels, previous preterm/low birth weight infant, history of previous fetal death, or maternal age less than 10 years." (p. 65)

Because they provided a table (Table 10-5) with the statistical results, these were not provided in the text. If the results of comparing mother's age, for example, had been presented in text, the discussion would have been presented as follows: There was a significant difference in mother's age ($t = 18.08$, $df = 1$, $p = .001$) between mothers living in rural areas and mothers living in urban areas.

The phrase ($t = 18.08$, $df = 1$, $p = .001$) tells you that the value of t obtained from calculating the *t*-test was 18.08, the degrees of freedom (df) was 1, and the results were significant since $p = .001$ is below the .05 cutoff. The t value, 18.08, has no meaning other than to determine the level of significance on a statistical table. In Table 10-5, the authors provide the mean (M) and standard deviation (SD) for each variable, as well as the t value and the p value. Providing this information allows another researcher to check the accuracy of the authors' analyses, to perform a power analysis, or to use the data in a meta-analysis. Because the authors used more than one *t*-test to examine data in the same sample, there is an increased risk of a Type I error.

TABLE 10-5. Comparison of Prenatal and Demographic Factors in Rural and Urban Samples

Variable	Rural (N = 364)		Urban (N = 415)		t	p
	M	*SD*	*M*	*SD*	*t*	*p*
Mother's age	22.03	4.88	23.61	5.33	18.08	<.001
Weeks gestation 1st visit	17.55	8.09	20.13	7.57	20.80	<.001
Gravidae	2.29	1.35	2.61	1.56	9.00	<.003
Birthweight (g)	3229	585	3335	583	6.21	<.02
Weeks gestation at delivery	39.06	2.05	39.37	1.84	4.65	<.03
Total # prenatal visits	8.34	4.30	8.86	3.33	3.56	<.06
Parity	1.02	1.14	0.90	1.19	1.32	<.25

From Alexy, B., Nichols, B., Heverly, M. A., & Garzon, L. (1997). Prenatal factors and birth outcomes in the Public Health Service: A rural/urban comparison. *Research in Nursing & Health, 20*(1), 65. ©1997. Reprinted by permission of John Wiley and Sons, Inc.

Pearson's Product-Moment Correlation

Pearson's product-moment correlation is a parametric test used to determine relationships among variables. *Bivariate correlation* measures the extent of relationship between two variables. Data are collected from a single sample, and measures of the two variables to be examined must be available for each subject in the data set. Less commonly, data are obtained from two related subjects, such as breast cancer incidence in mothers and daughters. Correlational analysis provides two pieces of information about the data: the nature of a relationship (positive or negative) between the two variables and the magnitude (or strength) of the relationship. Scatterplots are sometimes presented to illustrate the relationship graphically. The outcomes of correlational analyses are symmetrical rather than asymmetrical. "Symmetrical" means that there is no indication from the analysis of the direction of the relationship. One cannot say from the analysis that variable A leads to or causes variable B or that B causes A.

Interpretation of Results

The outcome of the Pearson product-moment correlation analysis is a correlation coefficient (*r*) value between −1 and +1. This *r* value indicates the degree of relationship between the two variables. A value of 0 indicates no relationship. A value of −1 indicates a perfect negative (inverse) correlation. In a negative relationship, a high score on one variable is related to a low score on the other variable. A value of +1 indicates a perfect positive relationship. In a positive relationship, a high score on one variable is related to a high score on the other variable. A positive correlation also exists when a low score on one variable is related to a low score on the other variable. As the negative or positive values of *r* approach 0, the strength of the relationship decreases. Traditionally, an *r* value of .1 to .3 is considered a weak relationship; .4 to .5 a moderate relationship; and above .5 a strong relationship (Burns & Grove, 1997). However, this interpretation depends to a great extent on the variables being examined and the situation in which they were observed. Therefore, interpretation requires some judgment on the part of the researcher.

When Pearson's correlation coefficient is squared (r^2), the resulting number is the percentage of variance explained by the relationship. Even when two variables are related, values of the two variables will not be a perfect match. For example, if two variables show a strong positive relationship, a high score on one variable can be expected to be associated with a high score on the other variable. However, a subject who has the highest score on one value will not necessarily have the highest score on the other variable. There will be some variation in the relationship of scores on the two variables for individual subjects. The amount of variation is indicated by r^2 and is expressed as a percentage. The author might state that the relationship of the two variables as expressed by r^2 explained 43% of the variance of scores in the two variables. This means that 57% of the variation in scores is due to something other than the relationship studied, perhaps variables not examined in the study.

There has been a tendency to disregard weak correlations in nursing research. This could result in overlooking a relationship that may have some meaning within nursing knowledge when examined in the context of other variables. This situation, which is similar to a Type II error, commonly occurs for three reasons. First, many nursing measurements are not powerful enough to detect fine discriminations. Some instruments may not detect extreme scores, and a relationship may be stronger than indicated by the crude measures available. Second, correlational studies must have a wide range of scores for relationships to be detected. If the study scores are homogeneous or the sample is small, relationships that exist in the population will not show up as clearly in the sample. Third, in many cases, bivariate analysis does not provide a clear picture of the dynamics in the situation. A number of variables can be linked through weak correlations, but together they provide increased insight into situations of interest. Statistical procedures (such as regression analysis) are available for examining the relationships among multiple variables concurrently.

Testing the Significance of a Correlation Coefficient

In order to infer that the sample correlation coefficient applies to the population from which the sample was taken, statistical analysis must be performed to determine whether the coefficient is significantly different from zero (no correlation). With a small sample, a very high correlation coefficient can be nonsignificant. With a very large sample, the correlation coefficient can be statistically significant when the degree of association is too small to be clinically significant. Therefore, in judging the significance of the coefficient, one must consider both the size of the coefficient and its statistical significance.

Berg, Dunbar-Jacob, and Sereika (1997) reported the results of correlation in a study of self-management of adults with asthma. In the study, two measures of adherence to the asthma protocol used in the study were correlated. One measure was the MDI Chronolog, a monitoring device designed to house a metered dose inhaler. Each time the inhaler was used, a microswitch was activated and the Chronolog recorded the date and time. The memory of the MDI Chronolog stored the date and time of each triggered activation within 4 seconds. These data were downloaded into a computer for storage and analysis. In a journal of daily asthma concerns, subjects were asked to provide information about medication-taking behavior daily. A correlational analysis was performed between the median value obtained from the MDI Chronolog and the median value obtained from the subject's reports of daily medication-taking behavior. The results are reported as follows:

> "When self-reported compliance and chronolog compliance was examined, median chronolog compliance was 37.5% as compared with a median asthma diary compliance of 93.1%. A modest correlation was documented between the two measures ($r = .44$). Of all subjects, 50% misrepresented their self-reported compliance—which suggests that self-report overestimates compliance with inhaled medications." (p. 233)

Tables are sometimes used to report the results of correlations, particularly when several variables have been correlated.

Topp, Estes, Dayhoff, and Suhrheinrich (1997) used a table (Table 10-6) to present the results of multiple correlations in a study of postural control, strength, and mood among older adults. Three protocols were used to measure postural control. The first two protocols measured postural control as a percentage of postural sway while the subjects stood still on the stable support surface of a computerized forceplate. Measures were collected both with eyes open and with eyes closed. Higher numbers indicated increased postural sway and poorer postural control. The third protocol measured stability while subjects shifted their center of gravity by leaning at the hips and/or ankles. Ankle and knee strength were measured using a Microfet (Hoggan Health Industries, Draper, UT) hand-held dynamometer with a 2-inch-diameter concave pressure distributing plate. "Subject mood was assessed by the Mood Rating Scale (MRS) which measures mood precursors to attention among older adults" (p. 14). Correlations were performed among the variables of age, mood, and strength. Correlational results for a number of variables presented in table form are referred to as a "correlation matrix." The reader could determine the percentage of variance explained by each relationship by squaring the value shown in Table 10-6.

continued

TABLE 10-6. Correlations Between Postural Control and Age, Strength, and Mood

| | | Postural Control | | |
| | | Postural Sway with | | Number of Targets Attained Set at 75% |
	Age	Eyes Opened	Eyes Closed	
Limits of Stability				
Strength				
Ankle dorsiflexion	−.07	−.32	−.21	.03
Ankle plantar flexion	−.28	−.28	−.25	−.03
Knee extension	−.05	−.05	−.03	.08
Mood				
Total mood	−.05	−.45*	−.35	.34
Alertness	−.11	−.50*	−.44*	.47*
Contentedness	−.17	−.25	−.11	.12
Calmness	.38*	−.18	−.12	−.05
Age		−.13	−.23	−.26

* = Pearson r correlation is significant at $p < .05$ level.
From Topp, R., Estes, P. K., Dayhoff, N., & Suhrheinrich, J. (1997). Postural control and strength and mood among older adults. *Applied Nursing Research, 10*(1), 15, with permission.

Analysis of Variance

Analysis of variance (ANOVA) tests for differences between means. ANOVA is more flexible than other analyses in that it can examine data from two or more groups. There are many types of ANOVA, some developed for analysis of data from complex experimental designs, such as those using blocking or repeated measures. Rather than focusing on differences between means, ANOVA tests for differences in variance. One source of variance is the variance within each group because individual scores in the group will vary from the group mean. This variance is referred to as the *within-group* variance. Another source of variation is variation of the group means around the grand mean, which is referred to as the *between-group* variance. One could assume that if all the samples were drawn from the same population, there would be little difference in these two sources of variance. When these two types of variance are combined, they are referred to as the *total* variance. The test for ANOVA is always one-tailed.

Interpretation of Results

The results of an ANOVA are reported as an *F* statistic. The *F* distribution table is used to determine the level of significance of the *F* statistic. If the *F* statistic is equal to or greater than the appropriate table value, there is a significant difference between the groups. If only two groups are being examined, the location of a significant difference is clear. However, if more than two groups are under study, it is not possible to determine from the ANOVA exactly where the significant differences lie. One cannot assume that all the groups examined are significantly different. Therefore, post-hoc analyses are conducted to determine the location of the differences among groups. The frequently used post-hoc tests are Bonferroni's procedure, Newman-Keuls' test, Tukey's Honestly Significantly Different (HSD) test, Scheffé's test, and Dunnett's test.

Russell and Champion (1996), in their study of home safety practices of mothers with preschool children, reported the results of an ANOVA to examine the effect of birth position on the mother's use of home safety practices. Would the parent be more careful and use more safety practices with their first child and then relax the use of these safety practices with later children, or would the parent learn from previous experience and thus use more safety practices with the second and third children? The authors report their findings as follows:

> "Birth position was analyzed across families of each target child. Birth position, which was categorized as youngest, middle, or oldest, was significant using ANOVA for both hazard accessibility and hazard frequency ($F = 8.73$, $df = 2,131$, $p \leq .001$). Post hoc analysis using Scheffé indicated that the oldest group was significantly different from the youngest and middle group. When the target child was the oldest, frequency of hazards in the home increased." (p. 61)

The value of F has no meaning other than to determine the level of significance on a statistical table. The p value (.001) indicates a significant difference in hazards in relation to age group. Because ANOVA is based on decision theory, the p value of .001 is not viewed as more important than a p value of .05. Each of these is interpreted as indicating that a decision that the groups are different is warranted. Note that because three groups were used, a post-hoc analysis was performed to determine the location of significant differences.

Sometimes, ANOVA results are reported in a table. Froman and Owen (1997) used a table to report the results of an ANOVA in their study designed to provide information on the validity of the AIDS Attitude Scale. They proposed that pediatric nurses would have more positive attitudes (higher empathy, lower avoidance) than adult care nurses. They administered the instrument to 28 pediatric nurses and 36 adult care nurses. Half of each group worked in an intensive care unit (ICU) and the other half worked on a floor setting. Table 10-7 presents their findings in an ANOVA summary table. The three sources of variance analyzed in ANOVA (between groups, within groups, and total) are given, as are the degrees of freedom (*df*) for each source of variance. The sum of squares (SS) and mean square (MS), values used in the process of performing

TABLE 10-7. ANOVA Summaries for Avoidance and Empathy

Dependent Variable	Source	SS	df	MS	F
Avoidance	Patient age	0.01	1	0.01	0.02
	Intensity	1.07	1	1.07	2.19
	Age × int.	2.02	1	2.02	4.15*
	Error	29.25	60	0.49	
Empathy	Patient age	0.59	1	0.59	1.63
	Intensity	0.79	1	0.79	2.19
	Age × int.	1.96	1	1.96	5.43*
	Error	21.66	60	0.36	

*$p < .05$.
From Froman, R. D., & Owen, S. V. (1997). Further validation of the AIDS Attitude Scale. *Research in Nursing & Health, 20*(2), 166. ©1997. Reprinted by permission of John Wiley and Sons, Inc.

an ANOVA, are provided. With these values, an individual could recalculate the *F* value to verify its accuracy. The *p* value is indicated by an asterisk beside the *F* value if the value is significant at the .05 level. Two ANOVAs were performed, one with Avoidance as the dependent variable and one with Empathy as the dependent variable. The authors discuss their results as follows.

"The results of the ANOVAs conducted in validity study 2 reveal a more complex relationship than had been expected, showing a joint effect of intensity of care and patient age on attitude. With further consideration, this finding is understandable in the context of construct validity. Nurses caring for children, regardless of their own risk of exposure, maintain similarly therapeutic and accepting attitudes. These attitudes are adequately sturdy and young patients are sufficiently attractive to counteract influences on attitude that might result from increased risks associated with ICU care. Nurses caring for noncritically ill adults (those experiencing illnesses requiring hospitalization but not fully debilitated) hold similar attitudes. Nurses in the non-ICU setting are likely to interact with their adult AIDS patients and know them as individuals. It is only the combination of adult patients and ICU setting, with its assumed advanced illness condition, that is associated with notably negative attitudes. In discussing these findings with practicing nurses they were not surprised at such results. Their interpretation, put simply, was that adult AIDS patients in ICU settings are repellent as a result of many diseases associated with AIDS (e.g., Kaposi's sarcoma, pneumocystic pneumonia). They are usually uncommunicative either because of apparatus (i.e., ventilator) or disease processes. Given these characteristics, the adult ICU AIDS patients lose opportunity to elicit the accepting attitudes that pediatric patients or alert adult patients experience." (Froman & Owen, 1997, p. 167)

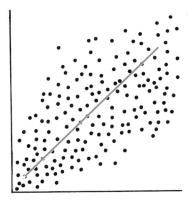

FIGURE 10-9
Overlay of scatterplot and best fit line.

Regression Analysis

Regression analysis is used to predict the value of one variable when we know the value of one or more other variables. The variable to be predicted is referred to as the "dependent variable." The dependent variable is usually measured at the interval level. The results of the analysis need to explain as much of the variance in the value of the dependent variable as possible. Variables used to predict values of the dependent variable are referred to as "independent variables." If there is more than one independent variable, the analysis is referred to as "multiple regression." In regression analysis, the symbol for the dependent variable is Y; the symbol for the independent variable(s) is X. Scatterplots and a bivariate correlation matrix are often developed prior to regression analysis to examine the relationships that exist in the variables. The purpose of the regression analysis is to develop a "line of best fit" that will best reflect the values illustrated on the scatterplot. The line of best fit is often illustrated as an overlay on the scatterplot (Fig. 10-9). Many types of regression analyses have been developed to analyze various types of data. One type, logistic regression, developed to predict values of a dependent variable measured at the ordinal level, is being used with increasing frequency in nursing studies.

Interpretation of Results

The outcome of a regression analysis is the regression coefficient R. When R is squared (R^2), it indicates the amount of variance in the data that is explained by the equation. When more than one independent variable is being used to predict values of the dependent variable, R^2 is sometimes referred to as the "coefficient of multiple determination." The test statistic used to determine the significance of a regression coefficient may be t or F. Small sample sizes decrease the possibility of obtaining statistical significance. In reporting the results of a regression analysis, the R^2 value and the t or F values are documented.

The calculated coefficient values may also be expressed as an equation. Many studies using regression analysis are complex, including multiple independent variables and involving more than one regression procedure. Understanding the discussion of complex results requires reading each sentence carefully for comprehension before proceeding to the next sentence.

Craft and Moss (1996) used regression analysis in their study of the accuracy of infant emesis volume assessment. In their study, carefully measured amounts of baby formula were poured on receiving blankets. Nurses and nursing students were asked to estimate the volume poured on each of 20 receiving blankets. Each nurse examined the blankets in the same order so that the researchers could determine if accuracy changed as the number of blankets examined by each nurse increased. Error was calculated as the difference between the volume actually poured on the blanket and the volume estimated by the nurse. The authors report the results of the regression analysis as follows:

> "Analysis with stepwise multiple regression using relative error per subject as the dependent measure showed that subject practice status (student versus practicing nurse), the nature of subject clinical experience, and number of displays assessed for weight accounted for a significant proportion of variance (Table 10-8). Nurses from large newborn nurseries underestimated 23% to 30%, whereas nurses from units with sick toddlers had a lower percentage of underestimation (M = −.13). These data show that the nature of experience, rather than the length of experience, could be important. Only a small portion of the variance (R^2 = .19) in mean relative error per subject was accounted for by the variables studied, indicating the need for further study of other variables that must also influence the accuracy of visual assessment in emesis volume determination." (p. 6)

TABLE 10-8. Stepwise Multiple Regression of Independent Variables on Mean Relative Error

Variable	R	R^2	R^2 Increase	F	p
Subject practice role (student vs. practicing nurse)	.26	.07	.07	7.55	.007
Nature of clinical practice	.36	.13	.06	7.53	.001
Number of displays assessed for weight	.36	.19	.06	7.21	.001

From Craft, M. J., & Moss, J. (1996). Accuracy of infant emesis volume assessment. *Applied Nursing Research, 9*(1), 6, with permission.

Other Statistical Procedures

Nurse researchers are using a variety of statistical techniques to examine complex multivariate data. Two of these, analysis of covariance (ANCOVA) and factor analysis, are briefly described. For discussion of additional types of statistical analyses, see Burns and Grove (1997).

Analysis of Covariance

Analysis of covariance (ANCOVA) allows the researcher to examine the effect of a treatment apart from the effect of one or more potentially confounding variables (see Chapter 3 for a discussion of confounding variables). Potentially confounding variables commonly of concern include pretest scores and variables such as age, education, social class, and anxiety level. These variables would be confounding if they were not measured and if their effect on study variables were not statistically removed prior to the planned statistical analyses by performing regression analysis prior to performing ANOVA. This strategy removes the effect of differences between groups that is due to a confounding variable. Once this effect is removed, the effect of the treatment can be examined more precisely. This technique is sometimes used as a method of statistical control when it is not possible to design the study to control for potentially confounding variables. However, control through careful planning of the design is more effective than statistical control.

ANCOVA may be used in pretest-posttest designs in which differences occur in groups on the pretest. For example, individuals who achieve low scores on a pretest tend to have lower scores on the posttest than those whose pretest scores were higher, even if the treatment had a significant effect on posttest scores. Conversely, if an individual achieves a high pretest score, it is doubtful that the posttest will indicate a strong change as a result of the treatment. ANCOVA maximizes the capacity to detect differences in such cases.

Factor Analysis

Factor analysis examines interrelationships among large numbers of variables and disentangles those relationships to identify clusters of variables that are most closely linked. Intellectually, you might do this by identifying categories and sorting the variables according to your judgment of the most appropriate category. Factor analysis sorts the variables into categories according to how closely related they are to the other variables. Closely related variables are grouped together into a "factor." Several factors may be identified within a data set. Once the factors have been identified mathematically, the researcher must interpret the results by explaining why the analysis grouped the variables in a specific way. Statistical results will indicate the amount of variance in the data set explained by a particular factor and the amount of variance in the factor explained by a particular variable. Factor analysis aids in the identification of theoretical constructs; it is also used to confirm the accuracy of a theoretically developed construct. For example, a theorist might state that the concept (or construct) "hope" consisted of the elements (1) anticipation of the future, (2) belief that things will work out for the best, and (3) optimism. Ways could be developed to measure these three elements, and a factor analysis could be conducted on the data to determine whether subject responses clustered into these three groupings. Factor analysis is frequently used in the process of developing measurement instruments, particularly those related to psychological variables such as attitudes, beliefs, values, and opinions. The instrument operationalizes a theoretical construct. Factor analysis can also be used to attempt to sort out meaning from large numbers of questions on survey instruments.

Judging Statistical Suitability

Multiple factors are involved in determining the suitability of a statistical procedure for a particular study. These include (1) the purpose of the study; (2) hypotheses, questions, or objectives; (3) design; and (4) level of measurement. Determining the suitability of various statistical procedures for a particular study is not straightforward. Regrettably, there is not usually one "right" statistical procedure for a particular study.

IN CRITIQUING suitability, you must not only be familiar with the statistical procedure used in the study but must also compare that procedure with others that could have been used, perhaps to greater advantage. You must judge whether the procedure was performed appropriately and the results interpreted correctly.

Evaluating statistical procedures requires that you make a number of judgments regarding the nature of the data and what the researcher wanted to know. You need to determine (1) whether the data for analysis were treated as nominal, ordinal, or interval; (2) the number of groups in the study; and (3) whether the groups were dependent or independent. In *independent groups,* the selection of one subject is totally unrelated to the selection of other subjects. For example, if subjects are randomly assigned to treatment and control groups, the groups are independent. In *dependent groups,* subjects or observations selected for data collection are related in some way to the selection of other subjects or observations. For example, if subjects serve as their own control by using the pretest as a control, the observations (and therefore the groups) are dependent. Also, if matched pairs of subjects are used for control or treatment groups, the observations are dependent. For example, in a study of twins, one twin might be placed in the control group and the other in the treatment group. Because they are twins, they are matched on several variables.

One approach to judging the appropriateness of an analysis technique for a critique is to use an algorithm, which directs you by gradually narrowing the number of appropriate statistical procedures as you make judgments about the nature of the study and the data. An algorithm that has been helpful in judging the appropriateness of statistical procedures is presented in Figure 10-10. This algorithm identifies four factors related to the appropriateness of a statistical procedure: the research question, level of measurement, design, and type of sample. To use the algorithm in Figure 10-10, (1) determine whether the research question focuses on differences (I) or associations (relationships) (II), (2) determine the level of measurement (A, B, or C), (3) select the design listed that most closely fits the study you are critiquing (1, 2, or 3), and (4) determine whether the study samples are independent (a), dependent (b), or mixed (c). Follow the lines on the algorithm through your selections to identify the appropriate statistical procedure.

Interpreting Statistical Outcomes

To be useful, the evidence from data analysis must be carefully examined, organized, and given meaning. Evaluating the entire research process, organizing the meaning of the results, and forecasting the usefulness of the findings, all of which are involved in interpretation, require high-level intellectual processes. In this segment of a study, the researcher translates the results of analysis into findings and then interprets them by attaching meaning to the findings.

Within the process of interpretation are several intellectual activities that can be isolated and explored, including examining evidence, forming conclusions, considering implications, exploring the significance of the findings, generalizing the findings, and suggesting further studies. This information is usually included in the final section of published studies, which often is entitled "Discussion."

Types of Results

Interpretation of results from quasi-experimental and experimental studies is traditionally based on decision theory, with five possible results: (1) significant results that are in keeping with those predicted by the researcher, (2) nonsignificant results, (3) significant results that are opposite those predicted by the researcher, (4) mixed results, and (5) unexpected results. In critiquing a study, you need to indicate which of these types of results were found.

Significant and Predicted Results

Significant results are in keeping with those predicted by the researcher and support the logical links developed by the researcher between the framework, questions, variables, and measurement tools. However, you need to consider

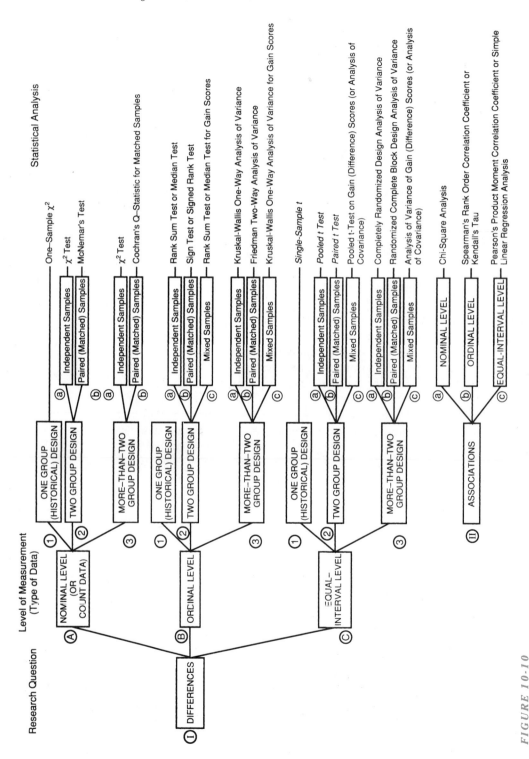

FIGURE 10-10

Algorithm for choosing a statistical test. (From Knapp, R. B. [1985]. *Basic Statistics for Nurses.* Albany, NY: Delmar. Reproduced by permission.)

the possibility of alternative explanations for the positive findings. What other elements could possibly have led to the significant results?

Nonsignificant Results

Nonsignificant (or inconclusive) *results,* often referred to as "negative results," could be a true reflection of reality. In this case, the reasoning of the researcher or the theory used by the researcher to develop the hypothesis is in error. If so, the negative findings are an important addition to the body of knowledge. The results could also be a Type II error due to inappropriate methods, a biased sample, a small sample, problems with internal validity, inadequate measurement, weak statistical measures, or faulty analysis. If so, the reported results could introduce faulty information into the body of knowledge (Angell, 1989). Negative results do not mean that no relationships exist among the variables; they indicate that the study failed to find any. Nonsignificant results provide no evidence of either the truth or the falsity of the hypothesis.

Significant and Unpredicted Results

Significant results opposite those predicted indicate flaws in the logic of both the researcher and the theory being tested. However, if the results are valid, they are an important addition to the body of knowledge. An example would be a study in which social support and ego strength were proposed to be positively related. If the study showed that high social support was related to low ego strength, the result would be opposite that predicted.

Mixed Results

Mixed results are probably the most common outcome of studies. In this case, one variable may uphold predicted characteristics while another does not, or two dependent measures of the same variable may show opposite results. These differences may be due to methodology problems, such as differing reliability or sensitivity of two methods of measuring variables. The mixed results may also indicate the need to modify existing theory.

Unexpected Results

Unexpected results are usually relationships found between variables that were not hypothesized and not predicted from the framework being used. Most researchers examine as many elements of data as possible in addition to those directed by the questions. These findings can be useful in theory development or modification of existing theory and in the development of later studies. In addition, serendipitous results are important as evidence in developing the implications of the study. However, serendipitous results must be dealt with carefully in considering meaning because the study was not designed to examine these results.

Findings

Results in a study are translated and interpreted; then they become *findings,* which are a consequence of evaluating evidence. Although much of the process of developing findings from results occurs in the mind of the researcher, evidence of the thinking can be found in published research reports.

IN CRITIQUING a study, you need to identify the findings and evaluate the linkages between statistical results and the findings expressed by the researcher.

Milligan, Flenniken, and Pugh's (1996) study, "Positioning intervention to minimize fatigue in breastfeeding women," presents the following hypothesis, results, and findings.

Hypothesis

"It was hypothesized that postpartum women who breastfeed in the side-lying position would report less fatigue symptoms than women in the sitting position." (p. 68)

Results

"To compare fatigue scores for each position (sitting and side-lying), a paired *t* test was used. Paired *t* tests are commonly used when one dependent measure (fatigue) is compared within the same sample of subjects under different sets of circumstances (two positions) (LoBiondo-Wood & Haber, 1994). In the 14 subjects who delivered vaginally, the average number of fatigue symptoms was 5.7 after breastfeeding in the sitting position and 3.7 after feeding in the side-lying position." (p. 69)

Findings

"This represents a significant difference in fatigue levels between the two breastfeeding positions ($t = 2.2, df = 13, p < .05$)." (p. 69)

Conclusions

Conclusions are a synthesis of the findings. In forming conclusions, the researcher uses logical reasoning, creative formation of a meaningful whole from pieces of information obtained through data analysis and findings from previous studies, receptivity to subtle clues in the data, and consideration of alternative explanations of the data. One of the risks in developing conclusions is going beyond the data—that is, forming conclusions that are not warranted by the data. This occurs more frequently in published studies than one would like to believe.

IN CRITIQUING a study, you need to identify the conclusions and judge whether they are warranted by the data.

Milligan and colleagues (1996) concluded that "Subjects experienced considerably less fatigue symptoms after using the side-lying position rather than the sitting position to breastfeed. The side-lying position may be generally more restful, may exert less pressure on the perineum (Olkin, 1987), or may require less effort to hold the infant (Riordan & Auerbach, 1993)" (p. 70). As can be seen in this example, the findings are related to findings from previous research and theoretical literature.

Considering Implications

Implications are the meanings of conclusions for the body of nursing knowledge, theory, and practice. Implications are based on but are more specific than conclusions, and they provide specific suggestions for implementing the findings. For example, the researcher might suggest how nursing practice should be modified. If a study indicated that a specific solution was effective in decreasing stomatitis, the implications would state how care for patients with stomatitis should be modified.

IN CRITIQUING a study, you need to identify the implications indicated by the researcher. In addition, you may be able to identify implications not considered by the author.

Milligan and colleagues' (1996) study suggested these implications:

"Nurse recognition of conditions and attitudes that enhance success of breastfeeding is critical. . . . Increased emphasis on the restfulness of the side-lying position for breastfeeding can easily be included in routine postpartum nursing practice or home nursing visit." (p. 70)

Exploring the Significance of Findings

The significance of a study is associated with its importance to the nursing body of knowledge. Significance is not a dichotomous characteristic because studies contribute in varying degrees to the body of knowledge. Significance may be associated with the amount of variance explained, control in the study design to eliminate unexplained variance, or detection of statistically significant differences. To the extent possible at the time the study is reported, the researcher is expected to clarify the significance.

A few studies, referred to as "landmark studies," become important referent points in the discipline (Johnson, 1972; Lindeman & Van Aernam, 1971; Passos & Brand, 1966; Williams, 1972). The true importance of a particular study may not become apparent for years after publication. However, there are some characteristics associated with the significance of studies. Significant studies make an important difference in peoples' lives; it is possible to generalize the findings far beyond the study sample so that the findings have the potential of affecting large numbers of people. The implications of significant studies go beyond concrete facts to abstractions and lead to the generation of theory or revisions of existing theory. A very significant study has implications for one or more disciplines in addition to nursing. The study is accepted by others in the discipline and is frequently referenced in the literature. Over a period of time, the significance of a study is measured by the number of studies it generates.

IN CRITIQUING a study, you need to judge the significance of the study and indicate factors that make it significant.

Clinical Significance

The findings of a study can have *statistical significance* but not *clinical significance*. Clinical significance is related to the practical importance of the findings. However, there is no common agreement in nursing about how to evaluate the clinical significance of a finding. The effect size can be used to determine clinical significance. For example, one group of patients might have a body temperature 1°F higher than that of another group. Data analysis might indicate that the two groups are statistically significantly different, but the findings have no clinical significance. The difference is not sufficiently important to warrant changing the patient's care. However, in many studies, it is difficult to judge how much change would constitute clinical significance. In studies testing the effectiveness of a treatment, clinical significance could be judged based on the proportion of subjects who showed improvement or the extent to which subjects returned to normal functioning. But how much improvement would subjects need to demonstrate for the findings to be considered clinically significant? There are also questions about who should judge clinical signifi-cance—the patients and their families, the clinician/researcher, or society at large. At this point in the development of nursing knowledge, clinical signifi-cance is ultimately a value judgment (LeFort, 1993).

IN CRITIQUING a study, you need to evaluate its clinical significance.

Generalizing the Findings

Generalization extends the implications of the findings from the sample stud-ied to a larger population. The findings may be extended from the situation studied to a larger situation. For example, if the study was conducted on diabetic patients, it may be possible to generalize the findings to persons with other illnesses or to well individuals. In the study by Milligan and col-leagues (1996) the authors cautioned that "The findings of this study must be interpreted in [the] context of the sample and study procedures. The small sample consisted of mostly white, well-educated adults who experi-enced normal operative or vaginal deliveries and healthy infants. These women were given a choice of which position to feed first. The intervention was provided by a lactation consultant" (p. 70).

How far can generalizations be made? From a very narrow perspective, one cannot really generalize from the sample on which the study was done; any other sample is likely to be different in some way. Those with a conservative view consider generalization particularly risky if the sample was not randomly selected. According to Kerlinger (1986), unless special precautions are taken and efforts made, the research results are frequently not representative and thus not generalizable. Most nurse researchers are not this conservative in making generalizations.

Empirical generalizations are based on accumulated evidence from many studies and are important for the verification of theoretical statements or the development of new theory. Empirical generalizations are the base of a science and contribute to scientific conceptualization. Nursing has few empirical gener-alizations at this time.

IN CRITIQUING a study, you need to determine the populations to which the re-searcher has generalized and judge the appropriateness of the generalization. You may be able to identify other populations to which the findings should be generalized.

Suggesting Further Studies

In every study, the researcher gains knowledge and experience that can be used to design a better study next time. Therefore, the researcher will often make suggestions for future studies that emerge logically from the present study. Recommendations for further study may include replications or repeating the design with a different or larger sample. Recommendations may also include hypotheses to further test the framework in use.

IN CRITIQUING a study, you need to identify the researcher's recommendations for future research. You may be able to make additional recommendations.

Milligan and colleagues (1996) made the following recommendations for future research:

"Future research could build on the results obtained in this preliminary study using a larger, more diverse population, an intervention provided by professional nurses (as opposed to [a] certified lactation consultant), and by adding random assignment of treatment order." (p. 70)

SUMMARY

To critique a quantitative study, the nurse needs to be able to (1) identify the statistical procedures used; (2) judge whether these statistical procedures were appropriate to the hypotheses, questions, or objectives of the study and to the data available for analysis; (3) comprehend the discussion of data analysis results; (4) judge whether the author's interpretation of the results is appropriate; and (5) evaluate the clinical significance of the findings. There are several stages to quantitative data analysis: (1) preparation of the data for analysis; (2) description of the sample; (3) testing the reliability of measurement methods; (4) exploratory analysis of the data; (5) confirmatory analyses guided by the hypotheses, questions, or objectives; and (6) post-hoc analyses.

One needs to understand the concepts of statistical theory in order to critique research effectively. Probability theory, which is deduc-

tive, is used to explain a relationship, the probability of an event's occurring in a given situation, or the probability of accurately predicting an event. Decision theory, which is inductive, assumes that all of the groups in a study (such as experimental and control groups) used to test a particular hypothesis are components of the same population in relation to the variables under study. The researcher must provide evidence that there is a difference between the groups. To test the assumption of no difference, a cutoff point is selected prior to data collection. The cutoff point, referred to as alpha (α), or the level of significance, is the probability level at which the results of statistical analysis are judged to indicate a statistically significant difference between the groups. A statistical inference is a conclusion or judgment based on evidence. A generalization is information applied to a general situation that has been acquired from a specific instance. In research, one infers from the study findings obtained from a specific sample to a more general population, using information obtained through statistical analyses.

The normal curve is a theoretical frequency distribution of all possible values in a population. Levels of significance and probability are based on the logic of the normal curve. Hypotheses usually assume that extreme scores, which fall in the tails of the normal curve, result because the group with the extreme score does not belong to the same population. A Type I error occurs when the null hypothesis is rejected when it is true; the risk of a Type I error is indicated by the level of significance. A Type II error occurs when the null hypothesis is regarded as true when it is false. Type II errors are often a consequence of flaws in the research methods. Power is the probability that a statistical test will detect a significant difference that exists. The risk of a Type II error can be determined using power analysis. Degrees of freedom in-

volve the freedom of a score's value to vary given the other existing scores' values and the established sum of these scores. Degrees of freedom are often indicated in reporting statistical results.

Summary statistics include frequency distributions, measures of central tendency, and measures of dispersion. Statistical procedures frequently used to test hypotheses include the chi-square test of independence, *t*-test, Pearson's product-moment correlation, analysis of variance, and regression analysis. Judging statistical suitability in a critique requires that you be familiar with the statistical procedure used in the study. You must judge whether the procedure was performed appropriately and the results interpreted correctly. In the discussion section of the research report, the researcher examines evidence, forms conclusions, considers implications, explores the significance of the findings, generalizes the findings, and suggests further studies. In critiquing a study, you need to evaluate the appropriateness of the researcher's discussion.

REFERENCES

Alexy, B., Nichols, B., Heverly, M. A., & Garzon, L. (1997). Prenatal factors and birth outcomes in the Public Health Service: A rural/urban comparison. *Research in Nursing & Health, 20*(1), 61–70.

Angell, M. (1989). Negative studies. *New England Journal of Medicine, 321*(7), 464–466.

Berg, J., Dunbar-Jacob, J., & Sereika, S. M. (1997). An evaluation of a self-management program for adults with asthma. *Clinical Nursing Research, 6*(3), 225–238.

Burns, N., & Grove, S. K. (1997). *The practice of nursing research: Conduct, critique, and utilization* (3rd ed.). Philadelphia: Saunders.

Cohen, J. (1988). *Statistical power analysis for the behavioral sciences* (2nd ed.). New York: Academic Press.

Craft, M. J., & Moss, J. (1996). Accuracy of infant emesis volume assessment. *Applied Nursing Research, 9*(1), 2–8.

Froman, R. D., & Owen, S. V. (1997). Further validation of the AIDS Attitude Scale. *Research in Nursing & Health, 20*(2), 161–167.

Johnson, J. E. (1972). Effects of structuring patients' expectations on their reactions to threatening events. *Nursing Research, 21*(6), 499–503.

Kerlinger, F. N. (1986). *Foundations of behavioral research* (3rd ed.). New York: Holt, Rinehart & Winston.

LeFort, S. M. (1993). The statistical versus clinical significance debate. *Image: Journal of Nursing Scholarship, 25*(1), 57–62.

Lindeman, C. A., & Van Aernam, B. (1971). Nursing intervention with the presurgical patient—The effects of structured and unstructured preoperative teaching. *Nursing Research, 20*(4), 319–332.

LoBiondo-Wood, G., & Haber, J. (1994). *Nursing research* (3rd ed.). St. Louis: Mosby.

LoBiondo-Wood, G., Williams, L., Wood, R. P., & Shaw, B. W. (1997). Impact of liver transplantation on quality of life: A longitudinal perspective. *Applied Nursing Research, 10*(1), 27–32.

Milligan, R. A., Flenniken, P. M., & Pugh, L. C. (1996). Positioning intervention to minimize fatigue in breastfeeding women. *Applied Nursing Research, 9*(2), 67–70.

Olkin, S. (1987). *Positive pregnancy fitness.* New York: Avery.

Passos, J. Y., & Brand, L. M. (1966). Effects of agents used for oral hygiene. *Nursing Research, 15*(3), 196–202.

Riordan, J., & Auerbach, K. G. (1993). *Breastfeeding and human lactation*. Boston: Jones and Bartlett.

Russell, K. M., & Champion, V. L. (1996). Health beliefs and social influence in home safety practices of mothers with preschool children. *Image: Journal of Nursing Scholarship, 28*(1), 59–64.

Slakter, M. H., Wu, Y. B., & Suzaki-Slakter, N. S. (1991). *, **, and ***, statistical nonsense at the .00000 level. *Nursing Research, 40*(4), 248–249.

Topp, R., Estes, P. K., Dayhoff, N., & Suhrheinrich, J. (1997). Postural control and strength and mood among older adults. *Applied Nursing Research, 10*(1), 11–18.

Tukey, J. W. (1977). *Exploratory data analysis*. Reading, MA: Addison-Wesley.

Williams, A. (1972). A study of factors contributing to skin breakdown. *Nursing Research, 21*(3), 238–243.

Introduction to Qualitative Research

OBJECTIVES

Completing this chapter should enable you to:

1. *Describe the scientific rigor associated with qualitative research.*
2. *Differentiate the purposes of the four types of qualitative research.*
3. *Examine the research processes used in phenomenology, grounded theory, ethnography, and historical research.*
4. *Describe the use of a decision trail, a qualitative research strategy.*
5. *Examine the data collection issues for a qualitative study, including the relationships between the researcher and the participants and the reflections of the researcher on the meanings obtained from the data.*

RELEVANT TERMS

Auditability
Bracketing
Coding
Decision trail
Emic approach
Ethnographic research
Ethnonursing research
Etic approach
External criticism
Grounded theory research
Historical research

Internal criticism
Phenomenological research
Primary source
Qualitative research
Reflexive thought
Researcher–participant relationships
Rigor
Secondary source
Storytakers
Storytelling

Q*ualitative research* is a systematic, subjective approach used to describe life experiences and give them meaning (Leininger, 1985; Munhall, 1989; Silva & Rothbart, 1984). Qualitative research is not a new idea in the social or behavioral sciences (Baumrind, 1980; Glaser & Strauss, 1967; Kaplan, 1964; Scheffler, 1967). However, nursing's interest in qualitative research is relatively recent, having begun in the late 1970s.

The terminology used in qualitative research and the methods of reasoning are different from those of more traditional quantitative research methods and are reflections of different philosophical orientations. The specific philosophical orientation of each approach directs the research method. Although each qualitative approach is unique, there are many commonalities.

In this chapter, we introduce you to some of the qualitative research approaches commonly used in nursing and their contributions to nursing knowledge. To facilitate comprehension of these methods, the logic underlying the qualitative approach is explored. A general overview of the following qualitative approaches is presented: phenomenological research, grounded theory research, ethnographic research, and historical research. The methods used to collect, analyze, and interpret qualitative data are described. The content should assist you in reading and comprehending published qualitative studies and applying their findings to your clinical practice.

The Logic of Qualitative Research

Qualitative research focuses on understanding the whole, which is consistent with the holistic philosophy of nursing (Baer, 1979; Leininger, 1985; Ludemann, 1979; Munhall, 1982b, 1989; Munhall & Boyd, 1993). Within a holistic framework, qualitative research is a means of exploring the depth, richness, and complexity inherent in phenomena. In addition, qualitative research is useful in understanding such human experiences as pain, caring, powerlessness, and comfort.

The qualitative approaches are based on a world view that has the following beliefs: (1) There is not a single reality. Reality, based on perceptions, is different for each person and changes over time. (2) What we know has meaning only within a given situation or context. The reasoning process used in qualitative research involves putting pieces together perceptually to make wholes. From this process, meaning is produced. However, because perception varies with the individual, many different meanings are possible (Munhall & Boyd, 1993).

Frameworks are used in a different sense in qualitative research than they are in quantitative studies because the goal is not theory testing. Nonetheless, each type of qualitative research is guided by a particular philosophical stance. The philosophy directs the questions that are asked, the observations that are made, and the approach to interpretation of data (Munhall, 1982a, 1988, 1989). These philosophical bases and their methods, developed outside of nursing, will likely undergo evolutionary changes within nursing.

The data from qualitative studies are subjective and incorporate the perceptions and beliefs of the researcher and the participants (Eisner, 1981; Leininger, 1985). The findings from a qualitative study lead to understanding a phenomenon in a particular situation and are not generalized in the same way as those of quantitative studies. However, understanding the meanings of a phenomenon in a particular situation gives insights that can be applied more broadly. The insights from qualitative studies can guide nursing practice and aid in the important process of theory development for building nursing knowledge (Schwartz-Barcott & Kim, 1986).

Qualitative research provides a process through which we can examine a phenomenon outside of traditional views. The earliest and perhaps most dramatic demonstration of the influence qualitative research can have on nursing practice was the 4-year study conducted by Glaser and Strauss (1965, 1968, 1971), who initiated the use of grounded theory research methods for health-related studies. Their study, which described the social environment of dying patients in hospitals, was reported in three books—*Awareness of Dying, Time for Dying,* and *Status Passage*. At that time, the traditional view was that people could not cope with knowing that they were dying. The environment of care was designed to protect the patient from that knowledge. Glaser and Strauss examined the meanings that protective social environment had for the patient; the study changed our perception. Instead of protecting, we saw the traditional care of the dying as creating loneliness and isolation. We began to see the patient in a new light, and our care began to change. Kübler-Ross (1969), perhaps influenced by the work of Glaser and Strauss, then began her studies of the dying, using an approach similar to that of phenomenology. From this new orientation to care for the dying, hospice care began to develop, and now, more than 30 years later, the environment of care for the dying has changed.

Approaches to Qualitative Research

Four common approaches to qualitative research used in nursing are presented in this chapter: phenomenological, grounded theory, ethnographic, and historical. In some ways, these approaches differ greatly. Ethnographic and historical research are broad and are the accepted methodologies for a discipline. The worldview of phenomenology is more unique and is controversial. However, in each approach, the purpose is to examine meaning, and the unit of analysis is a word or phrase rather than a numerical value.

Each approach is based on a philosophical orientation that influences the interpretation of the data. Thus, it is critical to understand the philosophy on which the method is based. Each approach is discussed in relation to its philosophical orientation and nursing knowledge, and a nursing study is provided to illustrate each methodology.

Phenomenological Research

Phenomenology is both a philosophy and a research method. The purpose of *phenomenological research* is to describe experiences as they are lived—in phenomenological terms, to capture the "lived experience" of study participants. The philosophical positions taken by phenomenological researchers are very different from those common in nursing's culture and research traditions and thus are difficult to understand. However, discussions of this philosophical stance, appearing more frequently in the nursing literature, are introducing a broader audience to these ideas (Anderson, 1989; Leonard, 1989; Munhall, 1989; Salsberry, Smith, & Boyd, 1989).

Philosophical Orientation

Phenomenologists view the person as integral with the environment. The world is shaped by and shapes the self. Reality is considered subjective; thus, an experience is seen as unique to the individual. This is considered true even of the researcher's experiences in collecting data for a study and analyzing them. "Truth is an interpretation of some phenomenon; the more shared that interpretation is, the more factual it seems to be, yet it remains temporal and cultural" (Munhall, 1989, p. 22). Heideggerian phenomenologists believe that the person is a self within a body. Thus, the person is referred to as "embodied." "Our bodies provide the possibility for the concrete actions of self in the world" (Leonard, 1989, p. 48). The person has a world that is "the meaningful set of relationships, practices, and language that we have by virtue of being born into a culture" (Leonard, 1989, p. 43). The person is situated as a consequence of being shaped by his or her world and thus is constrained in the ability to establish meanings by language, culture, history, purposes, and values. Thus, the person has only situated freedom, not total freedom. A person's world is so pervasive that generally it is not noticed unless some disruption occurs. Not only is the world of each person different, but each person's concerns are qualitatively different. The body, world, and concerns, which are unique to each person, are the context within which that person can be understood. The person experiences *being* within the framework of time. This is referred to as "being-in-time." The past and the future influence the now and thus are part of being-in-time (Leonard, 1989).

Nursing Knowledge and Phenomenological Research

Phenomenology is the philosophical base for three nursing theories: Parse's (1981) Theory of Man-Living-Health, Paterson and Zderad's (1976) Theory of Humanistic Nursing, and Watson's (1985) Theory of Caring. The broad research question that phenomenologists ask is, "What is the meaning of one's lived experience?" Being a person is self-interpreting; therefore, the only reliable source of information to answer this question is the person. Understanding human behavior or experience, which is a central concern of nursing, requires that the person interpret the action or experience for the researcher; the researcher must then interpret the explanation provided by the person. Boyd (1993) suggests that the long-range goal should be that of "making phenomenology work well for us in nursing research—that is, of extrapolating nursing research methodology from phenomenology. Phenomenology invites this kind of effort and insists on an openness that can protect us from reducing such ideas about method to dogma" (p. 99).

Example Study

One of the most significant nursing studies conducted using the phenomenological method is Benner's (1984) work, from which emerged the critical description of nursing practice presented in her book, *From Novice to Expert.* This study was funded by a grant from the Department of Health and Human

continued

Services, Division of Nursing, at a time when external funding for qualitative research was almost unheard of.

In Benner's study, the phenomenon to be explored was the experience of clinical practice. The researcher develops a research question, which involves the consideration of two factors (expressed as questions): "(1) What are the necessary and sufficient constituents of this feeling or experience? (2) What does the existence of this feeling or experience indicate concerning the nature of the human being?" (Omery, 1983, p. 55). Benner's research question was whether there were "distinguishable, characteristic differences in the novice's and expert's descriptions of the same clinical incident. If so, how could these differences, if identifiable from the nurses' descriptions of the incidents, be accounted for or understood?" (Benner, 1984, p. 14).

Benner conducted paired interviews with beginning nurses and nurses recognized for their expertise. Twenty-one pairs of nurses were selected from three hospitals in which preceptors were used to orient new graduates. Each member of the pair, one a preceptor and one a new graduate, was interviewed separately about patient-care situations they had experienced together. Interviews and participant observation were also conducted with additional nurses, including 51 experienced nurse clinicians, 11 new graduates, and 5 senior nursing students. Individual interviews, small-group interviews, and participant observation were conducted at six hospitals. Before the interviews, participants were given written explanations of the kinds of clinical descriptions of interest to the researchers. Interviews were tape-recorded and transcribed.

Benner's (1984) data analysis was an interpretative strategy based on Heideggerian phenomenology. She describes the procedure as follows.*

"The interviews and participant-observer records were read independently by the research team members, and interpretations of the data were compared and consensually validated. Each interpretation was accepted only if there was agreement in labeling and interpreting the major competency demonstrated and only if it was effective in describing skilled practice." (p. 16)

Benner's (1984) structural explanation of her findings was presented as five stages of gaining experience in clinical practice, which describe the nurse in a particular clinical situation as a novice, an advanced beginner, competent, proficient, or expert. The stages identified are based on the Dreyfus Model of Skill Acquisition.

Stage 1: Novice

"Beginners have had no experience of the situations in which they are expected to perform. To give them entry to these situations and

*From *From novice to expert* by Patricia Benner. Copyright 1984 by Addison-Wesley Publishing Company. Reprinted by permission.

allow them to gain the experience so necessary for skill development, they are taught about the situations in terms of objective attributes such as weight, intake and output, temperature, blood pressure, pulse, and other such objectifiable, measurable parameters of a patient's conditions—features of the task that can be recognized without situational experiences. Novices are also taught context-free rules to guide action in respect to different attributes." (pp. 20–21)

Stage 2: Advanced Beginner

"Advanced beginners are ones who can demonstrate marginally acceptable performance, ones who have coped with enough real situations to note (or to have pointed out to them by a mentor) the recurring meaningful situational components. . . . Aspects, in contrast to the measurable, context-free attributes or the procedural lists of things to do that are learned and used by the beginner, require prior experience in actual situations for recognitions. Aspects include overall, global characteristics that can be identified only through prior experience." (p. 22)

Stage 3: Competent

"Competence, typified by the nurse who has been on the job in the same or similar situations two to three years, develops when the nurse begins to see his or her actions in terms of long-range goals or plans of which he or she is consciously aware. The plan dictates which attributes and aspects of the current and contemplated future situation are to be considered most important and those which can be ignored. Hence, for the competent nurse, a plan establishes a perspective, and the plan is based on considerable conscious, abstract, analytic contemplation of the problem." (p. 26)

Stage 4: Proficient

"Characteristically, the proficient performer perceives situations as wholes rather than in terms of aspects, and performance is guided by maxims. [Maxims are cryptic instructions passed on by experts. Maxims make sense only if the person already has a deep understanding of the situation (p. 10).] Perception is the key word here. The perspective is *not* thought out but 'presents itself' based upon experience and recent events. Proficient nurses understand a situation as a whole because they perceive its meaning in terms of long-term goals." (p. 27)

continued

Stage 5: Expert

"The expert performer no longer relies on an analytic principle (rule, guideline, maxim) to connect her or his understanding of the situation to an appropriate action. The expert nurse, with an enormous background of experience, now has an intuitive grasp of each situation and zeros in on the accurate region of the problem without wasteful consideration of a large range of unfruitful, alternative diagnoses and solutions." (p. 32)

Benner (1984) also identified seven domains of practice: (1) the helping role, (2) the teaching-coaching function, (3) the diagnostic and patient-monitoring function, (4) effective management of rapidly changing situations, (5) administering and monitoring therapeutic interventions and regimens, (6) monitoring and ensuring the quality of health care practices, and (7) organizational and work-role competencies. Nursing competencies representative of each domain were identified.

Grounded Theory Research

Grounded theory research is an inductive technique that emerged from the discipline of sociology. The term "grounded" means that the theory that developed from the research has its roots in the data from which it was derived.

Philosophical Orientation

Grounded theory is based on symbolic interaction theory, which holds many views in common with phenomenology. George Herbert Mead (1934), a social psychologist, was a leader in the development of symbolic interaction theory. Symbolic interaction theory explores how people define reality and how their beliefs are related to their actions. Reality is created by attaching meanings to situations. Meaning is expressed in terms of symbols such as words, religious objects, and clothing. These symbolic meanings are the basis for actions and interactions. However, symbolic meanings are different for each individual, and we cannot completely know the symbolic meanings of another individual. In social life, meanings are shared by groups and are communicated to new members through socialization processes. Group life is based on consensus and shared meanings. Interaction may lead to redefinition and new meanings and can result in the redefinition of self. Because of its theoretical importance, the interaction is the focus of observation in grounded theory research (Chenitz & Swanson, 1986).

Grounded theory has been used most frequently to study areas in which little previous research has been conducted and to gain a new viewpoint in familiar areas of research. However, because of the quality of theory generated through this method, further theory testing is not usually needed to enhance its usefulness.

Nursing Knowledge and Grounded Theory Research

Artinian (1988) has identified four qualitative modes of nursing inquiry within grounded theory, each used for different purposes: descriptive mode, discovery mode, emergent fit mode, and intervention mode. The descriptive mode provides rich detail and must precede all other modes. This mode, ideal for the beginning researcher, answers such questions as What is going on? How are activities organized? What roles are evident? What are the steps in a process? What does a patient do in a particular setting? The discovery mode leads to the identification of patterns in life experiences of individuals and relates the patterns to each other. Through this mode, a theory of social process, referred to as "substantive theory," is developed that explains a particular social world. The emergent fit mode is used when substantive theory has been developed in order to extend or refine this existing theory. This mode enables the researcher to focus on a selected portion of the theory, to build on previous work, or to establish a research program around a particular social process. The intervention mode is used to test the relationships in the substantive theory. The fundamental question for this mode is How can I make something happen in such a way as to bring about new and desired states of affairs? This mode demands deep involvement on the part of the researcher/practitioner.

Example Study

One significant study using a grounded theory approach that is relevant to clinical nursing practice is Fagerhaugh and Strauss's (1977) study of the politics of pain management. This study emerged from the previous work of Glaser and Strauss in the care of the dying (Glaser & Strauss, 1965, 1968; Strauss & Glaser, 1970) and chronic illness care (Strauss, 1975; Strauss et al., 1984). The study of pain involved 5 researchers and 2 years of systematic observations in 20 wards, 2 clinics, and 9 hospitals. The purposes of the study were to (1) develop an approach to pain management that was radically different from established approaches and (2) develop a substantive theory about "what happens in hospitals when people are confronted with pain and attempt to deal with it." The research questions were, "Under what conditions is pain encountered by staff?" and "How will it be handled?" (Fagerhaugh & Strauss, 1977, p. 13).

In their pain study, Fagerhaugh and Strauss (1977) observed a variety of situations in which pain was a common phenomenon. The areas studied included an intensive care unit for severe burns, a cardiac care unit, an obstetrics ward, a physical rehabilitation unit, a neurology and neurosurgery

continued

unit, a routine surgery unit, a medical ward, an x-ray department, an emergency department, a kidney transplant unit, and a cancer ward. The following excerpt is from the report of the grounded theory study on pain. It focuses on a description of the sampling process and demonstrates the care and detailed thought that must go into the development of sampling categories.

"On all these wards we made 'internal comparisons' along the theoretical dimensions. That is, we continued our theory-directed sampling: for instance, high-pain regimens versus low-pain regimens; experienced inflicters of regimen pain versus new inflicters; delivering mothers who had the fathers supporting their efforts to endure pain versus those who had no such supporting or controlling agents. Meanwhile, we were also looking at an activity that spanned separate wards and which would maximize variables as they related to pain infliction. We followed a number of personnel who drew blood from patients. We observed some who were very experienced, some who were not; some who were able to work in a leisurely fashion, some who were not; some who met "first-time" patients, others who met patients very experienced at this particular procedure; some who encountered patients with much ongoing pain and some who did not; some who had recently had experiences with accusations of incompetence and some who had not." (p. 308)

The core categories that evolved in the study were pain work, pain trajectories, legitimation, balancing, and accountability. Pain work was further classified into relieving pain, handling pain expression, diagnosing the meaning of pain, inflicting pain, minimizing or preventing pain, patients enduring pain, and the staff members' controlling their own reactions to the patient's response to pain. The patient's cooperation in the pain work and negotiation between the staff and the patient were identified as important factors. An example of negotiation is described by Glaser (1973).

"'This won't take long,' I said to her. . . . 'It's not going to hurt. . . . I think I can inject it right into the IV tubing and not have to stick you.'
She looked unconvinced.
'Honestly I won't stick you unless I have to.'" (p. 130)

Pain trajectories were divided into expected and unexpected trajectories. For example, an expectant mother would have a very different pain trajectory from that of a person with intractable back pain.

"An unexpected trajectory—unexpected for a given ward, that is—carries a potential for staff and patient disturbance and ward upset. Both the sentimental order and the work order of the ward are threatened. . . . Patients with an unexpected or atypical trajectory tend to be labeled as 'uncooperative' or 'difficult,' and relations be-

tween them and the staff are likely to grow progressively worse."
(Fagerhaugh & Strauss, 1977, pp. 22–23)

The researchers also concluded that the pain trajectory was influenced by the patients' illnesses, their previous experience with pain, the medical care they were receiving, and their social history. They observed that the nursing and medical staff seldom knew anything about the patient's pain trajectory other than what was currently occurring.

Assessing and legitimating pain was also an important factor. Staff often suspected patients of claiming more pain than they had or of claiming pain when they had none. This left patients in the position of attempting to convince the staff that they were actually having the pain they claimed to have (legitimating). The staff and patients were often involved in the process of balancing priorities during pain work. Decisions were based on what the staff considered to be most important.

"The staff members may not always agree among themselves, and the balancing done by the patient may not agree with the staff's. Patient and staff may even opt for opposite choices, disagreeing over the value of living a bit longer versus enduring terrible pain. They may be balancing quite different considerations. The staff may be balancing more work versus quicker pain relief, while the patient may be balancing pride in not complaining about pain versus difficulty of enduring it without more medication." (p. 25)

In terms of accountability, the researchers found that staff members did not consider pain work a major priority, and they tended to be more concerned with controlling patients' expression of pain than the experience of pain.

As can be seen from the study described, grounded theory research examines a much broader scope of dimensions than is usually possible with quantitative research. The findings can be intuitively verified by the experiences of the reader. The clear, cohesive description of the phenomenon can allow greater understanding and thus more control of our nursing practice.

Fagerhaugh and Strauss (1977) concluded the following from their study.

"Genuine accountability concerning pain work could only be instituted if the major authorities on given wards or clinics understood the importance of that accountability and its implications for patient care. They would then need to convert that understanding into a commitment that would bring about necessary changes in written and verbal communication systems. This kind of understanding and commitment can probably come about only after considerable nationwide discussion, such as now is taking place about terminal care, but that kind of discussion seems to lie far in the future." (p. 27)

Ethnographic Research

Ethnographic research was developed by anthropologists as a mechanism for studying cultures. The word "ethnographic" means "portrait of a people." Many nurses involved in this type of research obtained their doctoral preparation in anthropology and have used the techniques to examine issues related to culture that are of interest in nursing.

Philosophical Orientation

Anthropology, which began at about the same time nursing did (in the mid-nineteenth century), seeks to understand people—their ways of living, believing, and adapting to changing environmental circumstances. Culture, the most central concept to anthropology, is "a way of life belonging to a designated group of people . . . a blueprint for living which guides a particular group's thoughts, actions, and sentiments . . . all the accumulated ways a group of people solve problems, which are reflected in the people's language, dress, food, and a number of accumulated traditions and customs" (Leininger, 1970, pp. 48–49). The purpose of anthropological research is to describe a culture by examining these various cultural characteristics.

Anthropologists study people's origin, past ways of living, and ways of surviving through time. "The Australian aborigine, who lives in a non-technological society and a harsh natural environment, is as important an area of study in furthering a broad understanding of man as is contemporary Western man, who lives in a highly technological modern world" (Leininger, 1970, p. 7). Anthropologists may study cultures in remote parts of the world, in modern cities, and in modern rural areas. By comparing these cultures, they gain insights that increase our ability to predict the future directions of cultures and the forces that guide their destiny or that may provide opportunities to influence the direction of cultural development (Leininger, 1970).

Culture is both material and nonmaterial. Material culture consists of all created objects associated with a given group. Nonmaterial culture consists of other aspects of culture, such as symbolic referents, the network of social relations, and the beliefs reflected in social and political institutions. Symbolic meaning, social customs, and beliefs cannot be touched or stored in a museum; thus, they are not material, but they are essential elements of cultures. Cultures also have ideals that the people hold as desirable, even though they do not always live up to these standards. Anthropologists seek to discover the many parts of a whole culture and how these parts are interrelated so that a picture of the wholeness of the culture evolves (Leininger, 1970). Ethnographic research is used in nursing not only to increase ethnic cultural awareness but also to enhance the provision of quality health care for persons of all cultures. There are two basic research approaches in anthropology: emic and etic. The *emic approach* involves studying behaviors from within the culture; the *etic approach* involves studying behavior from outside the culture and examining similarities and differences across cultures.

Nursing Knowledge and Ethnographic Research

A group of nurse scientists, influenced by Leininger's Theory of Transcultural Nursing, have developed an ethnographic research strategy for nursing. They refer to this strategy as *ethnonursing research*. Ethnonursing "focuses mainly on observing and documenting interactions with people of how these daily life conditions and patterns are influencing human care, health, and nursing care practices" (Leininger, 1985, p. 238). However, a number of nurse anthropologists not associated with the ethnonursing orientation are also providing important contributions to the nursing body of knowledge.

Example Study

A study of how nurses define medication error ("Rules outside the rules for administration of medication: A study in New South Wales, Australia") is used to explain ethnographic research (Baker, 1997). The purpose of this ethnomethodological study was to improve understanding of how nurses within the culture of hospital nursing practice define or redefine medication error.

In the brief literature review, Baker described Barker and McConnell's (1962) benchmark study reporting that the medication error rate of nurses was 1 in 10. The number of errors made was directly proportional to the number of medications administered by the nurse. These authors found that nurses were aware of only a few of the errors they made; of these recognized errors, they reported only a small number. Some studies found that as nurses became more experienced, they made fewer errors. Other studies indicated that experienced nurses made the same number of errors but reported fewer of them. A study by Frances (1980), which found that as nurses became more experienced, they seemed to redefine error, offered insight to Baker and raised a question that led her to conduct the present study: "If nurses do redefine error, what is the new definition?" (p. 155).

Baker (1997) spent 2 weeks on each of nine wards on morning, evening, and night shifts and included time on weekends and public holidays. The total time spent was 18 weeks. She used participant observation, formal and informal interviews, written documents, and participation in shift reports. Some nurses did not wish to talk within the hospital so arrangements were made to meet with them outside of the hospital setting. Shift reports proved to be a "rich source of data because nurses frequently account for their actions in asides during these formal reports" (p. 156). Baker discussed outcomes in three groups.

"The first group of findings are called situated and embodied logics. These are the practices adopted by nurses in order to accomplish certain goals in particular situations. Although they are situated, they and similar practices may be widespread. They include ways

continued

of managing the medication trolley, reading between lines of medi-
cation-order and administration sheets, and using the medication
round for gathering information for other purposes. These situated
and embodied logics help nurses to be orderly in the complex practice world.

The second set of findings are called the criteria for redefinition
of error. This is a set of criteria nurses use to decide whether an
incident is a 'real' error. Of course every nurse is professionally
obliged to report errors, but if an error can be redefined, a medica-
tion-related incident becomes a nonerror that does not need to be
reported and no guilt is attached to it.

The third set of findings were serendipitous and included the
other uses to which nurses turn institutional rules with the purpose
of making their own lives orderly." (p. 156)

The following criteria were used by nurses to decide whether incidents
were errors.

- If it's not my fault, it is not an error.
- If everyone knows, it is not an error.
- If you can put it right, it is not an error.
- If a patient has needs which are more urgent than the accurate adminis-
  tration of medication, it is not an error.
- A clerical error is not a medication error.
- If an irregularity is carried out to prevent something worse, it is not an
  error.

To validate the conclusions she had made, Baker shared the results of her
analyses with the nurses who had participated in the study. They agreed
with Baker's findings.

Historical Research

Historical research examines events of the past. Many historians believe that
the greatest value of historical knowledge is increased self-understanding; in
addition, it increases nurses' understanding of their profession.

Philosophical Orientation

History is a science that dates back to the beginnings of humankind. The primary questions of history are Where have we come from?, Who are we?, and
Where are we going? Although the questions do not change, the answers do.

One of the assumptions of historical philosophy is that "there is nothing
new under the sun." Because of this assumption, the historian can search
throughout history for generalizations. For example, one can ask, What causes

wars? A historian could search throughout history for commonalities in various wars and develop a theoretical explanation of the causes of wars. The questions asked, the factors a historian selects to look for throughout history, and the nature of the explanation in a historical study are all based on a worldview (Heller, 1982). Another assumption of historical philosophy is that one can learn from the past. The philosophy of history is a search for wisdom in which the historian examines what has been, what is, and what ought to be. Historical philosophers have attempted to identify a developmental scheme for history to explain all events and structures as elements of the same social process.

Nursing Knowledge and Historical Research

Christy (1978) asks, "How can we in nursing today possibly plan where we are going when we don't know where we have been nor how we got here?" (p. 9). One criterion of a profession is that there is knowledge of the history of the profession that is transmitted to those entering the profession. Until recently, historical nursing research has not been a valued activity, and few nurse researchers had the skills or desire to conduct it. Therefore, our knowledge of our past is sketchy. However, there is now a growing interest in the field of historical nursing research (Sarnecky, 1990). Lusk (1997) suggests that

"Topics should be significant, with the potential to illuminate or place a new perspective on current questions, thus contributing to scholarly understanding. Topics should also be feasible in terms of data and resource availability. Finally, topics should be intriguing and capable of sustaining a researcher's interest." (p. 355)

Examples from Historical Nursing Research

The researcher may spend much time reading related literature before making a final decision about the precise topic. Waring (1978) conducted her doctoral dissertation using historical research to examine the idea of the nurse experiencing a "calling" to practice nursing. She described the extensive process of developing a precise topic as follows.

"Originally my idea was to pursue concepts in the area of Puritan social thought and to relate concepts such as altruism and self-sacrifice to nursing. Two years after the formulation of this first idea, I finally realized that the topic was too broad. Reaching that point was slow and arduous but quite essential to the development of my thinking and the prospectus that developed as an outcome. When I first began the process, it seemed that I might have to abandon the topic 'calling.' Now, since the clarification and tightening up of

continued

my title and the clarification of my study thesis, I open volumes fearing that I will find yet another reference, once overlooked. It is only recently that I have become convinced that there was a needle in the haystack and that I had indeed found it." (pp. 18–19) [Waring's original title was "American nursing and the concept of the calling."]

Developing Research Questions

After the topic has been clearly defined, the researcher will identify the questions to be examined during the research process. These questions tend to be more general and analytical than those found in quantitative studies. Evans (1978), then a doctoral student, describes the research questions she developed for her historical study.

"I propose to study the nursing student. Who was this living person inside the uniform? Where did she come from? What were her experiences as a nursing student? I use the word 'experience' in terms of the dictionary definition of 'living through.' What did she live through? What happened to her and how did she respond, or react, as the case may be? What was her educational program like? We have a pretty good notion of what nurse educators and others thought about the educational program, but what about it from the students' point of view?

What were the functions of rituals and rites of passage such as bed check, morning inspection, and capping? What kind of person did the nursing student tend to become in order to successfully negotiate studenthood? What are the implications of this in terms of her own personal and professional development and the development of the profession at large?" (p. 16)

Developing an Inventory of Sources

The next step is to determine whether sources of data for the study exist and are available. Many of the materials for historical research are contained in private archives in libraries or are privately owned. One must obtain written permission to gain access to library archives. Private materials are often difficult to ferret out, and when they are discovered, access may again be a problem.

Historical materials in nursing, such as letters, memos, handwritten materials, and mementos of significant leaders in nursing, are being discarded because no one recognizes their value. The same is true of materials related to the history of institutions and agencies with which nursing has been involved. Christy (1978) states, "It seems obvious that interest in the preservation of historical materials will only be stimulated if there is a concomitant interest in the value of historical research" (p. 9). Sometimes when such material is found, it is in such poor condition that much of the data are unclear or completely lost. Christy (1978) describes one of her experiences in searching for historical data as follows.

"M. Adelaide Nutting and Isabel M. Stewart are two of the greatest leaders we have ever had, and their friends, acquaintances, and former students were persons of tremendous importance to developments in nursing and nursing education throughout the world. Since both of these women were historians, they saved letters, clippings, manuscripts—primary source materials of inestimable value. Their friends were from many walks of life: physicians, lawyers, social workers, philanthropists—supporters and nonsupporters of nursing and nursing interests. Miss Nutting and Miss Stewart crammed these documents into boxes, files, and whatever other receptacles were available and—unfortunately—some of these materials are this very day in those same old boxes.

When I began my research into the archives in 1966, the files were broken, rusty, and dilapidated. Many of the folders were so old and ill-tended that they fell apart in my hands, the ancient paper crumbled into dust before my eyes. My research was exhilaratingly stimulating, and appallingly depressing at the same time; stimulating due to the gold mine of data available, and depressing as I realized the lack of care provided for such priceless materials. In addition, there was little or no organization, and one had to go through each document, in each drawer, in each file, piece by piece. . . . The boxes and cartons were worse, for materials bearing absolutely no relationship to each other were simply piled, willy-nilly, one atop the other. Is it any wonder that it took me eighteen months of solid work to get through them?" (pp. 8–9)

Determining the Validity and Reliability of Data

The validity and reliability concerns in historical research are related to the sources from which data are collected. The most valued source of data is the primary source. A *primary source* is material most likely to shed true light on the information the researcher seeks. For example, material written by a person who experienced an event or letters and other mementos saved by the person being studied are primary source material. A *secondary source* is written by someone who previously read and summarized the primary source material.

History books and textbooks are secondary source materials. Primary sources are considered more valid and reliable than secondary sources. "The presumption is that an eyewitness can give a more accurate account of an occurrence than a person not present. If the author was an eyewitness, he is considered a primary source. If the author has been told about the occurrence by someone else, the author is a secondary source. The further the author moves from an eyewitness account, the less reliable are his statements" (Christy, 1975, p. 191). Historical researchers use primary sources whenever possible.

The historical researcher must consider the validity and reliability of primary sources used in the study. To determine this, the researcher uses principles of historical criticism.

> "One does not merely pick up a copy of Grandmother's diary and gleefully assume that all the things Grandma wrote were the unvarnished facts. Grandmother's glasses may at times have been clouded, at other times rose-colored. The well-prepared researcher will scrutinize, criticize, and analyze before even accepting its having been written by Grandma! And even after the validity of the document is established, every attempt is made to uncover bias, prejudice, or just plain exaggeration on Grandmother's part. Healthy skepticism becomes a way of life for the serious historiographer."
> (Christy, 1978, p. 6)

Two strategies have been developed to determine the authenticity and accuracy of the source: external and internal criticism. *External criticism* determines the validity of source material. The researcher needs to know where, when, why, and by whom a document was written. This may involve verifying the handwriting or determining the age of the paper on which it was written. Christy (1975) describes some difficulties she experienced in establishing the validity of documents.

> "An interesting problem presented by early nursing leaders was their frugality. Nutting occasionally saved stationery from hotels, resorts, or steamship lines during vacation trips and used it at a later date. this required double checking as to her exact location at the time the letter was written. When she first went to Teachers College in 1907, she still wrote a few letters on Johns Hopkins stationery. I found this practice rather confusing in early stages of research."
> (p. 190)

Internal criticism involves examination of the reliability of the document. The researcher must determine possible biases of the author. To verify the accuracy of a statement, the researcher should have two independent sources that provide the same information. In addition, the researcher should ensure that he or she understands the statements made by the writer because words and their meanings change across time and across cultures. It is also possible to read into a document a meaning not originally intended by the author. This is most likely to happen when one is seeking a particular meaning. Sometimes words can be taken out of context (Christy, 1975).

Collecting the Data

Data collection may require months or years of dedicated searching for pertinent material. Occasionally, one small source may open a door to an entire new field of facts. In addition, there is no clear, obvious end to data collection. By examining the research guide, the researcher must make the decision to discontinue collection of data. These facets of data collection are described by Newton (1965) as follows.

> "The search for data takes the researcher into most unexpected nooks and corners and adds facet after facet to the original problem. It may last for months or years or a decade. Days and weeks may be fruitless and endless references may be devoid of pertinent material. Again, one minor reference will open the door to the gold mine of facts. The search becomes more exciting when others know of it and bring possible clues to the investigator. The researcher cultivates persistence, optimism, and patience in his long and sometimes discouraging quest. But one real 'find' spurs him on and he continues his search. Added to this skill is the training in the most meticulous recording of data with every detail complete, and the logical classification of the data." (p. 23)

Writing the Research Report

Historical research reports do not follow the traditional formalized style characteristic of much research. The studies are designed to attract the interest of the reader and may appear to be deceptively simple. The untrained eye may not recognize the extensive work that was required to write the paper. Christy (1975) explains as follows.

> "The reader is never aware of the painstaking work, the careful attention to detail, nor the arduous pursuit of clues endured by the writer of history. Perhaps that is why so many nurses have failed to recognize historiography as a legitimate research endeavor. It looks so easy." (p. 192)

Qualitative Research Methodology

This section presents a more detailed description of the methodologies commonly used in qualitative studies. In some ways, the methods used are no different from those used in quantitative studies. The researcher must select a topic; state the problem or question; justify the significance of the study; design the study; identify sources of data, such as subjects; gain access to those sources of data; select subjects or other sources for study; gather data; describe, analyze, and interpret the data; and develop a written report of the results. There are, however, methods unique to qualitative studies and sometime to specific types of qualitative research. Research reports of qualitative studies tend to focus on study results and seldom spell out in great detail the methods used to reach the conclusions. However, understanding some of the unique methods used by qualitative researchers will help you appreciate the work involved in conducting such a study. This section includes selection of participants (subjects), data collection methods, data management, and data analysis. The achievement of rigor in qualitative research will be explored.

Selection of Participants (Subjects)

Subjects in qualitative studies are referred to as "participants." Participants may volunteer to be involved in the study or be selected by the researcher because of their particular knowledge, experience, or views related to the study. Qualitative researchers use purposive sampling methods rather than probability or convenience sampling. The researcher may select individuals typical in relation to the phenomenon under study or may intentionally seek out individuals who are different in some way from other participants in order to get diverse perspectives. The sampling technique of "snowballing," in which the researcher asks participants to suggest individuals known to them who could provide information useful to the study, is commonly used. Decisions regarding sample size are different from those in quantitative studies and are based on needs related to the purposes of the study. Usually the number of subjects is small in comparison to the number used in quantitative studies. In case studies, one subject may be used (Sandelowski, 1996). A study of 6 to 10 subjects is not unusual. However, studies seeking maximum variation to examine a complex phenomenon or to develop a theory may require larger samples. The decision to stop seeking new subjects is made when the researcher ceases learning new information (informational redundancy) or when theoretical ideas seem complete (theoretical saturation) (Sandelowski, 1995).

The historical researcher seeks sources of information about the event being studied. These sources may include individuals who have experienced the event, but in most cases, the sources are written or film documentation. The researcher develops an inventory of sources and determines the validity and reliability of data from those sources.

Researcher–Participant Relationships

One of the important differences between quantitative and qualitative research lies in the relationships between the researcher and the individuals being studied (participants). The nature of these *researcher–participant relationships* has an impact on the data collected and their interpretation. These people are not research subjects in the usual sense of the word, but rather colleagues. The researcher must have the support and confidence of these individuals in order to complete the research. Therefore, maintaining these relationships is of the utmost importance. In many qualitative studies, the researcher observes social behavior and may interact socially with the participants.

In varying degrees, the researcher influences the individuals being studied and, in turn, is influenced by them. The mere presence of the researcher may alter behavior in the setting. This involvement, considered a source of bias in quantitative research, is thought by qualitative researchers to be a natural and necessary element of the research process. The researcher's personality is a key factor in qualitative research. Skills in empathy and intuition are cultivated; the researcher must become closely involved in the subject's experience in order to interpret it. It is necessary for the researcher to be open to the perceptions of the participants rather than to attach his or her own meaning to the experience. Participants often assist in determining research questions, guiding data collection, and interpreting results. The ethnographic researcher must become very familiar with the culture being studied by active participation in it and by extensive questioning. The process of becoming immersed in the culture involves gaining increasing familiarity with aspects of the culture such as language; sociocultural norms; traditions; and other social dimensions, including family, communication patterns (verbal and nonverbal), religion, work patterns, and expression of emotion. Immersion also involves gradually increasing acceptance of the researcher into the culture. However, although ethnographic researchers must be actively involved in the culture they are studying, they must avoid "going native," which will interfere with both data collection and analysis. In going native, the researcher becomes a part of the culture and loses all objectivity, along with the ability to observe clearly.

In addition to the role the qualitative researcher takes in the relationship, expectations of the study must be carefully considered. The researcher's aims and means need to be consistent with those of the participants. For example, if the researcher's desire is to change the behavior of the participants, this must also be their desire.

Data Collection Methods

The most common data collection methods used in qualitative studies are observation, interviewing, and examination of written text. These three methods, as they are used in qualitative studies, are described in the following sections.

Observation

Observation is a fundamental method of gathering data for qualitative studies. The aim is to gather firsthand information in a naturally occurring situation. The researcher functions in the learning mode with the question What is going on here? It is important for the researcher to look carefully as well as to listen. In most cases, the activities being observed are routine to the participants. The researcher will focus on details related to the routine. The process of activities may be as important to note as the discrete events. Unexpected events occurring during routine activities may be significant and are carefully noted. As in any event of observing, the qualitative researcher will attend to some aspects of the situation while disregarding others. The researcher's focus on particular aspects of the situation may increase as insights about "what is going on" occur (Silverman, 1993).

Historians may observe film, videotapes, photographs, or artistic representations of historical events. The historian must recognize that these sources are limited to information the photographer or artist selectively chooses to reveal. Important elements of the event may not be photographed or may be edited out. In some cases, film that has been edited out of finished products has been preserved and may be sought by historians. The breakdown of the Communist countries has provided a treasure trove of archived films that can be used to provide important historical insights into a variety of aspects of people's lives, including factors related to health.

Various strategies may be used to record information about the observations. In some cases, the researcher will take detailed handwritten notes while observing. In other cases, the researcher may focus entirely on the observational experience to avoid missing something meaningful and, immediately following the observation, may make detailed notes. Another useful strategy is to videotape the events occurring, allowing careful observation and detailed note-taking at a later time.

Class Exercise in Qualitative Observation. Divide the class into groups. Select a familiar site such as a grocery store checkout stand, a hospital lobby, or the university bookstore. Arrange for each member of the group to observe activities at the site independently. Take notes of the observations without discussing your observations with others. Save your notes for a discussion and analysis exercise later in the chapter.

Interviews

There are differences in interviews conducted for a qualitative study and those conducted for a quantitative study. In qualitative studies, the interview format is more likely to be open-ended. Although the researcher defines the focus of the interview, there is no fixed sequence of questions. The questions addressed in interviews tend to change as the researcher gains insights from previous interviews and/or observations. Respondents are allowed, even encouraged, to raise important issues not addressed by the researcher. In some cases, groups of individuals, which may be referred to as "focus groups," are interviewed.

During the interview, the researcher and the participant are actively engaged in constructing a version of the world. The process of interviewing is performed so that a deep mutual understanding is achieved. The focus is on obtaining an authentic insight into the participant's experiences. Rather than occurring at a single point in time, dialogue between researcher and participant may continue at intervals across weeks or months. This decreases the problem of fleeting relationships in which respondents may have little commitment or may provide only information they believe the researcher wishes to hear (Silverman, 1993).

Historical researchers may interview individuals who were participants in or observers of historical events. The focus of the interview may be validation of available information about the event, heretofore unknown details about the event, or the perspectives of individuals not previously heard from regarding the event. Historical events are generally considered to be constructed truths rather than factual. Individual perspectives on an event may provide additional insight into the event, but they are not expected to provide the truth of an event, which will never be known (and perhaps does not exist). Another strategy for collecting historical data is to interview individuals to construct biographies or to obtain the personal histories of a number of individuals in order to understand the evolving history of a region or institution.

Strategies used to record information from interviews include writing notes during the interview, writing detailed notes immediately after the interview, or recording the interview on tape.

Class Exercise in Qualitative Interviewing. Have each member of the class interview an individual about his or her experiences with and perceptions of being in a grocery store, a hospital lobby, or a university bookstore. Alternatively, ask each class member to interview an individual (faculty member, staff member, etc.) connected with the school of nursing in order to construct an oral history of the school. Record data from the interview for reference in later exercises.

Text as a Source of Qualitative Data

In qualitative studies, text is considered a rich source of data. Text may be written by participants on a particular topic at the request of the researcher. In some cases, these written narratives may be solicited by mail rather than in person. Text provided by participants may be a component of a larger study using a variety of sources of data. Text developed for other purposes—for example, from patient records or procedure manuals—can be accessed for qualitative analysis. Published text such as newspaper articles, magazine articles, books, or Internet materials can be used as qualitative data. Transcriptions of recorded interviews are commonly used in qualitative studies. In historical research, written descriptions of historical events, letters, and documents related to the event may be accessed for analysis. A historical study might examine the changing pattern of nursing practice in a selected area or of a nursing procedure by examining nursing textbooks published across time and journal articles describing that area of practice across time. Notes taken while reading written documents are important to the analysis process.

Class Exercise in Obtaining Textual Data for Qualitative Analysis. As a class, select a topic related to health or patient care, such as asthma, diabetes, or weight loss. Ask each member of the class to search the Internet for chat lines or discussion groups related to the selected problem. Print or download files of text written by individuals with the particular health problem and save them for an analysis exercise later in the chapter.

Data Management

Qualitative data analysis occurs concurrently with data collection rather than sequentially, as in quantitative research. Therefore, the researcher is attempting simultaneously to gather the data, manage a growing bulk of collected data, and interpret the meaning of the data. Volumes of data are gathered during a qualitative study. The researcher must develop means of storing the data in an organized manner. Traditionally, qualitative data collection and analysis have been performed manually. The researcher records the data on small bits of paper or note cards that are then carefully coded, organized, and filed at the end of a day of data gathering. It is easy to lose data in the mass of paper. Keeping track of connections between various bits of data requires meticulous record keeping. Some qualitative researchers believe that using the computer can make management and analysis of qualitative data quicker and easier, without the risk of losing touch with the data. The computer offers assistance in such activities as processing, storage, retrieval, cataloging, and sorting, leaving the analysis activities up to the researcher.

Data Analysis

Qualitative data analysis occurs in three stages: description, analysis, and interpretation. The descriptive stage is more critical in qualitative studies than in quantitative ones. Researchers are encouraged to remain in the descriptive mode for as long as possible prior to moving to analysis and interpretation. Because published qualitative studies tend not to describe the methodology in detail, many believe that qualitative research is free-wheeling. According to Coffey and Atkinson (1996):

> "There still seem to be too many students and practitioners who believe implicitly that qualitative research can be done in a spirit of careless rapture, with no principled or disciplined thought whatsoever. They collect data with little thought for research problems and research design, and they think that they will know what to do with the data once those data are collected. . . . [When they begin analysis] they find that things are not quite so simple." (p. 11)

Description

In the initial phases of a qualitative study, the researcher needs to become familiar with the data. This may involve reading and rereading notes and transcripts, recalling observations and experiences, listening to audiotapes, and viewing videotapes until the researcher becomes immersed in the data. Audiotapes contain more than words; they contain feeling, emphasis, and nonverbal communication, which are at least as important to communication as words. In phenomenology, this immersion in the data is referred to as "dwelling with the data." The initial purpose of this immersion is to address the question What is going on? An important methodological technique in grounded theory research is the constant comparative process, in which every piece of data is compared with every other piece.

During the data analysis process, a dynamic interaction occurs between the researcher's self and the data, whether the data are communicated orally or in writing. During this process, referred to as *reflexive thought*, the researcher explores personal feelings and experiences that may influence the study and integrates this understanding into the study. The process requires a conscious self awareness.

Drew (1989), in a paper describing her experiences conducting a phenomenological study of caregiving behaviors, describes the impact of relationships on her study as follows.

"A session with a person who had been willing to talk about his or her experiences with caregivers, and who had invested energy into the interview session, often generated for me a sense of doing something worthwhile, as well as a feeling that I would be competent to analyze the transcribed material in a meaningful way. This sense of competency dispelled any doubts about being an intruder. I became relaxed, unself-conscious, and more self-assured. However, an encounter with a person with blunt affect, abrupt answers, and

continued

a paucity of responses left me feeling awkward and self-conscious. A sense of doubt about the validity of my project encroached as I attempted to elicit that person's thoughts. At the time, my immediate reaction was to think that I had obtained nothing from these individuals, when in fact, as I was to discover later, the 'nothing' was something important that I was as yet unable to see.

It was at the point of discouragement about my interviewing skills that I became aware that I was mentally classifying interviews as either 'good' or 'bad,' depending on my emotional response to the subjects. Good interviews were those in which I felt effective as an interviewer and was able to facilitate the person's recounting of experiences with caregivers. I enjoyed the interaction and felt that we connected on some level that produced meaningful discussion about the topic of relationships between patient and caregiver.

Bad interviews, on the other hand, were those in which I could not seem to get subjects to talk about how they had experienced their caregivers. There seemed to be no questions that I could devise with which to explore feelings, either positive or negative, with them. They gave no indications of awareness of their feelings, or of feelings in others. Whereas the subjects of the good interviews were people I experienced as open, curious, and thoughtful, those of the bad interviews were experienced as distrustful and elicited in me a sense of anxiety and frustration; it seemed I could not get through to them. I felt inadequate as an interviewer and was ready to discard these interviews. Frustration and anxiety arose because I felt that I was not getting the information that I needed for the study.

Subsequently, I discovered that my feelings of frustration and inadequacy were causing me to overlook data and that when I could put them aside, new data that were rich in meaning became apparent. . . . This discovery was a powerful experience for me, affecting my approach to subsequent interviews and influencing analysis of data thereafter." (pp. 433–434)*

*Reprinted by permission of Sage Publications, Inc.

In some phenomenological research this critical thinking leads to *bracketing,* which is used to help the researcher avoid misinterpreting the phenomenon as it is being experienced by the participants. Bracketing is suspending or laying aside what the researcher knows about the experience being studied (Oiler, 1982). Other phenomenologists, especially those using Heideggerian phenomenology, do not bracket, but they do identify beliefs, assumptions, and preconceptions about the research topic. These are put in writing at the beginning of the study for self-reflection and external review. These procedures are intended to facilitate openness and new insights.

Initial efforts at analysis focus on reducing the large volume of data acquired in order to facilitate examination. This may involve "selecting, focusing, simplifying, abstracting, and transforming the data" (Miles & Huberman, 1994, p. 10). During data reduction, the researcher begins to attach meaning to elements of the data; discovers classes of things, persons, events, and properties; and notes regularities in the setting or the people. The researcher then classifies the elements in the data, either by using an established classification system or by developing a new one.

Transcribing Interviews. Tape-recorded interviews are generally transcribed word for word. Morse and Field (1995) provide the following instructions for transcribing a tape-recorded interview.

> "Pauses should be indicated by using dashes, and ellipses should indicate gaps or prolonged pauses. All expressions, including exclamations, laughter, crying, and expletives, are included in the text and separated from the verbal text with square brackets. Type the interviews single-spaced with a blank line between each speaker. A generous margin on both sides of the page permits the left margin to be used for coding and the researcher's own critique of the interview style, and the right margin to be used for comments regarding the content. . . . Ensure that all pages are numbered sequentially and that each page is coded with the interview number and the participant's number." (p. 131)

The researcher should listen to tape recordings as soon after an interview as possible, listening to the voice tone, inflection, and pauses of the researcher and the participant as well as to the content. While listening, the researcher is advised to read the written transcript of the tape and make notations of observations on the transcript (Morse & Field, 1995).

Codes and Coding. *Coding* is essentially a way of indexing or identifying categories in the data. A code is a symbol or abbreviation used to classify words or phrases in the data. Codes may be placed in the data at the time of data collection, when entering data into the computer, or during later examination of the data. The purpose of coding is to facilitate the retrieval of data segments by coding category. Used in this manner, coding simplifies and reduces the data (Coffey & Atkinson, 1996; Miles & Huberman, 1994). Coffey and Atkinson (1996) point out that "The nature of qualitative data means that data relating to one particular topic are not found neatly bundled together at exactly the same spot in each interview (and field-notes usually have even less predictable organization). The ability to locate stretches of data that, at least ostensibly, are 'about' the same thing is a valuable aspect of data management" (p. 35). Organization of data, selection of specific elements of the data for categories, and naming these categories will reflect the philosophical base of the study. Later in the study, coding may progress to the development of a taxonomy. For example, the researcher may develop a taxonomy of types of pain, types of patients, or types of patient education.

Morse and Field (1995) suggest that, in selecting elements of the data to code, the researchers note

1. "the kinds of things that are going on in the context being studied;
2. the forms a phenomenon takes; and
3. any variations within a phenomenon." (pp. 136–137)

Morse and Field (1995) suggest several innovative strategies for coding data. One approach is to use highlighter pens, with a different color for each major category. Another strategy, developed by Murdock (1971), is to assign each major category a number, which is inserted in the computerized text. Using this approach, a word or phrase in the text could easily have several codes indicated by numbers. Knafl and Webster (1988) suggest using colored markers, paper clips, index cards, or self-adhesive stickers to identify categories of data. Codes are often written in the margins. Then one can sort data by cutting the pages into sections according to codes. Each section can be taped or pasted onto an index card for filing. This procedure can be performed easily using computer programs for qualitative analysis, in which broad margins are available for coding. In this case, computerized data can be sorted by code into separate files for each code while identifiers such as data and source are retained.

Reflective Remarks. While the researcher records notes, other thoughts or insights emerge into his or her consciousness. These thoughts are generally included in the notes and are separated from the rest of the notes by ((double parentheses)). Later, they may need to be extracted and used for memoing (Miles & Huberman, 1994).

Marginal Remarks. As the notes are being reviewed, observations about them must be written immediately. These remarks are usually placed in the right-hand margin of the notes. The remarks often connect the notes with other parts of the data or suggest new interpretations. Reviewing notes can become boring, which is a signal that thinking has ceased. Making marginal notes assists the researcher in "retaining a thoughtful stance" (Miles & Huberman, 1994).

Data Displays. One approach to describing qualitative data is data displays. Displays are highly condensed and are equivalent to the summary tables of statistical outcomes developed in quantitative research. These data displays allow the researcher to convey succinctly the main ideas of the research. Codes can be used to organize the display. The strategies for achieving displays are limited only by the imagination of the researcher. Displays can be developed relatively easily using computer spreadsheets, graphics programs, or desktop publishing programs. For further information on displays, see Miles and Huberman (1994).

Marsh (1990) used a process-oriented matrix to test conclusions and an emergent theory from a qualitative study examining healthy lifestyle changes. Seven individuals who had made or were making lifestyle changes were interviewed; the focus was on the process of lifestyle change. Marsh's emergent theory describing the process of lifestyle change is as follows.

"An individual, aware of the need and desiring to alter his or her life style, makes one or more attempts to change over time. The attempts result in relapse. A self-monitoring process mediates between awareness of the individual's need to change and his or her relapses in the process of change. At some point tension mounts over the need to change. This tension, labeled 'readiness,' is characterized by a combination of personal and environmental variables, such as low self-esteem or support from significant others. Following readiness, the individual experiences a profound self-revelation. The revelation is characterized by a dramatic self-insight, a coming to as if shaken by a new understanding of reality. The revelation is followed by a belief system change about personal power, following which the individual makes and sustains a health life-style change. An individual who experiences no revelation remains in the initial pattern of attempted change and relapse. Revelation appeared to be the emerging core variable of the life-style change process." (p. 45)

To evaluate the trustworthiness of the emergent theory, all the data were examined for their fit in a matrix. Categories for the matrix were developed and decision rules established for inclusion of data within a category. Every subject was represented in the matrix. When a subject had made more than one lifestyle change, each change was represented separately in the matrix. The matrix is presented in Table 11-1.

Counting. Qualitative researchers tend to avoid the use of numbers. However, when judgments of qualities are made, counting occurs. The researcher states that a pattern occurs frequently or more often. Something is considered important or significant. These judgments are made in part by counting. If the researcher is counting, this should be recognized and planned. Counting can help researchers see what data they have, help verify a hypothesis, and help keep them intellectually honest. Qualitative researchers work by insight and intuition; however, their conclusions can be wrong. It is easier to see confirming

TABLE 11-1. Process-Oriented Matrix of Life-Style Change

Subject No.	Life-Style Change	Problem Awareness	Relapse	Readiness	Revelation	Belief-System Change	Behavioral Outcome	Predicted Future Outcome
1	Overeating*	In 8th grade, I was conscious of being overweight I need to do something for myself	I have no time to care for I have character defects I didn't want to commit and fail	My husband was supportive I got friend to go to meeting with me People at group were honest I want to live Success of others in group was inspirational	I can use my power along with God's power to conquer demon, overeating	I have strength in working with God; this gives me power and I can use it	60-lb weight loss sustained for 4.5 months, confident of continued success	Will sustain
2	Overeating*	I feel uncomfortable and short of breath	I tried all new diets My spouse supported my failure, both have poor will power	I got help from spouse I got help from group	I realized, if that woman can do it, so can I	I no longer need to eat to be happy	75-lb weight loss sustained over 1 year	Will sustain
	Alcohol	None	None	I got support from spouse I have low self-esteem I got group support— I went willingly, with no expectations	It suddenly hit: "I didn't like *me* anymore"	I have personal power I find support in group	Alcohol abstinence	Will sustain
	Smoking	I have a bad cough	I made two failed attempts	My father's health was bad I had a bad cough I really wanted to quit	None	I can do it by myself (strength from alcohol problem)	Sustained smoking cessation for several years	Will sustain
3	Overeating*	Eating is a sin—I love it, I hate it At a group I was obsessive/compulsive over food	I had many, many failures Food controls me. I have little control I tried groups; I like the support but can't keep with it	I have low self-esteem I am concerned for my child Group gives me hope and strength I have been depressed, I hate my life When I'm okay, everything else is	None	None	Repeated relapses	Escalation of readiness

4	Overeating*	I was a fat slob and an introvert since I was a small child	I wanted a magic cure with no responsibility	I felt depressed and suicidal / I have low life satisfaction / I'm a miserable, hurting person not in touch with self / I have low self-esteem / I joined group from fear of death / I felt group inspiration, I'm not alone	I realized I can control my life and it's okay to seek guidance from others "All of a sudden everything was pulled together"	Asked my higher power for strength and help (higher power = God = inner self) Food controlled me, now I can control it. I'm proud of me	Sustained 65-lb loss 8 months. Still needs group support, seeks reinforcement from others → Success if group support continued
5	Smoking*	I was tired of it / It was a hassle	I have no one to share problem with, no pats on back, no group support / I'm a failure	I'm joining groups to meet people in similar situation	None	None	Never got the group support sought / Another relapse → Success with right group
	Alcohol	I was sneaking / I was hiding problem from family	None	I feel concern and love from little sister	I was shaken by my little sister's concern / I suddenly knew I needed help	I want help at any cost / Group support will help; joined group 3–4 years old / I'm making written commitment	Reformed alcoholic, no backsliding, 3 years of sustained change → Will sustain
6	Smoking*	I was thinking about change / I feel scared, angry / I need a focus / My body and health are changing / It's filthy / I'm ambivalent	I made it convenient / I quit in past, started again / I want others to help	I am grasping a focus, letting others know once you start you need to keep going	None	None	Smoking cessation for 4 days / Has not told family or friends, is afraid of failure → Relapse
7	Smoking*	It's expensive / It's filthy / I risk getting cancer of the mouth	I've made many attempts / I'm angry / I don't want to give it up	I want group help / Support of my son helps / I'm concerned for effect of my smoking on my granddaughter and son	None	None	Relapse → Continued relapse
	Alcohol	I was hiding bottles / I was a closet drinker	I tried quitting for 6 years	I have low self-esteem	I realized no one could do it for me. I could do it by myself	I only have myself to blame / I'm the only one who can do anything about it	Alcohol abstinence 6 years → Will sustain

* Change currently being made. (Reprinted from *Advances in Nursing Science*, Vol. 12, No. 3, pp. 51–52, with permission of Aspen Publishers, Inc. © 1990.)

evidence than disconfirming evidence. Comparing insights by using numbers can be a good method of verification (Miles & Huberman, 1994).

Class Exercise in Describing Qualitative Research Findings. Work as groups to examine data obtained from observing, interviewing, and gathering textual data. Use codes and remarks to gain understanding of the content. Develop a matrix using the codes. Set aside time to present results to the class. Explore similarities and differences in findings of different class groups.

Analysis

Analysis goes beyond description, using methods to transform the data. Through this process, the researcher extends the data beyond the description. Using analysis, he or she identifies essential features and describes interrelationships among them (Wolcott, 1994). The emphasis in analysis is on identifying themes and patterns from the data. Coding, used earlier for description, also can be used to expand, transform, and reconceptualize data, thus providing opportunities for more diverse analyses. Coffey and Atkinson (1996) suggest that by "reading through data extracts, one might discover particular events, key words, processes, or characters that capture the essence of a piece" (p. 31).

Memoing is used to record insights or ideas related to notes, transcripts, or codes. Memos move the researcher toward theorizing and are conceptual rather than factual. They may link pieces of data or use a specific piece of data as an example of a concept. The memo may be written to someone else involved in the study or to oneself. The important thing is to value one's ideas and write them down quickly. Whenever an idea emerges, even if it is vague and not well thought out, it should be written down immediately. Although one might think that the idea is so clear in one's mind that it can be written later, the thought is soon forgotten and often cannot be retrieved. Memos should be dated, titled with the key concept discussed, and connected by codes with the field notes or forms that generated the thoughts (Miles & Huberman, 1994).

Storytelling. During observation and interviewing, the researcher may record stories shared by participants. Banks-Wallace (1998) describes a story as "an event or series of events, encompassed by temporal or spatial boundaries, that are shared with others using an oral medium or sign language. *Storytelling* is the process or interaction used to share stories. People sharing a story (storytellers) and those listening to a story (*storytakers*) are the main elements of storytelling" (p. 17). Stories can be instructive in understanding a phenomenon of interest. In some qualitative studies, the research may focus on gathering stories. Gathering stories enables health care providers to develop storytelling as a powerful means to increase insight and facilitate health promotion behaviors of clients. For example, Nwoga (1997) studied storytelling by African-American mothers in guiding their adolescent daughters in relation to sexuality. The stories used by these mothers, captured by Nwoga, could be useful in assisting other mothers struggling to help their daughters deal with sexuality issues.

Coffey and Atkinson (1996) discuss the importance of capturing stories in qualitative studies.

> "The story is an obvious way for social actors, in talking to strangers (e.g., the researcher), to retell key experiences and events. Stories serve a variety of functions. Social actors often remember and order their careers or memories as a series of narrative chronicles, that is, as [a] series of stories marked by key happenings. Similarly, stories and legends are told and retold by members of particular social groups or organizations as a way of passing on a cultural heritage or an organizational culture. Tales of success or tales of key leaders/ personalities are familiar genres with which to maintain a collective sense of the culture of an organization. The use of atrocity stories and morality fables is also well documented within organizational and occupational settings. Stories of medical settings are especially well documented (Atkinson, 1992; Dingwall, 1977). Here tales of professional incompetence are used to give warning of 'what not to do' and what will happen if you commit mistakes. . . . Narratives are also a common genre from which to retell or come to terms with particularly sensitive or traumatic times and events." (p. 56)

Narrative analysis is a qualitative means of formally analyzing stories. Using this method, the researcher "unpacks" the structure of the story. A story includes a sequence of events with a beginning, a middle, and an end. Stories have their own logic and are temporal (Coffey & Atkinson, 1996; Denzin, 1989). The structures can also be used to determine how people tell stories, how they shape the events they describe, how they make a point, how they "package" events and react to them, and how they communicate their stories to audiences. The structure used for narrative analysis as identified by Coffey and Atkinson (1996, p. 58) is as follows:

Structure	Question
Abstract	What is this about?
Orientation	Who? What? When? Where?
Complication	Then what happened?
Evaluation	So what?
Result	What finally happened?
Coda	Finish narrative

The abstract initiates the narrative by summarizing the point of the story or stating the proposition the narrative will illustrate. The orientation provides an introduction to the major events central to the story. The complication continues the narrative, describing complications in the event that make it a story, taking the form "Then what happened?" Evaluation is the point of the narrative, followed by the result, which gives the outcome or resolution of events. The coda ends the story and is a transition point at which talk may revert to other topics.

The narrative analysis can focus on social action embedded in the text or can examine the effect of the story. Stories serve a purpose. They may make a point or be moralistic. They may be success stories, or may be a reminder of what not to do or how not to be, with guidance in how to avoid the fate described in the story. The purpose of the story can be the starting point for a more extensive narrative analysis. Narrative analysis may examine multiple stories of key life events and gain greater understanding of the impact of these events; it may assist in understanding the relationship between social processes and personal lives; or it may be used to understand cultural values, meanings, and personal experiences. Issues related to power, dominance, and opposition can be examined. Through stories, silenced groups can be given voice (Coffey & Atkinson, 1996).

Coding is not used in narrative analysis. Coding breaks data up into separate segments and is not useful in analyzing a story. The researcher can lose the sense that informants are providing an account or a narrative of events.

Qualitative researchers may choose to communicate the findings of their study as a story. A story can be a powerful way to make a point. Stories can be presented from a variety of perspectives: chronological order, the order in which the story was originally presented, progressive focusing, focusing only on a critical or key event in the story, describing the plot and characters as one would stage a play, following an analytical framework, providing versions of an event from the stories of several viewers, or presenting the story as one would write a mystery story, thus appealing to problem-solvers.

Interpretation

During interpretation, the researcher offers his or her interpretation of what is going on. The focus is on understanding and explanation beyond what can be stated with certainty (Coffey & Atkinson, 1996; Wolcott, 1994). Interpretation may focus on the usefulness of the findings for clinical practice or may move toward theorizing.

As the study progresses, relationships among categories, participants, actions, and events begin to emerge. The researcher will develop hunches about relationships that can be used to formulate tentative propositions. Statements or propositions can be written on index cards and sorted into categories or entered into the computer (Miles & Huberman, 1994).

Using information in the matrix in Table 11-1, Marsh (1990) made the following interpretations.

"Subjects 1, 2, and 4 experienced revelation related to overeating, followed by a belief-system change. Each of these individuals had lost 60 to 75 pounds and had maintained the weight loss for 4.5 months to 1 year. Subject 3 experienced no revelation and had no success in weight loss. The matrix revealed patterns in the data that might have been overlooked." (p. 45)

For example, Marsh assumed that the belief-system change that occurred was a change in health beliefs. The matrix illustrated that the change was rather one of personal empowerment and involved beliefs about self, not about health.

As the data are collected and analyzed, the researcher gains increasing understanding of the dynamics involved in the process under study. This understanding might be considered a tentative theory. The first tentative theories are vague and poorly pieced together; some are altogether wrong. The best way to verify a tentative theory is to share it with others, particularly informants in the study situations. Informants have their own tentative theories, which have never been clearly expressed. The tentative theory needs to be expressed as a map. Developing a good map of the tentative theory is difficult and requires some hard work.

The validity of predictions developed in a tentative theory must be tested; however, finding effective ways to achieve this is difficult. Predictions are usually developed near the end of the study. Because the findings are often context-specific, the predictions must be tested on the same or a similar sample. One strategy suggested is to predict outcomes expected to occur 6 months after completion of the study. Six months later, these predictions can be sent to informants who participated in the study. The informants can be asked to respond to the accuracy of (1) the predictions and (2) the explanation of why the prediction was expected to occur (Miles & Huberman, 1994).

People easily—almost too easily—identify patterns, themes, and gestalts from their observations. The difficulty is in seeking *real* additional evidence of a pattern while remaining open to disconfirming evidence. Any identified pattern should be subjected to skepticism by the researcher and others (Miles & Huberman, 1994). Morse and Field (1995) state the following.

"The researcher must distinguish between representative cases and anecdotal cases. Representative cases appear with regularity and encompass the range of behaviors described within a category. The anecdotal case appears infrequently and depicts a small range of

continued

> events that are atypical of the larger group. . . . Negative cases are those episodes that clearly refute an emergent theory or proposition. Negative cases are important because they help to clarify additional causal properties that influence the phenomena under study (Denzin, 1978)." (p. 139)

Often during analysis, a conclusion is seen as plausible. It seems to fit; it makes good sense. When asked how he or she arrived at that point, the researcher may state that it "just feels right." These intuitive feelings are important in both qualitative and quantitative research. However, plausibility cannot stand alone. After plausibility must come systematic analysis. First, intuition occurs; then careful examination of the data is done to verify the validity of that intuition (Miles & Huberman, 1994).

Rigor in Qualitative Research

Scientific *rigor* is valued because it is associated with the worth of research outcomes, and studies are critiqued as a means of judging rigor. Qualitative research methods have been criticized for lacking rigor; however, this criticism has occurred because of attempts to judge the rigor of qualitative studies using rules developed to judge quantitative studies. Rigor needs to be defined differently for qualitative research because the desired outcome is different (Burns, 1989; Dzurec, 1989; Morse, 1989; Sandelowski, 1986). In quantitative research, rigor is reflected in narrowness, conciseness, and objectivity and leads to rigid adherence to research designs and precise statistical analyses. In qualitative research, rigor is associated with openness, scrupulous adherence to a philosophical perspective, thoroughness in collecting data, and consideration of all of the data in the subjective theory development phase. Evaluation of the rigor of a qualitative study is based, in part, on the logic of the emerging theory and the clarity with which it sheds light on the phenomenon studied. Lack of rigor in qualitative research is due to problems such as inconsistency in adhering to the philosophy of the approach being used, failure to get away from older ideas, poorly developed methods, inadequate time spent collecting data, poor observations, failure to give careful consideration to all the data obtained, and inadequacy of theoretical development from the data.

Decision Trails

The credibility of qualitative data analysis has been seriously questioned in some cases by the larger scientific community. The concerns expressed are related to the inability to replicate the outcomes of a study, even when using the same data set. To respond to this concern, some qualitative researchers have attempted to develop strategies by which other researchers, using the same data, can follow the logic of the original researcher and arrive at the same conclusions. Miles and Huberman (1994) refer to this strategy as a *decision trail;* Guba and Lincoln (1982) refer to it as *auditability.*

Developing a decision trail requires that the researcher establish decision rules for categorizing data, arriving at ratings, or making judgments. A decision rule might say, for example, that a datum would be placed in a specific category if it met specified criteria. Another decision rule might say that an observed interaction would be considered an instance of an emerging theoretical explanation if it met specific criteria. A record is kept of all decision rules used in the analysis of data. All raw data are stored so that they are available for review if requested. As the analysis progresses, the researcher documents the data, the decision rules on which each decision was based, and the reasoning behind each decision. Thus, evidence is retained to support the study conclusions and the emerging theory and is made available on request (Burns, 1989). However, Marshall (1984, 1985) cautioned against undermining the strengths of qualitative research with overly mechanistic data analysis. Marshall and Rossman (1989) expressed concern that efforts to increase validity will "filter out the unusual, the serendipitous—the puzzle that, if tended to and pursued, would provide a recasting of the entire research endeavor" (p. 113). Decision trails are not usually included as part of a published qualitative study. The author might state that a decision trail is available on request from another qualitative researcher.

SUMMARY

Qualitative research is a systematic, subjective approach used to describe life experiences and give them meaning. The terminology used in qualitative research and the methods of reasoning are different from those of more traditional quantitative research methods and are reflections of different philosophical orientations. Qualitative research focuses on understanding the whole, which is consistent with the holistic philosophy of nursing. The qualitative approaches are based on a worldview that has the following beliefs: (1) there is not a single reality and (2) what we know has meaning only within a given situation or context.

Frameworks are used in a different sense in qualitative research than they are in quantitative studies because the goal is not theory testing. Nonetheless, each type of qualitative research is guided by a particular philosophical stance. The data from qualitative studies are subjective, and incorporate the percep-tions and beliefs of the researcher and the participants. Four common approaches to qualitative research used in nursing are presented in this chapter: phenomenological, grounded theory, ethnographic, and historical. The purpose of phenomenological research is to describe experiences as they are lived—in phenomenological terms, to capture the "lived experience" of study participants. Grounded theory is based on symbolic interaction theory, which explores how people define reality and how their beliefs are related to their actions. Ethnographic studies seeks to understand people—their ways of living, believing, and adapting to changing environmental circumstances. The primary questions of history are Where have we come from?, Who are we?, and Where are we going?

In some ways, the methods used in qualitative research are no different from those used in quantitative studies. The researcher must select a topic; state the problem or question; justify the significance of the study; design the study; identify sources of data such as subjects; gain access to those sources of data; select subjects or other sources for study; gather data; describe, analyze, and interpret the data; and develop a written report of their results. There are, however, methods unique to qualitative studies and sometimes to specific types of qualitative research. Subjects in qualitative studies are referred to as participants. The relationship between the researcher and the individuals being studied is one of colleagues. The effectiveness of this relationship has an impact on the data collected and their interpretation. In many degrees, the researcher influences the individuals being studied and, in turn, is influenced by them. The researcher's aims and means need to be consistent with those of the participants. For example, if the researcher's desire is to change the behavior of the participants, this must also be their desire.

The most common data collection methods used in qualitative studies are observation, interviewing, and examination of textual data. Qualitative data analysis occurs concurrently with data collection rather than sequentially, as in quantitative research. Therefore, the researcher is attempting simultaneously to gather the data, manage a growing bulk of collected data, and interpret the meaning of the data. Qualitative data analysis occurs in three stages: description, analysis, and interpretation. The descriptive stage is more critical in qualitative studies than in quantitative ones. Researchers are encouraged to remain in the descriptive mode as long as possible prior to moving to analysis and interpretation. In the initial phases of a qualitative study, the researcher needs to become familiar with the data. This may involve reading and rereading notes and transcripts, recalling observation and experiences, listening to audiotapes, and viewing videotapes until the researcher becomes immersed in the data. During the data

analysis process, a dynamic interaction occurs between the researcher's self and the data, whether the data are communicated orally or in writing during this process, referred to as reflexive thought, the researcher explores personal feelings and experiences that may influence the study and integrates this understanding into the study. The process requires a conscious awareness of self.

Initial efforts of analysis are focused on reducing the large volume of data acquired in order to facilitate examination. Coding is used to index or identify categories in the data. One approach to describing qualitative data is data displays. Displays are highly condensed and are equivalent to the summary tables of statistical outcomes developed in quantitative research. Qualitative researchers tend to avoid the use of numbers. However, if the researcher is counting, this should be recognized and planned. Judgments in qualitative studies are made in part by counting. Analysis goes beyond description, using methods to transform the data. Through analysis, the researcher identifies essential features and describes interrelationships among them. In analysis, the emphasis is on identifying themes and patterns from the data. Stories obtained during data gathering may be analyzed using narrative analysis. During interpretation, the researcher offers his or her interpretation of what is going on. The focus is on understanding and explanation beyond what can be stated with certainty. Interpretation may focus on the usefulness of the findings for clinical practice or may move toward theorizing.

Qualitative research methods have been criticized for lack of rigor; however, this criticism has occurred because of attempts to judge the rigor of qualitative studies using rules developed to judge quantitative studies. In qualitative research, rigor is associated with openness, scrupulous adherence to a philosophical perspective, thoroughness in collecting data, and consideration of all of the data in the subjective theory development phase. Evaluation of the rigor of a qualitative study is based, in part, on the logic of the emerging theory and the clarity with which it sheds light on the phenomenon studied.

The credibility of qualitative data analysis has been seriously questioned in some cases by the larger scientific community. The concerns expressed are related to the inability to replicate the outcomes of a study, even when using the same data set. To respond to the concern, some qualitative researchers have developed strategies referred to as decision trails by which other researchers, using the same data, can follow the logic of the original researcher and arrive at the same conclusions. Developing a decision trail requires that the researcher establish decision rules for categorizing data, arriving at ratings, or making judgments. As the analysis progresses, the researcher documents the data and the decision rules on which each decision was based and the reasoning that entered into each decision.

REFERENCES

Anderson, J. M. (1989). The phenomenological perspective. In J. M. Morse (Ed.), *Qualitative nursing research: A contemporary dialogue* (pp. 15–26). Rockville, MD: Aspen.

Artinian, B. A. (1988). Qualitative modes of inquiry. *Western Journal of Nursing Research, 10*(2), 138–149.

Atkinson, P. (1992). The ethnography of a medical setting: Reading, writing and rhetoric. *Qualitative Health Research, 2*(4), 451–474.

Baer, E. D. (1979). Philosophy provides the rationale for nursing's multiple research directions. *Image, 11*(3), 72–74.

Baker, H. M. (1997). Rules outside the rules for administration of medication: A study in new South Wales, Australia. *Image: Journal of Nursing Scholarship, 29*(2), 155–158.

Banks-Wallace, J. (1998). Emancipatory potential of storytelling in a group. *Image: Journal of Nursing Scholarship, 30*(1), 17–22.

Barker, K., & McConnell, W. (1962). The problems of detecting medication errors in hospitals. *American Journal of Hospital Pharmacy, 19*(8), 360–369.

Baumrind, D. (1980). New directions in socialization research. *American Psychologist, 35*(7), 639–652.

Benner, P. (1984). *From novice to expert: Excellence and power in clinical nursing practice.* Menlo Park, CA: Addison-Wesley.

Boyd, C. O. (1993). Phenomenology: The method. In P. L. Munhall & C. O. Boyd (Eds.), *Nursing Research: A qualitative perspective* (pp. 99–132). New York: National League for Nursing Press, Pub. No. 19-2535.

Burns, N. (1989). Standards for qualitative research, *Nursing Science Quarterly, 2*(1), 44–52.

Chenitz, W. C., & Swanson, J. M. (1986). Qualitative research using grounded theory. In W. C. Chenitz & J. M. Swanson (Eds.), *From practice to grounded theory: Qualitative research in nursing* (pp. 3–15). Menlo Park, CA: Addison-Wesley.

Christy, T. E. (1975). The methodology of historical research: A brief introduction. *Nursing Research, 24*(3), 189–192.

Christy, T. E. (1978). The hope of history. In M. L. Fitzpatrick (Ed.), *Historical studies in nursing* (pp. 3–11). New York: Teachers College Press.

Coffey, A., & Atkinson, P. (1996). *Making sense of qualitative data.* Thousand Oaks, CA: Sage.

Denzin, N. K. (1978). *Sociological methods: A sourcebook* (2nd ed.). New York: McGraw-Hill.

Denzin, N. K. (1989). *Interpretive interactionism.* Newbury Park, CA: Sage.

Dingwall, R. (1977). Atrocity stories and professional relationships. *Sociology of Work and Occupations, 4*(4), 371–396.

Drew, N. (1989). The interviewer's experience as data in phenomenological research. *Western Journal of Nursing Research, 11*(4), 431–439.

Dzurec, L. C. (1989). The necessity and evolution of multiple paradigms for nursing research. *Advances in Nursing Science, 11*(4), 69–77.

Eisner, E. W. (1981). On the differences between scientific and artistic approaches to qualitative research. *Educational Researcher, 10*(4), 5–9.

Evans, J. C. (1978). Formulating an idea. In M. L. Fitzpatrick (Ed.), *Historical studies in nursing* (pp. 15–17). New York: Teachers College Press.

Fagerhaugh, S., & Strauss, A. (1977). *Politics of pain management: Staff-patient interaction.* Menlo Park, CA: Addison-Wesley.

Frances, G. (1980). Nurses' medication errors: A new perspective. *Supervisor Nurse, 11*, 11–13.

Glaser, B. G. (1973). *Ward four hundred two.* New York: George Braziller.

Glaser, B. G., & Strauss, A. (1965). *Awareness of dying.* Chicago: Aldine.

Glaser, B. G., & Strauss, A. (1967). *The discovery of grounded theory: Strategies for qualitative research.* Chicago: Aldine.

Glaser, B. G., & Strauss, A. (1968). *Time for dying.* Chicago: Aldine.

Glaser, B. G., & Strauss, A. (1971). *Status passage.* London: Routledge & Kegan Paul.

Guba, E. G., & Lincoln, Y. S. (1982). *Effective evaluation.* Washington, DC: Jossey-Bass.

Heller, A. (1982). *A theory of history.* London: Routledge & Kegan Paul.

Kaplan, A. (1964). *The conduct of inquiry: Methodology for behavioral science.* New York: Chandler.

Knafl, K. A., & Webster, D. C. (1988). Managing and analyzing qualitative data: A description of tasks, techniques, and materials. *Western Journal of Nursing Research, 10*(2), 195–218.

Kubler-Ross, E. (1969). *On death and dying.* New York: Macmillan.

Leininger, M. M. (1970). *Nursing and anthropology: Two worlds to blend.* New York: Wiley.

Leininger, M. M. (1985). *Qualitative research methods in nursing.* Orlando, FL: Grune & Stratton.

Leonard, V. M. (1989). A Heideggerian phenomenologic perspective on the concept of the person. *Advances in Nursing Science, 11*(4), 40–55.

Ludemann, R. (1979). The paradoxical nature of nursing research. *Image, 11*(1), 2–8.

Lusk, B. (1997). Historical methodology for nursing research. *Image: Journal of Nursing Scholarship, 29*(4), 355–359.

Marsh, G. W. (1990). Refining an emergent life-style-change theory through matrix analysis. *Advances in Nursing Science, 12*(3), 41–52.

Marshall, C. (1984). Elites, bureaucrats, ostriches, and pussycats: Managing research in policy settings. *Anthropology and Education Quarterly, 15*(3), 235–251.

Marshall, C. (1985). Appropriate criteria of trustworthiness and goodness for qualitative research on education organizations. *Quality and Quantity, 19*(4), 353–373.

Marshall, C., & Rossman, G. B. (1989). *Designing qualitative research.* Newbury Park, CA: Sage.

Mead, G. H. (1934). *Mind, self and society,* Chicago: University of Chicago Press.

Miles, M. B., & Huberman, A. M. (1994). *Qualitative data analysis: An expanded sourcebook* (2nd ed.). Beverly Hills, CA: Sage.

Morse, J. M. (1989). Qualitative nursing research: A free-for-all? In J. M. Morse (Ed.), *Qualitative nursing research: A contemporary dialogue* (pp. 14–22). Rockville, MD: Aspen.

Morse, J. M., & Field, P. A. (1995). *Qualitative research methods for health professionals* (2nd ed.). Thousand Oaks, CA: Sage.

Munhall, P. L. (1982a). Nursing philosophy and nursing research: In apposition or opposition? *Nursing Research, 31*(3), 176–181.

Munhall, P. L. (1982b). Ethical juxtapositions in nursing research. *Topics in Clinical Nursing, 4*(1), 66–73.

Munhall, P. L. (1988). Ethical considerations in qualitative research. *Western Journal of Nursing Research, 10*(2), 150–162.

Munhall, P. L. (1989). Philosophical ponderings on qualitative research methods in nursing. *Nursing Science Quarterly, 2*(1), 20–28.

Munhall, P. L., & Boyd, C. O. (1993). *Nursing research: A qualitative perspective.* New York: National League for Nursing Press, Pub. No. 19-2535.

Murdock, G. (1971). *Outline of cultural materials.* New Haven, CT: Human Relations Area Files Press.

Newton, M. E. (1965). The case for historical research. *Nursing Research, 14*(1), 20–26.

Nwoga, I. (1997). *Mother-daughter conversations related to sex-role socialization and adolescent pregnancy.* PhD dissertation, The University of Florida.

Oiler, C. (1982). The phenomenological approach in nursing research. *Nursing Research, 31*(3), 178–181.

Omery, A. (1983). Phenomenology: A method for nursing research. *Advances in Nursing Science, 5*(2), 49–63.

Parse, R. R. (1981). *Man-living-health: A theory of nursing.* New York: Wiley.

Paterson, J. G., & Zderad, L. T. (1976). *Humanistic nursing.* New York: Wiley.

Salsberry, P. J., Smith, M. C., & Boyd, C. O. (1989). Dialogue on a research issue: Phenomenological research in nursing—Commentary and responses. *Nursing Science Quarterly, 2*(1), 9–19.

Sandelowski, M. (1986). The problem of rigor in qualitative research. *Advances in Nursing Science, 8*(3), 27–37.

Sandelowski, M. (1995). Sample size in qualitative research. *Research in Nursing & Health, 18*(2), 179–183.

Sandelowski, M. (1996). One is the liveliest number: The case orientation of qualitative research. *Research in Nursing & Health, 19*(6), 525–529.

Sarnecky, M. T. (1990). Historiography: A legitimate research methodology for nursing. *Advances in Nursing Science, 12*(4), 1–10.

Scheffler, I. (1967). *Science and subjectivity.* Indianapolis: Bobbs-Merrill.

Schwartz-Barcott, D., & Kim, H. S. (1986). A hybrid model

for concept development. In P. L. Chinn (Ed.), *Nursing research methodology: Issues and implementation* (pp. 91–101). Rockville, MD: Aspen.

Silva, M. C., & Rothbart, D. (1984). An analysis of changing trends in philosophies of science on nursing theory development and testing. *Advances in Nursing Science, 6*(2), 1–13.

Silverman, D. (1993). *Interpreting qualitative data: Methods for analysing talk, text and interaction.* Thousand Oaks, CA: Sage.

Strauss, A. L. (1975). *Chronic illness and quality of life.* St. Louis: Mosby.

Strauss, A. L., Corbin, J., Fagerhaugh, S., Glaser, B. G.,

Maines, D., Suczek, B., & Wiener, C. L. (1984). *Chronic illness and the quality of life* (2nd ed.). St. Louis: Mosby.

Strauss, A., & Glaser, B. G. (1970). *Anguish.* Mill Valley, CA: Sociology Press.

Waring, L. M. (1978). Developing the research prospectus. In M. L. Fitzpatrick (Ed.), *Historical studies in nursing* (pp. 18–20). New York: Teachers College Press.

Watson, J. (1985). *Nursing: Human science and human care: A theory of nursing.* Norwalk, CT: Appleton-Century-Crofts.

Wolcott, H. F. (1994). *Transforming qualitative data: Description, analysis, and interpretation.* Thousand Oaks, CA: Sage.

Critiquing Nursing Studies

Completing this chapter should enable you to:

1. *Define the term intellectual research critique.*
2. *Describe the basic guidelines that direct the conduct of a research critique.*
3. *Discuss the roles of nurses in conducting research critiques.*
4. *Describe the critical thinking phases used in the quantitative research critique process: comprehension, comparison, analysis, and evaluation.*
5. *Discuss the critique steps used in the four critical thinking phases: comprehension, comparison, analysis, and evaluation.*
6. *Conduct a critique of a research report.*
7. *Explore the critique process for qualitative research.*
8. *Discuss the standards used in critiquing qualitative studies: descriptive vividness, methodological congruence, analytical preciseness, theoretical connectedness, and heuristic relevance.*

Analysis phase

Analytical preciseness

Auditability

Comparison phase

Comprehension phase

Descriptive vividness

Evaluation phase

Heuristic relevance

Intellectual research critique

Methodological congruence

Rigor

Theoretical connectedness

*C*ritiquing research is essential for developing and refining nursing knowledge. However, the word "critique" is often linked with the word "criticize," which is frequently viewed as negative. In the arts and sciences, "critique" takes on another meaning; it is associated with critical thinking and appraisal and requires carefully developed intellectual skills. This type of critique is sometimes referred to as an "intellectual critique." An intellectual critique is directed not at the person who created but at the element of creation. For example, one might conduct an intellectual critique of an art object, an essay, or a study.

The idea of critique was introduced early in this textbook and woven throughout the chapters. As each step of the research process was introduced, guidelines were provided to direct the critique of that step in a research report. This chapter summarizes and builds upon previous critique content and provides direction for conducting critiques of studies. The elements of an intellectual critique of research are described, and nurses' roles in critiquing research are discussed. In addition, the phases of critical thinking used in the critique process for quantitative research (comprehension, comparison, analysis, and evaluation) are presented in detail. An example critique of a published quantitative study is provided. The chapter concludes with an introduction to the critique process for qualitative research.

Examining the Elements of an Intellectual Research Critique

An *intellectual research critique* involves careful examination of all aspects of a study to judge the strengths, weaknesses, meaning, and significance of the study. A quality study should focus on a significant problem, demonstrate sound methodology, produce credible findings, and have the capacity to be replicated by other researchers.

IN CRITIQUING a study, you need to address questions such as the following.

1. *Was the problem studied significant to generate or refine knowledge for nursing practice?*
2. *What are the major strengths of the study?*
3. *What are the major weaknesses of the study?*
4. *Was the methodology of the study sound?*
5. *Are the findings from the study an accurate reflection of reality or credible?*
6. *What is the significance of the findings for nursing practice?*
7. *Are the findings consistent with those from previous studies?*
8. *Can the study as conducted be replicated by other researchers?*

Answering these questions requires careful examination of the problem, purpose, literature review, framework, methods, results, and findings of the study.

The conduct of an intellectual critique involves applying some basic guidelines that are presented in Table 12-1. These guidelines stress the importance of critiquing the entire study and clearly, concisely, and objectively identifying the study's strengths and weaknesses. All studies have weaknesses or flaws; if all flawed studies were discarded, there would be no scientific base for practice. In fact, science itself is flawed. Science does not completely or perfectly describe, explain, predict, and control reality. However, improved understanding and increased ability to predict and control phenomena depend on recognizing the flaws in studies and in science. Additional studies can then be planned to minimize the weaknesses of earlier studies.

All studies have strengths as well as weaknesses. Recognizing these strengths is critical for generating scientific knowledge and using findings in practice. If only weaknesses are identified, nurses might discount the value of studies and refuse to invest time in examining research. The continued work of the researcher depends on the recognition of the study's strengths as well

TABLE 12-1. Guidelines for Conducting a Research Critique

1. *Read and critique the entire study.* A research critique involves examining the quality of all steps of the research process.
2. *Examine the organization and presentation of the research report.* The report should be complete, concise, clearly presented, and logically organized. A study should not include excessive jargon that is difficult for nonresearchers to read. The references need to be complete and presented in a consistent format.
3. *Examine the significance of the problem studied for nursing practice.* The focus of nursing studies needs to be on significant practice problems if a sound knowledge base is to be developed for the profession.
4. *Identify the strengths and weaknesses of a study.* All studies have strengths and weaknesses, so attention must be given to all aspects of the study.
5. *Be objective and realistic in identifying the study's strengths and weaknesses.* Be balanced in your critique of a study. Try not to be overly critical in identifying a study's weaknesses or overly flattering in identifying the strengths.
6. *Provide specific examples of the strengths and weaknesses of a study.* Examples provide evidence for your critique of the strengths and weaknesses of a study.
7. *Provide a rationale for your critique.* Include justifications for your critique and document your ideas with sources from the current literature. This strengthens the quality of your critique and documents the use of critical thinking skills.
8. *Suggest modifications for future studies.* Modifications in future studies will increase the strengths and decrease the weaknesses identified in the present study.
9. *Discuss the feasibility of replication of the study.* Is the study presented in enough detail to be replicated?
10. *Discuss the usefulness of the findings for practice.* The findings from the study need to be linked to the findings of previous studies. All these findings need to be examined for use in clinical practice.

as its weaknesses. If no study is good enough, why invest time conducting research? Points of strength in a study, added to points of strength from multiple other studies, slowly build a solid knowledge base for practice.

Two nursing research journals, *Scholarly Inquiry for Nursing Practice: An International Journal* and *The Western Journal of Nursing Research,* include commentaries (partial critiques) after a published research report. In these journals, authors receive critiques of their work and have an opportunity to respond to the critiques. Published critiques usually increase one's understanding of the study and one's ability to critique other studies. Another more informal critique of a published study might appear in a letter to the editor. Readers have the opportunity to comment on the strengths and weaknesses of published studies by writing to the editors of journals.

Nurses' Roles in Conducting Research Critiques

Research is critiqued to broaden understanding, improve practice, and provide a background for conducting a study. All nurses—including students, practicing nurses, educators, administrators, and researchers—need to critique research. Basic knowledge of the research process and the critique process is often provided early in professional nursing education at the baccalaureate level. More advanced critique skills are taught at the master's and doctorate levels. Critique skills increase as knowledge of the research process increases.

As a student, you are encouraged to critique published studies on relevant clinical topics to increase your understanding of the research process, promote your interest in reading research articles, and determine whether the findings are ready for use in practice. Critiques of studies by practicing nurses are essential for expanding understanding and making changes in practice. Nurses in practice constantly need to update their nursing interventions in response to current research knowledge. In addition, accrediting agencies for health care facilities require that policy and procedure manuals used to direct nursing care be based on research.

Educators critique studies to update their knowledge of research findings. This knowledge provides a basis for developing and refining content taught in classroom and clinical settings. Instructors and textbooks often identify the nursing interventions that were tested through research. Many educators who conduct studies critique research as a basis for planning and implementing their studies. Researchers often focus on one area and update their knowledge base by critiquing new studies in this area. The outcome of the critique influences the selection of research problems, identification of frameworks, development of methodologies, and interpretation of findings in future studies.

Understanding the Quantitative Research Critique Process

Critiquing research involves the use of a variety of critical thinking skills in the application of knowledge of the research process (Miller & Babcock, 1996). The research critique process includes four critical thinking phases: comprehension, comparison, analysis, and evaluation. These phases initially occur in sequence and presume accomplishment of the preceding steps. However, as your experience in research critique increases, you will probably perform several phases of this process simultaneously. Conducting a critique is a complex mental process that is stimulated by raising questions. Thus, relevant questions are provided for each phase of the critique process. The comprehension phase is covered separately because those new to critiquing start with this phase. The comparison and analysis phases are covered together because they often occur simultaneously in the mind of the person conducting the critique. Evaluation is covered separately because of the increased expertise required to perform this phase. Each of the critical thinking phases involves examination of the steps of the quantitative research process and identification of the strengths and weaknesses of these steps.

Phase 1: Comprehension

The *comprehension phase* is the first step in the research critique process. This critique phase involves understanding the terms and concepts in the report, as well as identifying the elements or steps of the research process, such as the problem, purpose, framework, and design. It is also necessary to grasp the nature, significance, and meaning of these steps in a research report.

Guidelines for Comprehension of a Research Report

First, review the abstract, read the entire study, and examine the references. Next, answer the following questions about the presentation of the study: Was the writing style clear and concise? Were the major sections of the research report (such as the literature review, framework, methods, results, and discussion) clearly identified? Were relevant terms clearly defined? (Burns & Grove, 1997; Phillips, 1986; Ryan-Wenger, 1992). You might underline terms you do not understand and look them up in the glossary at the back of this book. Next, you might read the article a second time and highlight or underline each step of the research process.

Comprehension Research Critique Guidelines

TO WRITE a beginning research critique that demonstrates comprehension of the study, concisely identify each step of the research process and briefly respond to the following questions. Do not answer the questions yes or no; rather, provide a rationale or include examples or content from the study to address these questions.

1. *What is the study problem?*
2. *What is the study purpose?*
3. *Is the literature review presented?*
   a. *Are relevant previous studies identified and described?*
   b. *Are relevant theories and models identified and described?*
   c. *Are the references current?*
   d. *Are the studies critiqued by the author?*
   e. *Is a summary of the current knowledge provided? This summary should include what is known and not known about the research problem.*
4. *Is a study framework identified?*
   a. *Is the framework explicitly expressed or must it be extracted from the literature review?*
   b. *Is a particular theory or model identified as a framework for the study?*
   c. *Does the framework describe and define the concepts of interest?*
   d. *Does the framework present the relationships among the concepts and relate them to the variables of the study?*
   e. *Is a map or model of the framework provided for clarity?*

continued

    f. If a map or model is not presented, develop one that represents the study's framework and describe it.

5. *Are research objectives, questions, or hypotheses used to direct the conduct of the study? Identify these.*

6. *Are the major variables or concepts identified and defined (conceptually and operationally)? Identify and define the appropriate variables included in the study:*
   a. Independent variables,
   b. Dependent variables, and/or
   c. Research variables or concepts

7. *What attributes or demographic variables are examined in the study?*

8. *Are the following elements of the sample described?*
   a. Sample criteria
   b. Method used to obtain the sample
   c. Sample size (indicate if a power analysis was conducted to determine sample size)
   d. Characteristics of the sample
   e. Sample mortality
   f. Type of consent obtained

9. *Is the research design clearly addressed?*
   a. Identify the specific design of the study.
   b. Does the study include a treatment? If so, is the treatment clearly described and consistently implemented?
   c. Are the extraneous variables identified and controlled?
   d. Were pilot study findings used to design the major study? Briefly discuss the pilot study and the findings. Indicate the changes made in the major study based on the pilot.

10. *Are the measurement strategies described?*
    a. Describe the methods of measurement, including the author of each instrument, how the instrument was developed, and how the instrument was used in the study.
    b. Identify the level of measurement achieved with each instrument.
    c. Describe the reliability of each instrument.
    d. Describe the validity of each instrument.

11. *How were study procedures implemented and data collected during the study?*

12. *What statistical analyses are included in the research report?*
    a. Identify the analysis techniques and indicate the purpose of each: description, determination of differences, examination of relationships.
    b. Are the statistics mainly descriptive, inferential, or both?
    c. List the statistical procedures used and their outcomes for each research objective, question, or hypothesis. If objectives, questions, or hypotheses are not stated, link the analysis techniques to the study purpose.

13. *What is the researcher's interpretation of the findings?*
    a. Are the results related to the study framework? If so, do the findings support the study framework?
    b. Which findings are consistent with those expected?

    c. *Which findings are unexpected?*
    d. *Are serendipitous findings described?*
    e. *Are the findings consistent with previous research findings?*
14. *What limitations of the study are identified by the researcher?*
15. *How does the researcher generalize the findings?*
16. *What implications do the findings have for nursing practice?*
17. *What suggestions are made for further studies?*
18. *What are the missing elements of the study?*
19. *Is the description of the study sufficiently clear to allow replication?*

Phases 2 and 3: Comparison and Analysis

Critical thinking phases 2 and 3 (comparison and analysis) are frequently done simultaneously when critiquing a study. The *comparison phase* requires knowledge of what each step of the research process should be like, and then the ideal is compared to the real. During the comparison phase, you need to examine the extent to which the researcher followed the rules for an ideal study. Examine the steps of the study, such as the problem, purpose, framework, methodology, and results, based on the content presented in Chapters 2–10 of this book. Did the researcher rigorously develop and implement the study? What are the strengths of the study? What are the weaknesses of the study?

    The *analysis phase* involves a critique of the logical links connecting one study element with another. For example, the presentation of the problem must provide background and direction for the statement of the purpose. In addition, the overall logical development of the study must be examined. The variables identified in the study purpose need to be consistent with the variables identified in the research objectives, questions, or hypotheses. These variables must be conceptually defined in light of the study framework. The conceptual definitions provide the basis for the development of the operational definitions. The study design must be appropriate for the investigation of the study purpose and for the specific objectives, questions, or hypotheses. The instruments used in the study must adequately measure the variables. The sample selected needs to be representative of the population identified in the problem and purpose. Analysis techniques need to provide results that address the purpose and the specific objectives, questions, or hypotheses. The findings from a study must be linked to the framework and the findings from previous research to determine the current knowledge of the study problem. The synthesis of these findings results in the formation of conclusions that can be generalized to individuals other than the study subjects. Depending on the quality of the findings, the researcher indicates the use of the findings in nursing practice. All these steps of the research process provide a basis for the identification of future research projects. As you can see, the steps of the research process need to be precisely developed and strongly linked to conduct a quality study.

Guidelines for Comparison and Analysis of a Research Report

To conduct the comparison and analysis steps, review Chapters 2–10 of this textbook and other sources on the steps of the research process (Burns & Grove, 1997; Munro, 1997; Phillips, 1986; Polit & Hungler, 1997). Then compare the steps in the study you are critiquing with the criteria established for each step in this textbook or other sources (Phase 2, comparison). Next, analyze the logical links among the steps of the study (Phase 3, analysis). The guidelines in this section will assist you in implementing the phases of comparison and analysis for each step of the research process. Questions relevant to analysis are identified; all other questions direct the comparison of the steps of the study with the ideal. Use these questions to determine how rigorously the steps of the research process were implemented in published studies. Indicate which steps are strengths and which ones are weaknesses. When labeling a step as a strength or weakness, provide examples from the study and/or state a rationale with documentation to support your conclusions. In addition, identify the strengths in the logical way the steps of the study are linked together or any breaks or weaknesses in the links of a study's steps.

Comparison and Analysis Research Critique Guidelines

THE WRITTEN critique will be a narrative summary of the strengths and weaknesses that you note in the study. The guidelines below will assist you in examining the significance of the problem, fit of the framework, rigor of the methodology, and quality and relevance of the findings in published studies.

1. *Research problem and purpose*
    a. *Is the problem sufficiently narrow in scope without being trivial?*
    b. *Is the problem significant and relevant to nursing?*
    c. *Does the purpose narrow and clarify the focus or aim of the study and identify the research variables, population, and setting?*
    d. *Was this study feasible to conduct in terms of money commitment; researchers' expertise; availability of subjects, facility, and equipment; and ethical considerations?*
2. *Literature review*
    a. *Is the literature review organized to demonstrate the progressive development of ideas through previous research? (Analysis)*
    b. *Is a theoretical knowledge base developed for the problem and purpose? (Analysis)*
    c. *Does the literature review provide a rationale and direction for the study? (Analysis)*
    d. *Does the summary of the current empirical and theoretical knowledge provide a basis for the study conducted?*
3. *Study framework*
    a. *Is the framework presented with clarity?*

    b. Is the framework linked to the research purpose? (Analysis)

    c. Would another framework fit more logically with the study? (Analysis)

    d. Is the framework related to nursing's body of knowledge? (Analysis)

    e. If a proposition from a theory is to be tested, is the proposition clearly identi-fied and linked to the study hypotheses? (Analysis)

4. Research objectives, questions, or hypotheses

    a. Are the objectives, questions, or hypotheses clearly and concisely expressed?

    b. Are the objectives, questions, or hypotheses logically linked to the research pur-pose? (Analysis)

    c. Are the research objectives, questions, or hypotheses derived from the frame-work? (Analysis)

5. Variables

    a. Are the variables reflective of the concepts identified in the framework? (Analysis)

    b. Are the variables clearly defined (conceptually and operationally) based on pre-vious research and/or theories?

    c. Is the conceptual definition of a variable consistent with the operational defi-nition? (Analysis)

    d. Are there uncontrolled extraneous variables that may have influenced the findings?

6. Design

    a. Was the best design selected to direct this study?

    b. Does the design provide a means to examine all of the objectives, questions, or hypotheses? (Analysis)

    c. Have the threats to design validity (statistical conclusion validity, internal va-lidity, construct validity, and external validity) been minimized?

    d. Is the design logically linked to the sampling method and statistical analyses? (Analysis)

    e. If a treatment is implemented, is it clearly defined conceptually and operation-ally? Is the treatment appropriate to examine the study purpose and hypothe-ses? (Analysis)

7. Sample, population, and setting

    a. Is the target population to which the findings will be generalized defined?

    b. Is the sampling method adequate to produce a sample that is representative of the study population?

    c. What are the potential biases in the sampling method?

    d. Is the sample size sufficient to avoid a Type II error?

    e. If more than one group is used, do the groups appear equivalent?

    f. Are the rights of human subjects protected?

    g. Is the setting used in the study typical of clinical settings?

8. Measurements

    a. Do the instruments adequately measure the study variables? (Analysis)

    b. Are the instruments sufficiently sensitive to detect differences between subjects?

    c. Is the reliability of the instruments adequate for use in the study?

    d. Is the validity of the instruments adequate for use in the study?

continued

    e. *Do the instruments need further research?*

    f. *Respond to the following questions, which are relevant to the measurement approaches used in the study.*

Scales and Questionnaires

    (1) *Are the instruments clearly described?*

    (2) *Are techniques to administer, complete, and score the instruments provided?*

    (3) *Is the reliability of the instruments described?*

    (4) *Is the validity of the instruments described?*

    (5) *Did the researcher examine the reliability and/or the validity of the instruments for the present sample?*

    (6) *If the instrument was developed for the study, is the instrument development process described?*

Observation

    (1) *Is what is to be observed clearly identified and defined?*

    (2) *Is interrater reliability described?*

    (3) *Are the techniques for recording observations described?*

Interviews

    (1) *Do the interview questions address concerns expressed in the research problem? (Analysis)*

    (2) *Are the interview questions relevant for the research purpose and objectives, questions, or hypotheses? (Analysis)*

    (3) *Does the design of the questions tend to bias subjects' responses?*

    (4) *Does the sequence of questions tend to bias subjects' responses?*

Physiologic Measures

    (1) *Are the physiologic measures or instruments clearly described? If appropriate, are the brand names (such as Space Labs or Hewlett-Packard) of the instruments identified?*

    (2) *Is the accuracy, selectivity, precision, sensitivity, and error of the physiologic instruments discussed?*

    (3) *Are the methods for recording data from the physiologic measures clearly described?*

 9. *Data collection*

    a. *Is the data collection process clearly described?*

    b. *Is the training of data collectors clearly described and adequate?*

    c. *Is the data collection process conducted in a consistent manner?*

    d. *Are the data collection methods ethical?*

    e. *Do the data collected address the research objectives, questions, or hypotheses? (Analysis)*

10. *Data analyses*

    a. *Are data analysis procedures clearly described?*

b.　*Do data analyses address each objective, question, or hypothesis?*

c.　*Are data analysis procedures appropriate to the type of data collected?*

d.　*Are the results presented in an understandable way?*

e.　*Are tables and figures used to synthesize and emphasize certain findings?*

f.　*Are the analyses interpreted appropriately?*

g.　*If the results were nonsignificant, was the sample size sufficient to detect significant differences? Was a power analysis conducted to examine nonsignificant findings?*

11.　*Interpretation of findings*

a.　*Are findings discussed in relation to each objective, question, or hypothesis? (Analysis)*

b.　*Are significant and nonsignificant findings explained?*

c.　*Were the statistically significant findings also examined for clinical significance?*

d.　*Does the interpretation of findings appear biased?*

e.　*Are biases in the study identified?*

f.　*Do the conclusions fit the results from the analyses? (Analysis)*

g.　*Are the conclusions based on statistically and clinically significant results? (Analysis)*

h.　*Did the researchers identify important study limitations?*

i.　*Are there inconsistencies in the report?*

Phase 4: Evaluation

During the *evaluation phase* of a research critique, the meaning and significance of the study findings are examined. The evaluation becomes a summary of the study's quality that builds on conclusions reached during the first three phases (comprehension, comparison, and analysis) of the critique. This level of critique might or might not be conducted by a baccalaureate nursing student. The level of critique accomplished during your educational program depends on the placement of your research course in the curriculum at either the junior or senior year and the number of credit hours that are devoted to research. The guidelines for the evaluation phase are provided for those of you who want to perform a more comprehensive critique of the literature as a basis for summarizing findings for use in practice.

Guidelines for Evaluation of a Research Report

The evaluation phase involves reexamining the findings, conclusions, limitations, implications for nursing, and suggestions for further study that are usually presented in the discussion section of a research report. You will need to determine the value of the findings generated for the development of nursing knowledge and for use in practice.

Evaluation Critique Guidelines

USING THE FOLLOWING questions as a guide, summarize the quality of the study, the accuracy of the findings, and the usefulness of the findings for nursing practice. The evaluation phase involves developing a summary of the study's quality. This summary is a narrative that is usually the last paragraph of a critique.

1. *How much confidence can be placed in the study findings? Are the findings an accurate reflection of reality?*
2. *Are the findings related to the framework?*
3. *Are the findings linked to the findings of previous studies?*
4. *What do the findings add to the current body of knowledge?*
5. *To what populations can the findings be generalized?*
6. *What research questions emerge from the findings? Are these questions identified by the researcher?*
7. *What is the overall quality of this study when the strengths and weaknesses are summarized? Could any of the weaknesses have been corrected?*
8. *Do the findings have potential for use in nursing practice?*

Example Critique of a Quantitative Study

An example critique is presented in this section and includes the four phases of comprehension, comparison, analysis, and evaluation. The article critiqued— "Oxygen uptake and cardiovascular response in patients and normal adults during in-bed and out-of-bed toileting" by Winslow, Lane, and Gaffney (1984)—precedes the example critique.

An initial critique might focus on comprehension and involve identification of the steps of the research process in the study. The comprehension critique might be written in outline format, with headings identifying the steps of the research process. A more in-depth critique includes not only the comprehension step but also the comparison, analysis, and evaluation phases. The example critique in this chapter includes all four phases; the comprehension, comparison, analysis, and evaluation steps are presented in narrative format. You might read the article and identify the steps of the research process, then try to list the strengths and weaknesses of the study, including the logical links among the study steps. You might want to use the questions in this chapter to develop a critique of this study that includes comprehension, comparison, and analysis. Then read the example critique that follows the article and compare it with the critique that you have developed. Doing your own initial critique and then reading the example critique can help you expand your critique skills.

CRITIQUE ARTICLE

Oxygen Uptake and Cardiovascular Response in Patients and Normal Adults During In-Bed and Out-of-Bed Toileting

Elizabeth Hahn Winslow, PhD, RN, Lynda Denton Lane, BSN, RN, and F. Andrew Gaffney, MD

*P*atients dislike using the bedpan and urinal while in bed and often insist that it would be easier and better for them to get out of bed to toilet. Little data are available about the physiologic costs of toileting. Therefore, we measured oxygen uptake (VO_2), peak heart rate (HR_{peak}), peak rate-pressure product (RPP_{peak}), rating of perceived exertion, and preference in 42 women who used the bedpan and bedside commode for urination and in 53 men who used the urinal while in bed and standing. The subjects included 26 healthy volunteers, 16 cardiac outpatients, 27 medical inpatients, and 26 acute post-myocardial infarction patients (two to 28 days postinfarction). No physiologically important differences were found between in-bed and out-of-bed toileting. Both in-bed and out-of-bed toileting produced small increases in energy cost and myocardial work over resting levels, with a mean $VO_2 < 1.6$ times resting VO_2, a mean $HR_{peak} < 100$ beats/min, and a mean $RPP_{peak} < 11,200$. The subjects clearly preferred getting out of bed to toilet. Out-of-bed toileting produces minimal energy expenditure and cardiac stress and can help reduce bed rest-induced orthostatic intolerance. In-bed toileting should be reserved for patients with specific contraindications to postural change.

Over 30 years ago Benton and co-workers[1] reported that using the bedpan required 50% greater energy cost above resting level than did using the bedside commode. Since then, many clinicians have recommended that the myocardial infarction (MI) patient use the bedside commode after hospital admission.[2-6] However, time-honored traditions change slowly, especially when only a single study of the topic is available. Many physicians still wait several days before permitting their acute MI

From Texas Women's University, Parkland Memorial Hospital, and the Pauline and Adolph Weinberger Laboratory for Cardiopulmonary Research, University of Texas Health Science Center, Dallas.

Supported in part by the American Association of Critical-Care Nurses' Clinical Research Award sponsored by IVAC.

Address for reprints: Elizabeth H. Winslow, PhD, RN, Clinical Evaluation and Development Department, Methodist Central Hospital, P.O. Box 22599, Dallas, TX 75265.

patients to use the bedside commode or stand beside the bed to urinate. patients often complain about this and insist that it would be easier and better for them to get out of bed to toilet.

To determine which toileting method is more appropriate for the acutely ill medical patient, one should consider both the total energy cost and also the approximate myocardial work of in-bed and out-of-bed toileting methods when performed by patients. Therefore, we measured oxygen uptake (VO_2), peak heart rate (HR_{peak}), peak rate-pressure product (RPP_{peak}) (systolic blood pressure × heart rate), rating of perceived exertion (RPE), and preference in 95 hospitalized and nonhospitalized adults during in-bed (bedpan and urinal) and out-of-bed (bedside commode and standing urinal) toileting. Data on which to base toilet method recommendations for the hospitalized patient are provided.

Materials and Methods

Subjects

The 42 women and 53 men (range 18–79 years) who volunteered for the study consisted of 26 healthy adults, 16 coronary artery disease patients who were participating in a supervised outpatient exercise program, 27 stable medical inpatients with a variety of cardiac and noncardiac disorders, and 26 stable acute MI inpatients who had their MI from two to 28 days earlier (8.81 ± 5 days [mean ± SD]) (Table I). Eight patients had their MI five days or less before the study began. Acute MI was established by history, clinical, electrocardiographic (ECG), and enzyme findings and by myocardial scintigraphy. Nineteen (73%) of the patients had transmural infarctions; seven (27%) had subendocardial infarctions. All medical and cardiac inpatients were ambulatory prior to hospitalization, and none had neural or musculoskeletal problems that would preclude standing unassisted. Six (37%) of the cardiac outpatients, seven (26%) of the medical

TABLE I. Subject Characteristics

Subject Group	Sex	N	Age (years ± SD)	Weight (kg ± SD)	Height (cm ± SD)
Healthy volunteers	Female	11	38 ± 13	65 ± 8	168 ± 4
	Male	15	29 ± 7	77 ± 8	177 ± 4
Cardiac outpatients	Female	6	62 ± 4	58 ± 10	157 ± 6
	Male	10	58 ± 5	76 ± 8	173 ± 3
Medical inpatients	Female	14	57 ± 15	72 ± 16	161 ± 9
	Male	13	51 ± 10	84 ± 17	175 ± 7
Acute MI inpatients	Female	11	63 ± 11	76 ± 18	164 ± 6
	Male	15	61 ± 12	84 ± 17	172 ± 9

N = number of subjects; SD = standard deviation; MI = myocardial infarction.

inpatients, and five (19%) of the acute MI patients were receiving propranolol at the time of the study. The research protocol was approved by the Institutional Review Board, and informed written consent was obtained from all subjects prior to the study.

Methods

Oxygen uptake during rest and toileting was determined by open-circuit, indirect calorimetry. The subject had a nose clip and mouthpiece in place. During the timed period, expired air was collected via a one-way respiratory valve (Daniels) and 64-inch plastic tubing into a 30 L (rest) or 150 L (toileting) bag (Douglas). A standard adjustable helmet held the mouthpiece and valve in a comfortable, secure position; the Douglas bag was tied to a rolling intravenous pole. Expired air volume was measured by a Collins Chain Compensated Gasometer (Tissot), and air composition was analyzed by mass spectrometer (Perkin-Elmer Medical Gas Analyzer 1100). The mass spectrometer was calibrated electronically and checked against gases of known concentration. Standard equations were used to derive VO_2.

Gas collection was begun immediately before toileting when the subject was supine and was stopped when the subject had resumed the supine position. A continuous ECG (lead II) was recorded during toileting. Peak HR was the most rapid HR observed during any 15-second period. Blood pressure was measured by cuff sphygmomanometer immediately before and after toileting and after each position change. In the eight coronary care unit (CCU) patients, blood pressure was taken before and after toileting only. After each toileting method, the subject selected a number from the Borg scale of perceived exertion.[7] After both toileting methods, the subject completed a questionnaire wherein he ranked each method for comfort, pleasantness, and ease.

Protocol

Oxygen uptake, HR, and RPP were determined during a three-minute supine rest period and during in-bed and out-of-bed toileting. A ten-minute rest period separated the randomly ordered toileting methods. Women used the bedpan and bedside commode for urinating; men used the urinal while lying in bed and while standing beside the bed. The subject simulated voiding if unable to void during the second toileting trial.

The toileting protocol simulated usual clinical conditions; therefore, toileting duration varied. The investigator assisted the women in lifting their hips for bedpan placement and removal, and placed the bedside commode in a standardized position beside the head of the bed. Subjects used their own techniques to get out of and back into bed and were not lifted by the investigator. The investigator left the room while the subject urinated and returned when given a signal from the subject. Subjects took as much time as they needed for urination.

Statistical Analysis

Oxygen uptake, HR, and RPP results were analyzed for each sex and group by repeated measures analysis of variance (ANOVA). Ratings of perceived exertion and preferences were analyzed by the Friedman two-way ANOVA by ranks. Spearman correlation coefficients were calculated for selected variables including VO_2, age, and toileting duration.

Results

Oxygen uptake, HR, and RPP results during rest and toileting are shown in Table II and Figures I, II, and III. During rest, VO_2 ranged from 2.15 to 4.52 ml/kg/min, HR from 44 to 104 beats/min, and RPP from 5,000 to 14,100. During toileting, VO_2 ranged from 2.77 to 5.84 ml/kg/min, HR_{peak} from 56 to 132 beats/min, and RPP_{peak} from 5,400 to 14,400.

During in-bed toileting, 14 subjects (15%) had a HR_{peak} of 100 beats/min or greater; during out-of-bed toileting, 19 subjects (21%) had a HR_{peak} of 100 beats/min or greater at some time during toileting. Only four subjects had a HR_{peak} over 108 beats/min. The subjects with the highest resting HRs had the highest HRs during toileting. The highest HRs observed during each study condition were 104, 120, and 132 beats/min during rest, bedpan use, and bedside commode use, respectively, in one elderly woman with atrial fibrillation and an uncontrolled ventricular response. None of the subjects experienced chest pain, shortness of breath, light-headedness, palpitations, or other signs or symptoms of cardiovascular distress during toileting.

Statistically significant differences in VO_2, HR, and RPP between in-bed and out-of-bed toileting were found within some groups of subjects ($p < .05$). These differences represent mean differences of less than 1 ml/kg/min, 8 beats/min, and 1,300 units in VO_2, HR_{peak}, and RPP_{peak}, respectively.

Analysis for differences among the four subject groups did not show any statistically significant differences in resting VO_2. However, during toileting, hospitalized patients generally had a significantly lower VO_2 value than did nonhospitalized subjects ($p < .05$). Heart rate and RPP responses during rest and toileting did not differ significantly among the four groups of female subjects; however, significant differences in cardiovascular response were found among some male groups. The hospitalized men generally had a significantly higher HR and RPP during rest and toileting than did nonhospitalized men ($p < .05$).

Mean duration for bedpan use (5.8 ± 1.5 min) did not differ significantly from that of bedside commode use (6.2 ± 1.4 min); however, duration for in-bed urinal use (3.6 ± 1.0 min) was significantly shorter than that of out-of-bed urinal use (5.2 min ± 0.9 min) ($p < .05$). Analysis for group differences did not show a significant difference in duration among the four male groups; the healthy women, however, had a significantly shorter duration than did the other three groups of women ($p < .05$).

TABLE 11. Mean Oxygen Uptake (V̇O$_2$), Heart Rate (HR), and Rate-Pressure Product (RPP) During Rest and Mean V̇O$_2$ Peak HR, and Peak RPP During In-Bed and Out-of-Bed Toileting

Subject	Activity	Women (W)			Men (M)		
		V̇O$_2$ (ml/kg/min ± SD)	HR (beats/min ± SD)	RPP (SBP × HR/100 ± SD)	V̇O$_2$ (ml/kg/min ± SD)	HR (beats/min ± SD)	RPP (SBP × HR/100 ± SD)
Healthy volunteers (W = 11, M = 15)	Rest	3.43 ± 0.42	66 ± 10	79 ± 15	3.67 ± 0.41	60 ± 7	72 ± 12
	In-bed	4.84 ± 0.71	84 ± 10	92 ± 14	4.78 ± 0.46	87 ± 10	79 ± 12
	Out-of-bed	4.66 ± 0.63	85 ± 9	91 ± 15	4.66 ± 0.52	84 ± 8	91 ± 14*
		(N = 11)	(N = 10)	(N = 11)	(N = 15)	(N = 12)	(N = 15)
Cardiac outpatients (W = 6, M = 10)	Rest	3.20 ± 0.35	65 ± 12	89 ± 25	3.56 ± 0.36	59 ± 8	75 ± 17
	In-bed	4.43 ± 0.57	81 ± 16	104 ± 30	4.72 ± 0.59	77 ± 11	86 ± 20
	Out-of-bed	4.36 ± 0.61	81 ± 17	103 ± 24	4.77 ± 0.47	77 ± 12	84 ± 15
		(N = 5)	(N = 6)	(N = 6)	(N = 9)	(N = 10)	(N = 10)
Medical inpatients (W = 14, M = 13)	Rest	3.14 ± 0.43	74 ± 14	97 ± 17	3.32 ± 0.37	73 ± 8	90 ± 13
	In-bed	3.91 ± 0.61	85 ± 15	111 ± 17	3.92 ± 0.53	89 ± 8	99 ± 18
	Out-of-bed	4.25 ± 0.79*	88 ± 16	105 ± 19	4.24 ± 0.42*	96 ± 9*	108 ± 21
		(N = 11)	(N = 14)	(N = 14)	(N = 12)	(N = 13)	(N = 13)
Acute MI inpatients† (W = 11, M = 15)	Rest	2.90 ± 0.65	77 ± 9	101 ± 26	3.22 ± 0.38	72 ± 7	89 ± 13
	In-bed	3.52 ± 0.59	89 ± 9	110 ± 22	3.78 ± 0.56	84 ± 12	94 ± 15
	Out-of-bed	3.84 ± 0.55	94 ± 9	109 ± 26	4.21 ± 0.42*	91 ± 9*	102 ± 15
		(N = 7)	(N = 11)	(N = 9)	(N = 11)	(N = 15)	(N = 15)

*In-bed vs. out-of-bed toileting ($p < .05$).

†Data from the eight coronary care unit patients (4W and 4M) are not included in V̇O$_2$ results because a modified V̇O$_2$ collection protocol was used (see text).

SD = standard deviation; SBP = systolic blood pressure; N = number of subjects; MI = myocardial infarction.

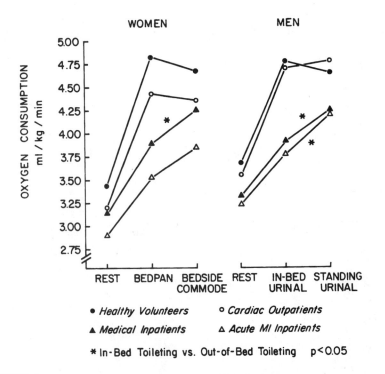

WOMEN   MEN

OXYGEN CONSUMPTION ml / kg / min

5.00
4.75
4.50
4.25
4.00
3.75
3.50
3.25
3.00
2.75

REST   BEDPAN   BEDSIDE   REST   IN-BED   STANDING
                  COMMODE   URINAL   URINAL

● *Healthy Volunteers*   ○ *Cardiac Outpatients*

▲ *Medical Inpatients*   △ *Acute MI Inpatients*

* In-Bed Toileting vs. Out-of-Bed Toileting   p<0.05

FIGURE I

Mean oxygen uptake during rest, in-bed toileting, and out-of-bed toileting in four groups of subjects. *In-bed toileting vs. out-of-bed toileting, $p < .05$. MI = myocardial infarction.

The rating of perceived exertion (RPE) results showed that in-bed toileting was perceived to require significantly more exertion than out-of-bed toileting ($p < .05$). However, most subjects considered both in-bed and out-of-bed toileting light exertion. The mode RPE scores were 9 (very light) for bedpan, bedside commode, and out-of-bed urinal and 11 (fairly light) for in-bed urinal. The median RPE scores were 11 for bedpan, 10 for bedside commode, 11 for in-bed urinal, and 9 for out-of-bed urinal. Both men and women reported significantly higher comfort, pleasantness, and ease of ranking ($p < .0005$) for out-of-bed toileting compared with in-bed toileting.

Discussion

Both in-bed and out-of-bed toileting methods produced small increases in energy cost over resting levels. When the energy cost results are expressed as multiples of the subject's resting VO₂ (METs), the energy costs of using the bedpan and bedside commode were 1.3 and 1.4 METs, respec-

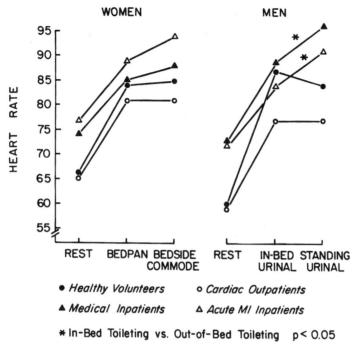

FIGURE II

Mean heart rate during rest and mean peak heart rate during in-bed and out-of-bed toileting in four groups of subjects. *In-bed toileting vs. out-of-bed toileting, $p < .05$. MI = myocardial infarction.

tively; and the energy costs of using the urinal while in bed and while standing were 1.2 and 1.3 METs, respectively. These results are comparable with those of Benton and co-workers,[1] who measured VO_2 in 15 cardiac subjects and 13 noncardiac subjects during simulated defecation in the bedpan and bedside commode and found that bedpan use required 1.6 METs and bedside commode use required 1.4 METs. The higher energy cost for bedpan use in the Benton study (1.6 METs) compared with that found in our study (1.3 METs) may be explained by differences in research protocol—the Benton subjects got on and off the bedpan unassisted, whereas our subjects received assistance.

The measured VO_2 values in Benton's study and ours are slightly lower than the actual VO_2 for toileting, because Benton measured VO_2 during toileting as well as during a recovery period following toileting, and we measured VO_2 during the entire toileting process, which included pauses for blood pressure measurement. When the blood pressure pauses were eliminated for the eight coronary care unit patients, the VO_2 values for in-bed and out-of-bed toileting were 4.3 and 4.6 ml/kg/min, respectively, for the women and 4.5 and 4.7 ml/kg/min, respectively, for the men. These results convert to 1.4 METs for bedpan use, 1.5 METs for

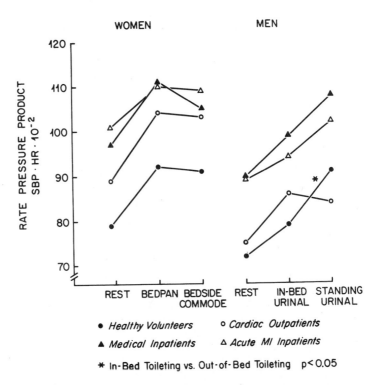

WOMEN   MEN

• *Healthy Volunteers*   ○ *Cardiac Outpatients*
▲ *Medical Inpatients*   △ *Acute MI Inpatients*
* In-Bed Toileting vs. Out-of-Bed Toileting   p< 0.05

FIGURE III

Mean rate-pressure product during rest and mean peak rate-pressure product during in-bed and out-of-bed toileting. SBP = systolic blood pressure; HR = heart rate; MI = myocardial infarction.

bedside commode use, 1.3 METs for using the urinal while in bed, and 1.4 METs for using the urinal while standing. Therefore, toileting produces low energy costs, and the differences in energy cost between in-bed and out-of-bed toileting, though statistically significant in some groups of subjects, appear clinically and physiologically unimportant.

The findings of Benton and co-workers[1] have been misunderstood and misquoted in several publications. Gordon[8] erroneously stated that bedside commode use required 3.6 kcal/min (approximately 3 METs) and bedpan use required 4.6 kcal/min (approximately 4 METs). Zohman and Tobias,[9] Acker,[10] the editors of *Exercise Equivalents,*[11] and others quote Gordon's numbers and thus perpetuate Gordon's misinterpretation of the Benton data. In *Exercise Equivalents,*[11] the energy cost of using a bedside commode (3 METs) is shown to be equal to that of scrubbing a floor, and the energy cost of using a bedpan (4 METs) is shown to be equal to that of beating a carpet. Close examination of the Benton data, however, shows that use of the bedpan and bedside commode require only about 1.5 times resting energy cost and not the three- to fourfold increase subsequently reported.

Our hospitalized patients generally had significantly lower VO_2 values during toileting than did the nonhospitalized subjects. Hospitalized patients also have been reported to have a significantly lower energy cost during bathing than did healthy volunteers.[12,13] Resting VO_2, adjusted for body weight, did not differ significantly among our four groups of subjects. Spearman rank correlation coefficients (r_s) were calculated to determine the relationship of toilet method VO_2 (ml/kg/min) to age and toileting duration. In nonhospitalized women, VO_2 during bedpan use correlated with toileting duration $(r_s = -.60, p = .01)$. In hospitalized men, age correlated with VO_2 during in-bed urinal use $(r_s = -.60, p = .002)$, and during standing urinal use $(r_s = -.41, p = .05)$. No other significant correlations were found. The meaning of the few significant correlations is unclear because of the lack of consistent trends. Conservation of effort may explain the hospitalized patients' lower energy expenditure, because in our study and in the bathing studies[12,13] the hospitalized patients appeared to move more slowly and deliberately than did the nonhospitalized subjects. However, none of the studies used matched groups; thus, other variables may also explain the VO_2 differences.

In addition to quantitating overall energy costs, we measured HR_{peak} and RPP_{peak} during toileting to estimate myocardial work.[14] The statistically significant differences in HR_{peak} and RPP_{peak} between in-bed and out-of-bed toileting in some groups of subjects represent increases of only 8% in HR and 15% in RPP. These differences are quite small and probably not of physiologic importance. The higher values in the hospitalized men can be explained by differences in conditioning, orthostatic tolerance, and the presence of arterial hypertension.

Benton and co-workers[1] recorded blood pressure, HR, and an ECG before, during, and after each toileting method but did not report the data because of their extreme variability. Singman and co-workers[15] recorded continuous ECGs during defecation in 51 CCU patients, including 23 with acute MI. Both bedpan (N = 15) and bedside commode (N = 48) were used. The ECGs were analyzed for ectopy and for changes in ST segments or of 10 beats/min or greater in HR. Only two patients had ECG changes other than an increased HR; the authors do not describe these changes. The finding that more patients increased HRs by 10 beats/min or more during bedside commode use than during bedpan use is an expected response to the upright posture. The virtual absence of ECG abnormalities supports our findings that the cardiovascular differences in bedpan and bedside commode use are physiologically insignificant.

Acute MI patients treated with strict bed rest for nine to 24 days have pronounced orthostatic intolerance during upright tilt or sitting posture; in contrast, orthostatic tolerance is not impaired in acute MI patients treated for seven to 18 days with modified bed rest—the patients performed active leg exercises, sat on the edge of the bed, and used the commode from the day of admission.[16] Signs of orthostatic intolerance develop after as little as six hours of bed rest[17] and progress as bed rest continues.[18] Orthostatic intolerance needs to be prevented in acute MI patients, because the postural changes in HR and blood pressure are potential causes of cerebral infarction and extension of MI.

Studies by Convertino and associates[19,20] show that orthostatic stress is the most important factor limiting exercise tolerance after bed rest and that exposure to gravitational stress for 3.5 hours daily may obviate much of the deterioration in cardiovascular performance resulting from bed rest. Getting the patient up for eating and toileting should provide the gravitational stress necessary to minimize bed rest-induced orthostatic intolerance.

The results of our study show that both in-bed and out-of-bed toileting methods produce minimal energy cost and cardiovascular stress for healthy volunteers, cardiac outpatients, stable medical inpatients, and stable inpatients who had an acute MI from two to 28 days earlier. Clinically or physiologically important differences were not found between staying in bed and getting out of bed to toilet. The subjects clearly preferred getting out of bed to toilet. Findings from other studies show that getting out of bed for short periods minimizes bed rest-induced orthostatic intolerance[16,20] and that the upright posture may even decrease myocardial oxygen demands.[21,22] In-bed toileting should be reserved for those patients with specific contraindications to postural changes. Thus, for medical patients without specific contraindications, we recommend out-of-bed toileting.

The authors thank Cathleen L. Michaels, MSN, PN, Ann McCash, BSN, RN, Jo Cole, MSN, RN, Robert Rude, MD, C. Gunnar Blomqvist, MD, and the nurses of the tenth floor, coronary care unit, and MILIS study at Parkland Memorial Hospital for assistance in the study; Kent Dana, MA, and Nancy Wilson, MS, at the University of Texas Health Science Center for statistical advice; and Carolyn Donahue for preparing the manuscript.

REFERENCES

1. Benton JG, Brown H, Rusk HA: Energy expanded by patients on the bedpan and bedside commode. *JAMA* 1950;144:1443–1447.
2. Gazes PC, Gaddy JE: Bedside management of acute myocardial infarction. *Am Heart J* 1979; 97:782–796.
3. Levine SA, Lown B: Armchair treatment of acute coronary thrombosis. *JAMA* 1952;148:1365–1369.
4. Newman LB, Wasserman, RR, Borden G: Productive living for those with heart disease: The role of physical medicine and rehabilitation. *Arch Phys Med Rehabil* 1956;37:137–149.
5. Niccoli A, Brammell HL: A program for rehabilitation in coronary heart disease. *Nursing Clin North Am* 1976;11:237–250.
6. Wenger NK: Rehabilitation of the patient with myocardial infarction: Responsibility of the primary care physician. *Primary Care* 1981;8:491–507.
7. Borg G: Perceived exertion: A note on history and methods. *Med Sci Sports* 1973;5:90–93.
8. Gordon EE: Energy costs of activities in health and disease. *Arch Intern Med* 1958;101:702–713.
9. Zohman LR, Tobis JS: *Cardiac Rehabilitation.* New York, Grune and Stratton, 1970.
10. Acker J: Early ambulation of post-myocardial infarction patients: Early activity after myocardial infarction, in Naughton JP, Hellerstein HK (eds): *Exercise Testing and Exercise Training in Coronary Heart Disease.* New York, Academic Press, 1973.
11. *Exercise Equivalents.* Denver Colorado Heart Association.
12. Gordon EE: Energy costs of various physical activities in relation to pulmonary tuberculosis. *Arch Phys Med* 1952;33:201–209.
13. Winslow EH, Gaffrey L: Oxygen consumption and cardiovascular responses in normal adults and acute myocardial infarction patients during basin bath, tub bath, and shower. *Nurs Res* (submitted for publication).

14. Kilamura K, Jorgensen CR, Gobel FL, Taylor HL, Wang Y: Hemodynamic correlates of myocardial oxygen consumption during upright exercise. *J Appl Physiol* 1972;32:516–522.
15. Singman H, Kinsella E, Goldberg E: Electrocardiographic changes in coronary care unit patients during defecation. *Vasc Surg* 1975;9:54–57.
16. Fareeduddin K, Abelmann WH: Impaired orthostatic tolerance after bed rest in patients with myocardial infarction. *N Engl J Med* 1969;280:345–350.
17. McCally M, Piemme TE, Murray RH: Tilt table responses of human subjects following application of lower body negative pressure. *Aerospace Med* 1966;37:1247–1249.
18. Chobanian AV, Lille RD, Tercyak A, Blevins P: The metabolic and hemodynamic effects of prolonged bed rest in normal subjects. *Circulation* 1974;49:551–559.
19. Convertino VA, Hung J, Goldwater D, DeBusk RF: Cardiovascular responses to exercise in middle-aged men after 10 days of bed rest. *Circulation* 1982;65:134–140.
20. Convertino VA, Sandler H, Webb P, Annis JF: Induced venous pooling and cardiorespiratory responses to exercise after bed rest. *J Appl Physiol* 1982;52:1342–1348.
21. Lecerof H: Influence of body position on exercise tolerance, heart rate, blood pressure, and respiration rate in coronary insufficiency. *Br Heart J* 1971;33:78–83.
22. Langou RA, Wolfson S, Olson EG, Cohen LS: Effects of orthostatic postural changes on myocardial oxygen demands. *Am J Cardiol* 1977;39:418–421.

Comprehension Phase

Example Critique

1. *Problem:* "Patients dislike using the bedpan and urinal while in bed and often insist that it would be easier and better for them to get out of bed to toilet. Little data are available about the physiologic costs of toileting" (Winslow et al., 1984, p. 462).*

2. *Purpose:* The researchers "measured oxygen uptake (VO_2), peak heart rate (HR_{peak}), peak rate-pressure product (RPP_{peak}) (systolic blood pressure × heart rate), rating of perceived exertion (RPE), and preference in 95 hospitalized and nonhospitalized adults during in-bed (bedpan and urinal) and out-of-bed (bedside commode and standing urinal) toileting" (p. 463).

3. *Literature review:* A minimal review of literature is presented at the beginning of the article. However, many studies are cited in the discussion section, where the findings from this study are compared and contrasted with the findings from previous studies (see the research article, p. 463). Often in clinical specialty journals, such as the *Journal of Cardiac Rehabilitation* and *Heart & Lung,* studies are cited in the discussion section so that findings can be synthesized to indicate the current knowledge in a problem area. Therefore, when critiquing the review of literature for a study, examine both the beginning of the article and the discussion section.

   The researchers cited several studies, but few focused on the effects of in-bed and out-of-bed toileting (Benton, Brown, & Rusk, 1950; Singman, Kinsella, & Goldberg, 1975). Because limited research has been done in this area, additional study is needed. The references range from

*Page numbers refer to the version of the article reprinted in this text.

continued

1950 to 1982; most were published in the 1970s. These sources are considered current because the study being critiqued was published in 1984. The findings from studies are synthesized to indicate briefly what is known and not known about the study problem.

4. *Framework:* The framework is not identified by the researchers and must be extracted from the literature review. The key concepts of toileting, acutely ill adults, healthy adults, rehabilitating adults, and energy cost were identified but not defined in the article. The researchers indicate that Levine's Conservation Model, specifically the energy conservation principle and the overload and progression principle of exercise physiology, provided the framework for this study (Winslow, January 1994, personal communication). Based on the review of literature and personal communication with the primary researcher, we developed the following map to identify the relationships among the concepts relevant to this study.

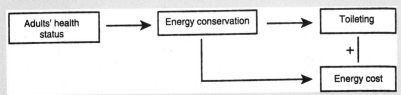

This map indicates that adults' health status (acutely ill, rehabilitating, or healthy) affects their use of energy conservation; their energy conservation affects their toileting and energy costs during toileting. Energy conservation involves the appropriate use of energy to prevent energy depletion and promote wholeness and integrity of the individual (Schaefer & Pond, 1991). Thus, acutely ill adults with depleted energy conserve their energy more than do healthy adults. Toileting increases energy costs, but ill individuals conserve their energy more than do healthy individuals during toileting. The more they conserve their energy, the smaller their energy costs during activities such as toileting. When individuals are ill, they need to use the most appropriate toileting method to prevent excessive energy costs.

The adults in this study were male and female healthy volunteers, cardiac outpatients, medical inpatients, and acute myocardial infarction (MI) inpatients. The toileting methods examined were the in-bed methods of bedpan and urinal and the out-of-bed methods of bedside commode and standing urinal. The energy costs for different types of individuals during toileting were examined by measuring the variables of VO_2, HR_{peak}, RPP_{peak}, *RPE, and toileting preference.*

5. The researchers did not include objectives, questions, or hypotheses.
6. *Variables:* The researchers identified and operationally defined the variables but did not provide conceptual definitions. The operational definition and a possible conceptual definition follow for each variable.

Independent Variables

Toileting Methods

Conceptual Definition. In-bed and out-of-bed toileting methods that require greater energy cost than a resting level.

Operational Definition. In-bed toileting is the use of the bedpan by women and the urinal by men to urinate while lying in bed. Out-of-bed toileting is the use of the bedside commode by women and the standing urinal by men to urinate.

Subjects' Health Status

Conceptual Definition. Adults with varying levels of health (acutely ill, rehabilitating, or healthy) conserve their energy appropriately during toileting to prevent energy depletion (Schaefer & Pond, 1991).

Operational Definition. Subjects with four levels of health were studied: healthy volunteers, cardiac outpatients, medical inpatients, and acute MI inpatients.

Dependent Variables

Oxygen Uptake (VO_2)

Conceptual Definition. The amount of oxygen used by the body during an activity.

Operational Definition. Oxygen uptake was "determined by open-circuit, indirect calorimetry. . . . Expired air volume was measured by a Collins chain compensated gasometer (Tissot), and air composition was analyzed by mass spectrometer (Perkin-Elmer Medical Gas Analyzer 1100). . . . Standard equations were used to derive VO_2" (Winslow et al., 1984, p. 464).

Peak Heart Rate (HR_{peak})

Conceptual Definition. The highest HR an adult reaches during an activity.

Operational Definition. "Peak HR was the most rapid HR observed during any 15-second period" (Winslow et al., 1984, p. 465).

Peak Rate-Pressure Product (RPP_{peak})

Conceptual Definition. The myocardial energy cost for an adult during an activity.

Operational Definition. A product of systolic blood pressure times HR. The highest RPP observed during toileting was defined as the RPP_{peak}.

Perceived Exertion

Conceptual Definition. An individual's perception of the energy cost during an activity.

continued

Operational Definition. The subjects selected "a number from the Borg Scale of Perceived Exertion" to indicate their perceived level of exertion during toileting (Winslow et al., 1984, p. 465).

Preferred Toileting Method

Conceptual Definition. The toileting method an individual liked best.

Operational Definition. "After both toileting methods, the subject completed a questionnaire wherein he ranked each method for comfort, pleasantness, and ease" (Winslow et al., 1984, p. 465).

7. *Attribute variables:* The attribute variables were gender, age, weight, height, medical diagnosis, date and type of MI, and current medications.
8. *Description of the sample*
   a. *Sample criteria:* The subjects were adult male and female volunteers who were either healthy individuals, coronary artery disease patients who were participating in a supervised outpatient exercise program, stable medical inpatients with a variety of cardiac and noncardiac disorders, or stable acute MI inpatients whose MI had occurred at least 2 days earlier. "Acute MI was established by history, clinical, electrocardiographic (ECG), and enzyme findings and by myocardial scintigraphy. . . . All medical and cardiac inpatients were ambulatory prior to hospitalization, and none had neural or musculoskeletal problems that would preclude standing unassisted" (Winslow et al., 1984, p. 464).
   b. *Sample size:* There were 95 hospitalized and nonhospitalized adult subjects. The authors did not indicate that power analysis was used to determine sample size.
   c. *Characteristics of the sample:* "The 42 women and 53 men (range 18–79 years) who volunteered for the study consisted of 26 healthy adults, 16 coronary artery disease patients . . . , 27 stable medical inpatients with a variety of cardiac and noncardiac disorders, and 26 stable acute MI inpatients who had their MI from two to 28 days earlier (8.81 ± 5 days [mean ± SD]). Eight patients had their MI five days or less before the study began. . . . Nineteen (73%) of the patients had transmural infarctions; seven (27%) had subendocardial infarctions. . . . Six (37%) of the cardiac outpatients, seven (26%) of the medical inpatients, and five (19%) of the acute MI patients were receiving propranolol at the time of the study" (Winslow et al., 1984, pp. 463–464). Some of the sample characteristics are also presented in a table (see Table I, p. 464).
   d. *Sample mortality:* No sample mortality was mentioned; data analyses included all 95 subjects.
   e. *Sampling method:* Nonprobability sample of convenience.

f. *Type of consent:* "The research protocol was approved by the Institutional Review Board, and informed written consent was obtained from all subjects prior to the study" (Winslow et al., 1984, p. 464).

9. *Research design:* The research design is not identified but appears to be a quasi-experimental repeated-measures design, in which each subject was exposed to both treatments (in-bed and out-of-bed toileting). The subjects were randomly assigned to an initial toileting method. The gas collections for VO_2 and HR were measured immediately before, during, and after each toileting method. Blood pressure for RPP was measured before and after each method of toileting (pretest and posttest). The Borg Scale of Perceived Exertion and the questionnaire for toileting preference were completed after each toileting method (posttest only).

   a. *Study procedures:* The following protocol was used to direct the study. "Protocol: Oxygen uptake, HR, and RPP were determined during a three-minute supine rest period and during in-bed and out-of-bed toileting. A ten-minute rest period separated the randomly ordered toileting methods. Women used the bedpan and bedside commode for urinating; men used the urinal while lying in bed and while standing beside the bed. The subjects simulated voiding if unable to void during the second toileting trial" (Winslow et al., 1984, p. 469).

   "The toileting protocol simulated usual clinical conditions; therefore, toileting duration varied. The investigator assisted the women in lifting their hips for bedpan placement and removal, and placed the bedside commode in a standardized position beside the head of the bed. Subjects used their own techniques to get out of and back into bed and were not lifted by the investigator. The investigator left the room while the subject urinated and returned when given a signal from the subject. Subjects took as much time as they needed for urination" (Winslow et al., 1984, p. 465).

   b. *Extraneous variables* are not specifically identified, but the researchers structured the sample criteria, treatment protocols, and data collection process to eliminate extraneous variables. For example, the medical diagnoses of patients were clearly documented, and all patients were ambulatory and had no neural or musculoskeletal problems that might interfere with the toileting treatments. The treatments were randomly implemented, and the protocols for the treatments and measurements were highly structured and consistently implemented.

   c. No *pilot study* was identified.

10. *Measurement strategies:* The researchers measured five variables—three (VO_2, HR_{peak}, and RPP_{peak}) with physiologic instruments, one (perceived exertion) with a self-report scale, and one (toileting preference) with a questionnaire.

continued

a. *VO₂* was "determined by open-circuit, indirect calorimetry. The subject had a nose clip and mouth piece in place. During the timed period, expired air was collected via a one-way respiratory valve (Daniels) and 64-inch plastic tubing into a 30 L (rest) or 150 L (toileting) bag (Douglas). . . . Expired air volume was measured by a Collins Chain Compensated Gasometer (Tissot), and air composition was analyzed by mass spectrometer (Perkin-Elmer Medical Gas Analyzer 1100). . . . Standard equations were used to derive VO_2" (Winslow et al., 1984, p. 464).

The measurement strategy produced ratio-level data. To demonstrate the precision and accuracy of the equipment, the "mass spectrometer was calibrated electronically and checked against gases of known concentration" (Winslow et al., 1984, p. 464).

b. HR_{peak} was identified using a continuous ECG (lead II) that was recorded during toileting. "Peak HR was the most rapid HR observed during any 15-second period" (Winslow et al., 1984, p. 465). This measurement strategy produced ratio-level data. The brand name of the ECG equipment and the precision, sensitivity, accuracy, and error of the equipment were not addressed.

c. RPP_{peak} was determined by multiplying systolic blood pressure times heart rate and selecting the highest RPP. "Blood pressure was measured by cuff sphygmomanometer immediately before and after toileting and after each position change" (Winslow et al., 1984, p. 465). This measurement strategy produced ratio-level data. The precision, sensitivity, selectivity, accuracy, and error of the blood pressure cuff and sphygmomanometer were not addressed. The manufacturer of this equipment was not identified.

d. *Perceived exertion* was measured using the Borg Scale of Perceived Exertion. The level of data is unclear but was probably ordinal because nonparametric tests for ordinal data (Friedman two-way analysis of variance [ANOVA] by ranks and Spearman correlation coefficients) were used for analysis. The validity and reliability of the Borg Scale are not discussed, but a reference article is cited.

e. *Preferred toileting method* was measured with a questionnaire that examined the comfort, pleasantness, and ease of each method. The data were probably ordinal because nonparametric tests were used to analyze the data. The development of this questionnaire was not discussed.

11. *Data collection procedures:* The data collection process was detailed in the methods and protocol sections of the article (pp. 464–465). Most of this content was presented in the measurement and design sections of this critique.

12. *Statistical analyses:* The analyses were descriptive and inferential. VO_2, HR, and RPP data were analyzed with descriptive statistics, including mean, range, and standard deviation. These results are presented in a

table (see Table II, p. 466). Graphs are also presented, allowing the reader to visualize the differences among the four groups (healthy volunteers, medical inpatients, cardiac outpatients, and acute MI inpatients) in VO_2 (see Fig. I), HR (see Fig. II), and RPP (see Fig. III) during rest, in-bed toileting, and out-of-bed toileting.

The inferential statistical analyses were conducted primarily to examine differences between in-bed and out-of-bed toileting methods for four groups of subjects. "Oxygen uptake, HR, and RPP results were analyzed for each sex and group by repeated measures analysis of variance. Ratings of perceived exertion and preferences were analyzed by the Friedman two-way ANOVA by ranks. Spearman correlation coefficients were calculated for selected variables including VO_2, age, and toileting duration" (Winslow et al., 1984, p. 465). The repeated measures ANOVA results indicated that "no physiologically important differences were found between in-bed and out-of-bed toileting. Both in-bed and out-of-bed toileting produced small increases in energy cost and myocardial work over resting levels, with a mean $VO_2 < 1.6$ times resting VO_2, a mean HR_{peak} 100 beats/min, and a mean $RPP_{peak} < 11,200$" (Winslow et al., 1984, p. 463).

13. *Interpretation of findings:* The findings from the study "show that both in-bed and out-of-bed toileting methods produce minimal energy cost and cardiovascular stress for healthy volunteers, cardiac outpatients, stable medical inpatients, and stable inpatients who had an acute MI from two to 28 days earlier. Clinically or physiologically important differences were not found between staying in bed and getting out of bed to toilet. The subjects clearly preferred getting out of bed to toilet" (Winslow et al., 1984, p. 471). These findings were expected and were consistent with the findings from Benton et al. (1950) and Singman et al. (1975).

An unexpected finding was that hospitalized patients had significantly lower VO_2 values than nonhospitalized patients. The researchers hypothesized that hospitalized patients with depleted energy reduce their energy expenditure during toileting. No serendipitous findings were identified. Because the study has no clearly designated framework, the findings were not linked to a framework.

14. *Limitations of the study:* Limitations are not identified.

15. *Generalization of findings:* "In-bed toileting should be reserved for patients with specific contraindications to postural change. . . . For medical patients without specific contraindications, we recommend out-of-bed toileting" (Winslow et al., 1984, p. 471).

16. *Implications for nursing:* Nurses are encouraged to get stable medical inpatients and stable inpatients who have had an acute MI out of bed to toilet. This toileting method has minimal energy cost, is preferred by patients, and minimizes bed rest-induced orthostatic intolerance.

continued

17. *Suggestions for further research:* The researchers provide no specific directions for further research.
18. *Missing elements of the study:* The study lacks a clearly expressed framework; reliability and validity information for one of the scales; precision, accuracy, and sensitivity information for some of the physiologic instruments; limitations; and recommendations for further research.
19. *Replication:* The study is sufficiently clear to replicate. Anyone planning replication should contact the researchers for clarification of parts of the data collection process and the research protocol and for more information regarding some of the measurement methods.

Comparison and Analysis Phases

This section discusses the strengths and weaknesses of the steps of the research process and the logical links among these steps. The title, abstract, problem, purpose, literature review, framework, methodology, results, and discussion elements of the article are critiqued.

Title and Abstract. The title, although a little long, clearly indicates the focus of the study. The abstract includes the study problem, purpose, sample size, sample characteristics, significant results, relevant findings, and implications of the findings for nursing practice. This relevant information is presented in a way that captures the attention of the reader.

Problem and Purpose. The problem is clearly identified in the abstract and in the first paragraph of the article. Determining the energy costs of different methods of toileting will provide direction in caring for hospitalized patients. Because toileting is the responsibility of nurses, this is a significant problem and requires investigation.

The purpose is expressed clearly in the abstract and in the second paragraph of the article. The purpose identifies the independent and dependent variables, the population, and the setting. The study was feasible to conduct because of (1) the clinical and research expertise of the investigators; (2) the financial support received for the study (see p. 462); (3) the availability of subjects, facilities, and equipment discussed in the methods section; (4) the cooperation of others (acknowledged at the end of the article); and (5) the ethical considerations given the subjects (informed consent) (Burns & Grove, 1997).

Literature Review. The literature review is brief because of the limited number of studies conducted in this area. Additional related research and theoretical sources might have been cited to indicate the current knowledge of the problem. However, journals often limit the length of an article, and researchers must cut information from the literature review and other sections of their research reports to meet publication requirements. A final summary of what is known and not known about the problem studied would have added clarity to the literature review.

Framework. The study lacks a clearly identified framework. The concepts relevant to the study are identified but not defined, and the relationships among the concepts should have been clarified and documented. The variables are clearly defined operationally but are neither conceptually defined nor linked to the concepts identified. The study findings, if linked to Levine's conservation model, could have added support to this model and to the understanding of energy conservation in healthy and ill adults (Schaefer & Pond, 1991).

Methods. The methods section is a major strength of the study. The sample size was large (95 subjects) and included a variety of subjects (healthy volunteers, cardiac outpatients, medical inpatients, and acute MI inpatients). The heterogeneity of the subjects increases the generalizability of the findings (Burns & Grove, 1997; Phillips, 1986). A limitation is that the study groups were of unequal size. The cardiac outpatient group had only 16 subjects, but the other three groups were fairly equal, with 26 to 27 subjects per group. The sampling method, sampling criteria, and sample characteristics are clearly presented. The study was examined by an Institutional Review Board, and informed written consent was obtained from the subjects.

The measurement methods seem appropriate for measuring energy cost, myocardial workload, perceived exertion, and preferred toileting method. The measurement of VO_2 is presented in detail, and the precision and accuracy of the equipment are described. The equipment (ECG, blood pressure cuff, and sphygmomanometer) for measuring HR and RPP are described, but the accuracy and precision of the equipment are not addressed (Gift & Soeken, 1988). Discussion of the Borg Scale of Perceived Exertion and the questionnaire used to measure toileting preference is limited; discussing the reliability and validity of these instruments would have strengthened the study.

The design is not identified, and the threats to design validity are not discussed. However, the study protocol clearly describes the implementation of the independent variables and the measurement of the dependent variables. The toileting protocol simulated usual clinical conditions, which increases the ability to generalize the findings to patients in clinical practice. The researchers did not indicate who collected the data. If more than one person collected data, the reliability or consistency of the data collection process must be addressed (Burns & Grove, 1997).

Results. The statistical techniques used to analyze data from the measurement of the five dependent variables are clearly identified. The analysis techniques (descriptive and inferential) were appropriate for the level of measurement of the variables (Burns & Grove, 1997; Munro, 1997). The purpose of the study is clearly addressed in the results section. The results are presented in narrative form, tables, and graphs to facilitate understanding.

Discussion. The expected and unexpected findings are explained and the statistical and clinical significance of the findings addressed (Burns & Grove, 1997). The findings are consistent with previous research, and this is documented. The generalization of the findings and their implications for nursing are clearly presented. The researchers could have strengthened the report by identifying the study limitations and providing suggestions for further research.

Evaluation Phase

This study examines a significant nursing problem and provides important findings that can be used in nursing practice. The findings are consistent with those of previous research (Benton et al., 1950; Singman et al., 1975) and seem to describe accurately the energy costs of toileting for hospitalized and nonhospitalized patients. Out-of-bed toileting is recommended for medical patients without specific contraindications. These findings can be generalized to stable medical inpatients and stable inpatients who had an acute MI.

The following questions might generate further research: What additional dependent variables might be measured to determine the energy costs during toileting? How might these dependent variables be measured? What are the best toileting methods for other types of patients? What are the energy costs for toileting in the bathroom? What are the energy costs for in-bed and out-of-bed toileting during defecation versus urination? Further research in these areas would strengthen the knowledge base regarding toileting and increase the usefulness of the findings for practice.

The strengths of this study greatly outweigh the weaknesses. The weaknesses regarding the framework, design, measurement methods, and suggestions for further research could easily be corrected in future studies. The findings support previous research and need to be used in practice to help determine optimal toileting methods for patients.

Introduction to the Critique Process for Qualitative Studies

Qualitative studies are appearing more frequently in nursing journals and are providing relevant information for nursing practice. Therefore, you need experience in critiquing qualitative as well as quantitative studies. However, critiquing a qualitative study involves a different approach. Strengths and weaknesses exist in both types of studies, but they vary. You need to know the potential weaknesses of qualitative studies and to be able to identify them in published studies.

A scholarly critique of qualitative studies includes a balanced evaluation of a study's strengths and weaknesses. Five standards have been proposed to evaluate qualitative studies: (1) descriptive vividness, (2) methodological congruence, (3) analytical preciseness, (4) theoretical connectedness, and (5) heuristic relevance (Burns, 1989). In the following sections, these standards and the threats to them are described.

Standard 1: Descriptive Vividness

To achieve *descriptive vividness,* the site, subjects (informants), experience of collecting data, and thinking of the researcher during the data collection process must be described so clearly that the reader has the sense of personally experiencing the event. Glaser and Strauss (1965) say that the researcher should "describe the social world studied so vividly that the reader can almost literally see and hear its people" (p. 9).

Threats to Descriptive Vividness

1. *Failure to include essential descriptive information.*
2. *Lack of clarity in description.*
3. *Lack of credibility in description (Beck, 1993).*
4. *Inadequate length of time at the site to gain the familiarity necessary for vivid description.*
5. *Inadequate observational skills.*
6. *No indication that the researchers validated the findings with the subjects (Beck, 1993).*
7. *Inadequate skills in writing descriptive narrative.*

Standard 2: Methodological Congruence

Evaluation of *methodological congruence* requires knowledge of the philosophy and the methodological approach the researcher used (see Chapter 11). Qualitative researchers need to identify the philosophy and methodological approach they used and to cite reference sources for additional information (Munhall, 1989). Methodological excellence has four dimensions: rigor in documentation, procedural rigor, ethical rigor, and auditability (Beck, 1993; Burns, 1989; Burns & Grove, 1997; Miles & Huberman, 1994).

Rigor in Documentation

Rigor in documentation requires clear, concise presentation of the following study elements: the phenomenon to be studied, significance of the phenomenon; study purpose, research questions, assumptions, philosophy, researcher credentials, context, role of the researcher, ethical implications, sampling methods, subjects, data-gathering strategies, data analysis strategies, theoretical development, conclusions, implications for practice, suggestions for further study, and literature review. The study elements or steps are examined for completeness and clarity, and any threats to rigor in documentation are identified.

Threats to Rigor in Documentation

1. Failure to present all elements or steps of the study.

2. Failure to present the elements of the study accurately or clearly.

Procedural Rigor

Another dimension of methodological congruence is the rigor of the researcher in applying selected procedures for the study. To the extent possible, the researcher needs to make clear the steps taken to ensure that data were accurately recorded and that the data obtained are representative of the data as a whole (Knafl & Howard, 1984).

When critiquing a qualitative study, you need to examine the description of the data collection process and the study findings for threats to procedural rigor.

Threats to Procedural Rigor

1. The researcher asked the wrong questions. The questions must tap the subjects' experiences, not their theoretical knowledge of the phenomenon (Kirk & Miller, 1986).

2. The subject (informant) might have misinformed the researcher; this can occur for several reasons. The informant might have had an ulterior motive for deceiving the researcher. Someone might have been present who inhibited free expression by the informant. The informant might have wanted to impress the researcher by giving the response that seemed most desirable (Dean & Whyte, 1958).

3. The informant did not observe the details requested or was not able to recall the event and substituted instead what he or she supposed happened (Dean & Whyte, 1958).

4. The researcher placed more weight on data obtained from well-informed, articulate, high-status informants (an "elite bias") than on data obtained from those who were less informed, less articulate, or low in status (Beck, 1993; Miles & Huberman, 1994).

5. The presence of the researcher distorted the event being observed (LeCompte & Goetz, 1982).

6. Insufficient data were gathered.

7. Insufficient time was spent gathering data.

8. The training of data collectors was insufficient.

9. The approaches for gaining access to the site or to subjects were inappropriate.

10. The selection of subjects was inappropriate (Miles & Huberman, 1994).

Ethical Rigor

Ethical rigor requires recognition and discussion by the researcher of the ethical implications related to the study. Consent is obtained from subjects and documented. The report must indicate that the researcher took action to ensure that the rights of subjects were protected during the study. As you critique the study, examine the data-gathering process and identify potential threats to ethical rigor.

Threats to Ethical Rigor

1. *Failure to inform the subjects of their rights.*
2. *Failure to obtain consent from the subjects.*
3. *Failure to ensure the protection of the subjects' rights.*

Auditability

A fourth dimension of methodological congruence is the rigorous development of a decision trail (Miles & Huberman, 1994). Guba and Lincoln (1982) refer to this dimension as *auditability.* The research report should be sufficiently detailed to allow a second researcher, using the original data and the decision trail, to arrive at conclusions similar to those of the original researcher.

Threats to Auditability

1. *The description of the data collection process was inadequate.*
2. *The records of raw data were not sufficient to allow judgments to be made.*
3. *The researcher failed to develop or identify the decision rules for arriving at ratings or judgments.*
4. *Other researchers were unable to arrive at similar conclusions after applying the decision rules to the data (Beck, 1993).*
5. *The researcher failed to record the nature of the decisions, the data on which they were based, and the reasoning that entered into the decisions (Beck, 1993; Burns, 1989).*

Standard 3: Analytical Preciseness

The analytical process in qualitative research involves a series of transformations during which concrete data are transformed across several levels of abstraction. The outcome of the analysis is a theory that imparts meaning to the phenomenon under study. The analytical process occurs primarily within the researcher's mind and is frequently poorly described in research reports. *Analytical preciseness* requires the researcher to make the intense effort needed to identify and record the decision-making processes through which the transformations are made.

Threats to Analytical Preciseness

1. *The interpretive theoretical statements developed do not correspond with the findings (Miles & Huberman, 1994).*
2. *The set of categories, themes, or theoretical statements fails to set forth a whole picture.*
3. *The hypotheses or propositions developed during the study cannot be verified by data.*
4. *Neither hypotheses nor propositions developed during the study are presented in the research report.*
5. *The study conclusions are not based on the data gathered (Burns, 1989).*

Standard 4: Theoretical Connectedness

Theoretical connectedness requires that the theoretical schema developed from the study be clearly expressed, logically consistent, reflective of the data, and compatible with the knowledge base of nursing.

Threats to Theoretical Connectedness

1. *The clarification of concepts is inadequate. For example, the concepts are inadequately identified and defined or the concepts are not validated by data.*
2. *The relationships among the concepts are not clearly expressed.*
3. *The proposed relationships among the concepts are not validated by data.*
4. *The theory developed during the study fails to yield a meaningful picture of the phenomenon under study.*
5. *A conceptual framework or map is not derived from the data.*
6. *No clear connection is made between the data and nursing frameworks.*

Standard 5: Heuristic Relevance

To be of value, the results of a study need *heuristic relevance* for the reader. This value is reflected in the reader's ability to recognize the phenomenon described in the study, its theoretical significance, its applicability to nursing practice, and its influence on future research. The dimensions of heuristic relevance include intuitive recognition, relationship to the existing body of knowledge, and applicability.

Intuitive Recognition

Intuitive recognition indicates that when individuals are confronted with the theory derived from the data, it has meaning within their personal knowledge base. They immediately recognize the phenomenon and its relationship to a theoretical perspective in nursing.

Threats to Intuitive Recognition

1. *The phenomenon is poorly described.*
2. *The reader lacks familiarity with the phenomenon.*
3. *The description is not consistent with common meanings or experiences.*

Relationship to the Existing Body of Knowledge

The existing body of knowledge, particularly the nursing theoretical perspective from which the phenomenon was approached, must be reviewed by the researcher and compared with the study findings. Similarities between the current knowledge base and the study findings add strength to the findings; reasons for differences should be explored by the researcher. When critiquing a study, you need to examine the strength of the link between the study findings and the current knowledge base.

Threats to the Relationship to the Existing Body of Knowledge

1. *The researcher failed to examine the existing body of knowledge.*
2. *The process studied was not related to nursing and health.*

Applicability

Nurses need to be able to integrate the research findings into their knowledge base and apply them in nursing practice. Also, the findings should contribute to theory development. You need to examine the discussion section of the research report for threats to applicability.

Threats to Applicability

1. *The findings are not relevant to nursing practice.*
2. *The findings are not important for the discipline of nursing; for example, they do not contribute to theory development.*

Conducting critiques of qualitative studies requires application of the five standards (descriptive vividness, methodological congruence, analytical preciseness, theoretical connectedness, and heuristic relevance) to determine the strengths and weaknesses of the study. The summary of strengths will indicate the researcher's adherence to the standards; the summary of weaknesses will indicate the potential threats to the integrity of the study.

SUMMARY

An intellectual critique of research involves careful examination of all aspects of a study to judge its strengths, weaknesses, meaning, and significance. The conduct of an intellectual critique involves the application of basic guidelines that stress the importance of critiquing the entire study and clearly, concisely, and objectively identifying the study's strengths and weaknesses. Research is critiqued to broaden understanding, improve practice, and provide a background for conducting a study. All nurses—including students, practicing nurses, nurse administrators, nurse educators, and nurse researchers—critique research.

The critical thinking phases applied in the quantitative research critique process include comprehension, comparison, analysis, and evaluation. Phase 1, comprehension, involves understanding the terms and concepts in the report, as well as identifying and grasping the nature, significance, and meaning of the study elements. Phase 2, comparison, requires knowledge of what each step of the research process should be; the ideal is compared with the real. Phase 3, analysis, involves critiquing the logical links connecting one study element with another. Phase 4, evaluation, involves examining the meaning and significance of the study using certain criteria. Each step of the critique process is described, and questions are provided to direct the critique. A quantitative research report is provided with a critique that includes the four phases of comprehension, comparison, analysis, and evaluation.

This chapter also provides an introduction to the critique process for qualitative research. The standards for critique of qualitative studies include descriptive vividness, methodological congruence, analytical preciseness, theoretical connectedness, and heuristic relevance. To achieve descriptive vividness, the site, subjects, experience of collecting data, and thinking of the researcher during the process must be presented so clearly that the reader has the sense of personally experiencing the event. Methodological congruence has four dimensions: rigor in documentation, procedural rigor, ethical rigor, and auditability. Analytical preciseness is essential to perform a series of transformations in which concrete data are transformed across several levels of abstraction. The outcome of the analysis is a theory that imparts meaning to the phenomenon under study. Theoretical connectedness requires that the theory developed from the study be clearly expressed, logically consistent, reflective of the data, and compatible with the knowledge base of nursing. Heuristic relevance includes intuitive recognition, relationship to the existing body of knowledge, and applicability. These standards and the threats to them are presented to guide the critique of qualitative studies.

REFERENCES

Beck, C. T. (1993). Technical Notes: Qualitative research: The evaluation of its credibility, fittingness, and auditability. *Western Journal of Nursing Research, 15*(2), 263–266.

Benton, J. G., Brown, H., & Rusk, H. A. (1950). Energy expended by patients on the bedpan and bedside commode. *Journal of the American Medical Association, 144*(17), 1443–1447.

Burns, N. (1989). Standards for qualitative research. *Nursing Science Quarterly, 2*(1), 44–52.

Burns, N., & Grove, S. K. (1997). *The practice of nursing research: Conduct, critique, and utilization* (3rd ed.) Philadelphia: Saunders.

Dean, J. P., & Whyte, W. F. (1958). How do you know if the informant is telling the truth? *Human Organization, 17*(2), 34–38.

Gift, A. G., & Soeken, K. L. (1988). Assessment of physiologic instruments. *Heart & Lung, 17*(2), 128–133.

Glaser, B., & Strauss, A. L. (1965). Discovery of substantive theory: A basic strategy underlying qualitative research. *American Behavioral Scientist, 8*(1), 5–12.

Guba, E. G., & Lincoln, Y. S. (1982). *Effective evaluation.* Washington, DC: Jossey-Bass.

Kirk, J., & Miller, M. L. (1986). *Reliability and validity in qualitative research.* Beverly Hills, CA: Sage.

Knafl, K. A., & Howard, M. J. (1984). Interpreting and reporting qualitative research. *Research in Nursing & Health, 7*(1), 17–24.

LeCompte, M. D., & Goetz, J. P. (1982). Problems of reliability and validity in ethnographic research. *Review of Educational Research, 52*(1), 31–60.

Miles, M. B., & Huberman, A. M. (1994). *An expanded sourcebook: Qualitative data analysis* (2nd ed.). Beverly Hills, CA: Sage.

Miller, M. A., & Babcock, D. E. (1996). *Critical thinking applied to nursing.* St. Louis: Mosby.

Munhall, P. L. (1989). Philosophical ponderings on qualitative research methods in nursing. *Nursing Science Quarterly, 2*(1), 20–28.

Munro, B. H. (1997). *Statistical methods for health care research* (3rd ed.). Philadelphia: Lippincott.

Phillips, L. R. F. (1986). *A clinician's guide to the critique and utilization of nursing research.* Norwalk, CT: Appleton-Century-Crofts.

Polit, D. F., & Hungler, B. P. (1997). *Essentials of nursing research: Methods, appraisal, and utilization* (4th ed.). Philadelphia: Lippincott.

Ryan-Wenger, N. M. (1992). Guidelines for critique of a research report. *Heart & Lung, 21*(4), 394–401.

Schaefer, K. M., & Pond, J. B. (1991). *Levine's Conservation Model: A framework for nursing practice.* Philadelphia: Davis.

Singman, H., Kinsella, E., & Goldberg, E. (1975). Electrocardiographic changes in coronary care unit patients during defecation. *Vascular Surgery, 9*(1), 54–57.

Winslow, E. H., Lane, L. D., & Gaffney, F. A. (1984). Oxygen uptake and cardiovascular response in patients and normal adults during in-bed and out-of-bed toileting. *Journal of Cardiac Rehabilitation, 4*(8), 348–354.

Using Research in Nursing Practice

Completing this chapter should enable you to:

1. *Define research utilization.*
2. *Explore ways to communicate research findings in nursing.*
3. *Discuss the importance of the WICHE and CURN research utilization projects.*
4. *Identify barriers to using research in nursing practice.*
5. *Discuss strategies to promote the use of research in nursing practice.*
6. *Describe Rogers's theory of utilization of research knowledge.*
7. *Discuss the importance of published research-based protocols and clinical practice guidelines in promoting the use of research findings in practice.*
8. *Use selected research knowledge in nursing practice.*

Cognitive clustering
Communication of research findings
Innovation
Innovators
Integrative review of research
Meta-analysis
Research-based protocol
Research utilization
Rogers's theory of research utilization
   Confirmation stage
     Continuance
     Discontinuance
       Disenchantment
         discontinuance
       Replacement discontinuance
   Decision stage
     Adoption
     Rejection
       Active rejection
       Passive rejection

Implementation stage
   Direct application
   Indirect effects
   Reinvention
Knowledge stage
Persuasion stage
   Compatibility
   Complexity
   Observability
   Relative advantage
   Trialability
Social system

*T*he expected outcome of nursing research projects is the use of the findings to improve practice. The preceding chapters of this textbook describe the steps of the research process, identify guidelines for critiquing studies, and present directions for summarizing research findings. Reading, critiquing, and summarizing research literature are essential steps in determining if the findings are ready for use in practice. During the last 20 years, many quality clinical studies have been conducted and replicated, providing research findings that are ready for use in practice. Thus, the next step is the communication of these research findings to nurses for use in their practice. Using research-based interventions, nurses can provide quality care, improve patient outcomes, and decrease health care costs. Thus, patients, nurses, and health care agencies benefit from making changes based on research. An understanding of the research utilization process will enable you to promote the use of research findings in your agency.

Although extensive research knowledge has been generated in nursing, only a limited amount of this knowledge is being used in practice (Bueno, 1998; Coyle & Sokop, 1990; Michel & Sneed, 1995). Thus, the purpose of this chapter is to assist you in using research findings to improve your practice. The concept of research utilization and the major nursing research utilization projects are introduced. The barriers to and the strategies for using research findings to improve practice are described, and a process for using research in your practice is provided. The chapter concludes with examples of how current research findings can be used in clinical practice.

What Is Research Utilization?

Research utilization is the process of communicating and using research-generated knowledge to make an impact on or a change in the existing practices in the health care system. The main elements of research utilization include summarizing knowledge generated through research; communicating the research knowledge to nurses, other health care professionals, policy makers, and consumers of health care; and achieving desired outcomes for patients, nurses, and health care agencies.

Summarizing Research Knowledge

Research or empirical knowledge is generated through the conduct of quality studies. Often several studies on a specific topic are conducted, and these findings need to be integrated in preparation for use in practice. The integration of findings from scientifically sound research to determine what is currently known is called *cognitive clustering*. Cognitive clustering is accomplished through integrative reviews and meta-analyses of nursing research. *Integrative reviews of research* are conducted to identify, analyze, and synthesize results from independent studies to determine the current knowledge of a particular topic. These reviews are published in a variety of research and clinical journals and in the *Annual Review of Nursing Research*. Chapter 4 provides guidelines for summarizing research findings and introduces the process for conducting an integrative review of the research literature.

Some researchers have gone beyond critique and integration of research findings to analysis and synthesis of studies' finding through meta-analyses. *Meta-analysis* involves the use of statistical analysis techniques to integrate and synthesize findings from completed studies to determine what is known about a particular research area (Massey & Loomis, 1988). This approach allows the application of scientific criteria to such factors as sample size, level of significance, and variables examined. Through the use of meta-analysis, you can determine the

1. overall significance of pooled data from several studies;
2. average of the effect size indicating the degree to which the null hypothesis is false or the degree to which the phenomenon is present in the population; and
3. relationships among the variables studied (Hunt, 1987; Smith & Stullenbarger, 1991).

Meta-analyses make it possible to be objective rather than subjective in evaluating research findings. This objectivity makes it possible to determine accurately the usefulness of findings for practice. Published integrative reviews and meta-analyses of nursing research can assist you in summarizing the research literature in a selected area. These summaries of the research literature identify the changes or innovations that need to be implemented in practice. An *innovation* is an idea or nursing intervention that is perceived as new (although it may not be) by you or the group of nurses adopting it. New interventions must be communicated in a clear, concise manner that will promote their use by practicing nurses.

Communicating Research Knowledge

The research utilization process involves communicating study findings from investigators to practicing nurses. *Communication of research findings* includes developing a research report and disseminating that report through presentations and publications to audiences of nurses, health care professionals, policy makers, and health care consumers. Research findings can be disseminated by one person communicating to another; by one individual communicating to several others; or by the use of mass media such as journals, books, newspapers, and television. Some strategies for communicating research findings to nurses, other health care professionals, policy makers, and consumers are outlined in Table 13-1.

Audience of Nurses and Other Health Care Professionals

Initially, nurse researchers usually communicate their study findings through presentations to nurses and other health care professionals at conferences and meetings. An increasing number of nursing organizations and institutions are sponsoring research conferences. The American Nurses Association and many of its state associations sponsor annual nursing research conferences. The members of Sigma Theta Tau, the international honor society for nursing, sponsor international, national, regional, and local research conferences. Specialty

TABLE 13-1. Audiences and Strategies for Communicating Research	
Audiences	*Strategies for Communication of Research*
Nurses	Presentations
	Nursing research conferences
	Clinical practice conferences and meetings
	Videotaped and audiotaped presentations from conferences and meetings
	In-service education programs
	Agency-based research committee
	Agency-based journal club
	Written Reports
	Research publication in professional journals
	Research publications in books
	Monographs from research and clinical conferences and meetings
	Theses and dissertations
	Nursing research newsletter
	Electronic databases (WWW)
Other health care providers	Presentations
	Professional conferences and meetings in other disciplines
	Interdisciplinary team meetings
	Written Reports
	Research publications in professional journals and books in other disciplines
	Interdisciplinary research newsletter
Policy makers	Presentations
	Presentations on health problems to state and federal legislators
	Written Reports
	Research reports developed for legislators
	Research reports published by funding agencies
	Electronic databases (WWW)
	Agency for Health Care Policy and Research (AHCPR) clinical practice guidelines
Health care consumers	Presentations
	Television and radio
	Community meetings
	Patient and family teaching
	Written Reports
	Newspaper
	News and popular magazines
	Electronic databases (WWW)

organizations and associations, such as the Oncology Nurses Society and the American Heart Association, also sponsor research conferences. For a variety of reasons, many practicing nurses and other health professionals are unable to attend research conferences. To increase the communication of research findings, conference sponsors provide audio- or videotapes of the research presentations. Some sponsors publish abstracts of studies with the conference proceedings or in specialty journals or make them available electronically on the World Wide Web (WWW).

Many nurse researchers not only present their studies at conferences but also publish their findings in nursing research journals, specialty practice journals, or other health professional journals. For example, Blegen, Goode, and Reed (1998) studied the relationships among the registered nurse (RN) skill mix and adverse patient outcomes of medication errors, patient falls, skin breakdown, patient and family complaints, infections, and deaths. These researchers found that the higher the RN skill mix, the lower the incidence of adverse occurrences on inpatient units, and they published their findings in *Nursing Research*. This study documents the significance of RN care to patient outcomes and needs to be communicated to practicing nurses, other health professionals, policy makers, and consumers.

Practicing nurses often hear about research findings at conferences or read about them in journals and then communicate the findings to other nurses working in their clinical agencies. Research findings can be communicated in clinical agencies through research committees, newsletters, in-service education programs, interdisciplinary team meetings, and electronic databases (such as E-mail). For example, Bueno (1998) described the positive impact of a research newsletter in a clinical agency to increase the understanding of the research process and to promote the communication of research findings.

Interpersonal communication involving face-to-face exchange has been extremely effective in making changes in nursing practice. The communication is most effective when the two interacting individuals have similar beliefs, values, education, social status, and professions (Rogers, 1995). For example, you might read the research findings of Blegen and colleagues (1998) about the effects of the RN skill mix on lowering the incidence of adverse occurrences for patients and communicate these findings to your closest coworkers. Together you and your colleagues might inform nursing administrators, physicians, and hospital administrators about the findings so that the RN skill mix for hospital units might be increased to promote positive outcomes for patients and their families.

Audience of Policy Makers and Consumers

Newspapers and television greatly increase the communication of research findings (see Table 13-1). Thus, Blegen and colleagues (1998) could greatly expand the communication of their findings by developing a news release based on their study. They might publish their research findings in an article in their state (Iowa) newspaper, such as the *Des Moines Register*. This article could then be picked up by other news services and published in papers across the country or presented on a local or national news program. Communicating research findings by mass media greatly increases the number of nurses, other health care professionals, policy makers, and potential health care consumers who are aware of the findings.

The federal government also strongly supports the conduct of research, the communication of research findings, and the use of findings to direct health care. The formation of the National Institute for Nursing Research (NINR) has significantly expanded the conduct of nursing research and the communication of findings. In 1989, the Agency for Health Care Policy and Research (AHCPR) was established to enhance the quality, appropriateness, and effectiveness of health care services and access to these services. This agency has promoted the conduct of patient outcomes research and has facilitated the dissemination and use of research findings in practice. To promote the communication of research findings, AHCPR formed a work group for the dissemination of patient outcomes' research. This work group included a variety of researchers and health practitioners, including nurses and physicians. The purpose of this group was to develop a plan for the dissemination of research findings that identified the audiences and strategies for communication of research. The audiences identified included consumers, health care practitioners, the health care industry, policy makers, researchers, and journalists. Media for the dissemination of research included printed materials provided through direct mail, technical journals, health journals, the popular press, and electronic media, with communication by radio, television, and the WWW (Goldberg et al., 1994).

Achieving Desired Outcomes in a Health Care System

The desired outcomes of research utilization are improving nursing care, promoting positive patient and family outcomes, and providing cost-effective services within a health care system. Research knowledge is invaluable for expanding the assessment, diagnosis, and intervention expertise of practicing nurses. For example, assessment tools have been developed to identify fall-prone patients, and research-based fall-prevention programs have been developed (Morse, 1993). Practice guidelines for the prediction and prevention of pressure ulcers have been developed and tested through research (Harrison, Wells, Fisher, & Prince, 1996). Several nursing studies have been conducted to identify effective nursing interventions for patients. For example, Foss-Durant and McAfee (1997) examined the efficacy, patient satisfaction, and cost outcomes of three oral care products (lemon glycerin swabs, an artificial saliva product, and tapwater applied with a toothette). They found that patients were satisfied with all three types of oral care and that the artificial saliva product performed slightly better in promoting the moistness of the oral mucosa. Effective, efficient nursing interventions identified through research can be implemented to promote positive patient outcomes and cost-effective care for health care agencies.

Research utilization occurs within a specific social system. A *social system* is a set of interrelated individuals who engage in joint problem-solving to accomplish a common goal or outcome (Rogers, 1995). Making a change in practice based on research might involve the nurses on a specific hospital unit, all the nurses in one hospital, or all the nurses in a corporation of hospitals. The larger social system requires more detailed communication and planning to use research knowledge to change practice. For example, the change might require review by several committees and approval by different administrators. The practice change of increasing the RN skill mix to decrease the incidence of adverse occurrences for patients might be started on a medical-surgical unit, then expanded to other units in the same hospital, and then implemented in other hospitals in a corporation (Blegen et al., 1998).

A social system has both a formal and an informal structure. The formal structure is related to authority and power. The informal structure is related to who interacts with whom under what circumstances. Health care systems, such as hospitals and primary care clinics, have leaders who are in favor of making changes (*innovators*) and those who are opposed. Some leaders are at the center of the system's interpersonal communication networks and tend to have extensive power in the system. When making research-based changes in nursing practice, you need the support of innovative nurses and of those who have power in the agency. The innovative nurses might be organized into a subcommittee for the purpose of making a change in practice. They could verbalize the need for change and role-model the change for other nurses. The significance of research utilization for nursing practice is evident, but nurses need to be provided a background for using research findings in their practice.

Research Utilization Projects in Nursing

The limited use of research findings in practice has been a problem in nursing for many years. To address this problem, some major research utilization projects were implemented. Two of these projects were the Western Interstate Commission for Higher Education (WICHE) regional nursing research development project and the Conduct and Utilization of Research in Nursing (CURN) project. These federally funded projects involved designing and implementing strategies to promote research use in practice. The projects' outcomes and implications for nursing are discussed in this section.

WICHE

The WICHE project, initiated in the mid-1970s, was the first major project to address research utilization in nursing. The 6-year project was directed by Krueger and colleagues (Krueger, 1978; Krueger, Nelson, & Wolanin, 1978) and was funded by the Division of Nursing. Members for this project were recruited from a variety of clinical agencies and educational institutions. The clinicians and educators were asked to participate in a workshop that focused on improving their skills in critiquing research. The participants selected research-based interventions that they were willing to implement in practice. These educators and clinicians developed detailed plans for using selected research findings in practice and functioned as change agents when the utilization projects were implemented in clinical agencies. At a second workshop, the participants reported the impact of using research findings in practice.

The WICHE project also included follow-up reports on the continuation of the research utilization activities at 3 and 6 months. These reports indicated that the WICHE project was successful in increasing the use of research findings in practice. Three reports from this project were published; the authors were Axford and Cutchen (1977), who developed a preoperative teaching program; Dracup and Breu (1978), who devised a care plan for grieving spouses and tested its effectiveness; and Wichita (1977), who developed a program to treat and prevent constipation in nursing home residents by increasing the fiber in their diets. One of the outcomes of the WICHE project was the realization that only a limited number of quality clinical studies had been conducted and that most of the findings were not ready for use in practice.

CURN

The CURN project facilitated the development of clinical protocols to direct the use of selected research findings in practice. Many of these protocols (with modifications) are used in practice today. This project was directed by Horsley and funded by the Division of Nursing (Horsley, Crane, & Bingle, 1978; Horsley, Crane, Crabtree, & Wood, 1983). The purpose of this 5-year (1975–1980) project was to increase the use of research findings in practice by communicating findings, facilitating organizational modifications necessary for implementation, and encouraging collaborative research that is directly useful in clinical practice. For this project, research utilization was viewed as an organizational process rather than as a process to be implemented by an individual nurse. From this perspective, research utilization required a decision by the clinical agency to implement research findings and the development of policies and procedures to guide the implementation process. The research utilization process included the following steps.

1. Identification and synthesis of multiple studies on a selected topic (research base)
2. Organization of the research knowledge into a solution or clinical protocol for practice
3. Transformation of the clinical protocol into specific nursing actions (innovations) that are used with patients
4. Clinical evaluation of the new practice to determine whether it produced the desired outcome (Horsley et al., 1983)

During this project, published clinical studies were critiqued for scientific merit, replication, and relevance to practice. Determining the relevance of the research for practice involved examining its clinical merit or significance in addressing patient problems, the extent to which the clinical control belonged to nursing, the feasibility of implementing a change in an agency, and an analysis of the cost-benefit ratio. In 1975, the research findings in the following 10 areas were considered worthy of implementation in practice.

1. Structured preoperative teaching
2. Reducing diarrhea in tube-fed patients
3. Preoperative sensory preparation to promote recovery
4. Preventing decubitus ulcers
5. Intravenous cannula change
6. Closed urinary drainage systems
7. Distress reduction through sensory preparation
8. Mutual goal setting in patient care
9. Clean intermittent catheterization
10. Pain: deliberative nursing interventions (CURN Project, 1981, 1982)

The participants in the CURN project developed protocols based on research findings in the 10 identified areas (Haller, Reynolds, & Horsley, 1979; Horsley et al., 1983). Each protocol detailed the implementation of a research-based nursing intervention. The protocols were implemented in clinical trials and evaluated for effectiveness. Based on the evaluations, a decision was made to reject, modify, or adopt the intervention. If the intervention was adopted, strategies were developed to extend this intervention to other appropriate nursing practice settings (Horsley et al., 1983).

Seventeen hospitals participated in the project. Each hospital identified a nursing unit as a site for the clinical trial and implemented one of the protocols. Data were collected before and after implementation of the protocols to determine the extent to which the findings were being used in practice. The effect of the protocols on patient outcomes was also evaluated. If the protocols produced positive patient outcomes, they were adopted and used in other units of the hospitals. Follow-up questionnaires were sent to the hospitals for a 4-year period to determine the long-term effect of the implementation of the research-based protocols on the organization. Pelz and Horsley (1981) reported that prior to the project, research utilization was low in all the hospitals. However, 4 years after the project, most of the hospitals were still performing the protocols. The clinical protocols developed during this project are available for use in your practice (CURN Project, 1981, 1982).

Barriers to Research Utilization

The WICHE and CURN projects were successful but limited in scope. Extensive additional research findings have been generated since the 1970s; thus, many more nurses in acute and primary care agencies need to use current findings in their practice. This was evident in a study by Brett (1987), who examined the extent to which selected nursing research findings were being used by practicing nurses. One of the findings concerned the positioning of patients during intramuscular injection, and research has demonstrated that "internal rotation of the femur during an injection into the dorsogluteal site, in either the prone or the side-lying position, results in reduced discomfort from the injection" (Brett, 1987, p. 346). Internal rotation of the femur is achieved by having the patient point the toes inward during an injection. Forty-four percent of the nurses were aware of this research finding, 34% were persuaded that it was useful for practice, and 29% were implementing it in practice sometimes, but only 10% were implementing it always.

Coyle and Sokop (1990) replicated Brett's (1987) study and found that 34% of the nurses surveyed were aware of the research finding about positioning during an injection and 21% were persuaded that the finding was useful for practice; however, only 4% used the intervention sometimes, and 22% used it always. Thus, only a small percentage of these nurses were using the knowledge about positioning during intramuscular injections even though it had been available for 15 years (Kruszewski, Lang, & Johnson, 1979).

The research finding about positioning during injections would be quite easy to implement in practice. The decision about positioning the patient during an injection could be made by the nurse alone; no physician's order would be needed. Administrative personnel would not have to give approval to make this change in practice. This nursing intervention would not increase costs or nursing time and would reduce the patient's discomfort during injections.

Why are many nurses not using research knowledge to improve their practice? The exact reasons are unknown, but several barriers to research utilization have been identified. They are related to the quality of the research findings, the characteristics of the nurses who need to use the findings in practice, and the characteristics of the organizations in which the research needs to be used. The barriers to research utilization are discussed in this section, and some possible solutions are identified.

Barriers Related to Research Findings

As noted in the WICHE project, many of the early studies in nursing (those conducted from the 1930s to the 1970s) did not focus on clinical problems. Thus, very little research knowledge was ready for use in practice before 1980. To overcome this barrier, many researchers focused their studies on clinical problems during the 1980s, and that focus has continued in the 1990s. Thus, the quantity and quality of clinical research studies are improving, and more findings are ready for use in practice.

Another barrier related to research findings is that many nursing studies lack replication. Two or three studies do not provide sound research findings that can be used in a variety of practice settings. Thus, studies need to be replicated or repeated in different settings with different populations to determine whether the findings are ready for use in practice. The different types of replication and their contribution to nursing knowledge are discussed in Chapter 4. The nursing profession now recognizes the significance of replication for the generation and refinement of nursing knowledge and supports the conduct of such studies. Replication studies are encouraged by the National Institute of Nursing Research (NINR), and funding is provided for replication research projects. More replication studies are presented at research conferences and published in research and clinical journals than in the 1980s. Funding for replication studies and opportunities for presentation and publication will increase the incidence of these studies.

Probably the most significant barrier is that researchers often communicate their findings using words that are difficult for practicing nurses to understand (Bock, 1990; Gould, 1986; Liehr & Houston, 1993). In addition, some research reports do not indicate how the findings from a study are useful in nursing practice. Efforts are now being made to overcome this communication barrier. Clinical journals are including more studies written for nurses in practice; the journals *Applied Nursing Research* and *Clinical Nursing Research* were developed to communicate studies to practicing nurses. To increase the use of findings in practice, all researchers need to present their findings clearly and understandably, with an emphasis on how the findings can be used in practice.

Barriers Created by Practicing Nurses

Serious barriers to research utilization are created by nurses in practice, many of whom do not value research and are unaware of or unwilling to read research reports. Often these nurses have inadequate education to read and critique studies and to use research findings in practice (MacGuire, 1990; Phillips, 1986; Walczak, McGuire, Haisfield, & Beezley, 1994). To overcome these barriers, nursing students are being taught the steps of the research process, skills of research critique, and the process for using research findings in practice. Baccalaureate nursing programs have increased the focus on research, and educators often encourage students to make changes in practice based on research findings. Textbooks and lectures often include knowledge generated from research.

Through conferences and in-service programs, practicing nurses are being taught the skills to critique research and to use research findings in practice. Some agencies are hiring nurse researchers to increase practicing nurses' knowledge of research and to help them use research findings in practice. The nurse researchers are also conducting studies to address clinical problems and are encouraging practicing nurses to be involved in these studies.

Barriers Created by Organizations

Any organization has forces that promote stability and oppose change as well as forces that promote change. Generally, organizations that have existed for a long time, value tradition, and have an authoritative management style oppose change. In this type of system, innovators are not valued and administrators support the institutional stance. These institutions often discourage making changes in practice by indicating that the changes are too time-consuming or costly, and those nurses proposing the changes are not rewarded for their innovativeness (Walczak et al., 1994). Practicing nurses as a group might need to identify a research-based change and then convince the administration that the change will improve patient outcomes with minimal or no cost to the institution.

Other organizations take pride in being innovative and actively encourage the use of new ideas. In these systems, management style and communication patterns facilitate the rapid spread of new ideas and support efforts to implement them. Resources needed for communicating and using research findings in practice are available, and innovators are nurtured in these systems.

Organizations in disarray also tend to be more receptive to change and to the adoption of innovations because the forces resisting change have weakened. Currently, the entire health care system is in disarray because of the changes in organization, settings, management styles, and mechanisms for health care delivery. Economic constraints in the health care system are greater now, but the potential for change has increased. Thus, opportunities for practicing nurses to implement research findings in practice may be greater. Many changes have occurred in nursing, but the changes were often imposed by external powers. Nursing has tended to be traditional and to rely on authorities; however, the values and norms of nursing as a social system are starting to change to support the use of research in practice. In addition, nurses are beginning to use research to shape health care delivery (Clinton, 1993; Fitzgerald, Hill, Santamaria, Howard, & Jadack, 1997).

Strategies for Using Research Findings in Practice

Most people believe that a good idea will sell itself; the word will spread rapidly, and the idea will quickly be used. Unfortunately, this is seldom true; several sound nursing research findings are not being widely used in practice. Research utilization is not a problem unique to nursing; many disciplines have experienced difficulties promoting change based on research knowledge. To address this problem, Rogers (1995) studied the processes for using research findings in society and developed a theory of research utilization. *Rogers's theory of research utilization* included a five-stage process: (1) knowledge, (2) persuasion, (3) decision, (4) implementation, and (5) confirmation. The *knowledge stage* is the first awareness of the existence of an innovation or a new idea for use in practice. During the *persuasion stage,* nurses form an attitude toward the innovation. A decision is then made in the *decision stage* to adopt or reject the innovation. The *implementation stage* involves using the new idea to change practice. During the *confirmation stage,* nurses seek reinforcement

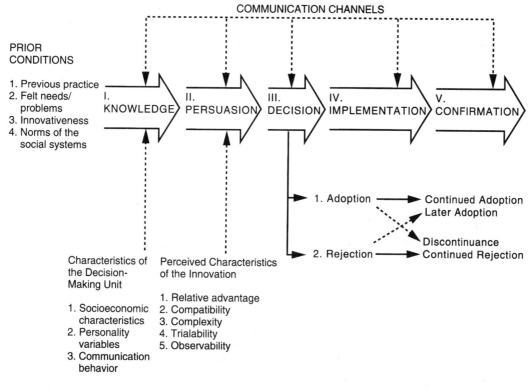

COMMUNICATION CHANNELS

PRIOR
CONDITIONS

1. Previous practice
2. Felt needs/
   problems
3. Innovativeness
4. Norms of the
   social systems

I.
KNOWLEDGE

II.
PERSUASION

III.
DECISION

IV.
IMPLEMENTATION

V.
CONFIRMATION

1. Adoption ———→ Continued Adoption
                  Later Adoption

                  Discontinuance
2. Rejection ———→ Continued Rejection

Characteristics of
the Decision-
Making Unit

1. Socioeconomic
   characteristics
2. Personality
   variables
3. Communication
   behavior

Perceived Characteristics
of the Innovation

1. Relative advantage
2. Compatibility
3. Complexity
4. Trialability
5. Observability

FIGURE 13-1

A model of stages of the innovation-decision process. (Reprinted with the permission of
The Free Press, an imprint of Simon & Schuster from DIFFUSION OF INNOVATIONS,
Fourth Edition by Everett M. Rogers. Copyright 1962, 1971, 1983, 1995 by The Free Press,
p. 162.)

of their decision and continue to adopt or reject the change in their practice.
Figure 13-1 presents a model of Rogers's innovation-decision process to promote the use of research findings. Rogers's model provided the basis for implementing the first nursing research utilization projects, WICHE and CURN. This
model, including its five essential stages of research utilization, is presented to
assist you in using research findings in your practice.

Knowledge Stage

Knowledge of research findings can be achieved by formal communication
through conference presentations, publications in clinical and research journals, and news releases on television and in newspapers. In addition, informal
communication within an agency from one nurse to another or among different
health professionals can be effective in increasing awareness of research knowl-

edge. Certain conditions influence the knowledge stage, such as previous practice, felt needs/problems, innovativeness, and norms of the social system. Dissatisfaction with previous practice can lead to recognizing the needs or problems that require change. A need might create a search for an innovation to improve practice; knowledge of a new idea also might create a need for change. For example, knowledge of a new treatment for pressure ulcers might create the need to change the existing treatment protocol.

Innovativeness is the degree to which an individual or agency is willing to adopt new ideas and make changes in practice (Rogers, 1995). Those who read research and want to make changes in practice are innovators. They actively promote change and encourage others to change, but the degree and speed of change depend on the norms of the agency. Norms are the expected behavior patterns within an agency or social system. Norms can serve as barriers to change or can facilitate change. When the norms of the social system are oriented to change, the leaders in the agency tend to be innovative and change is facilitated. When the norms are opposed to change, so are the agency leaders, thus creating barriers to change.

During the knowledge stage, it is necessary to examine the characteristics of the decision-making unit that is considering adoption of a research-based change. The decision-making unit might be an individual, a nursing unit, or the entire agency. The socioeconomic characteristics, personality variables, and communication behavior of the decision-making unit can support or interfere with the adoption of a new idea (see Fig. 13-1). Can the agency afford the change? Will the change save money? Examination of personality variables will indicate individuals' innovativeness and whether they will facilitate or resist change. Communication behavior, whether it is open and honest or closed and subversive, has a strong impact on the research utilization process.

Persuasion Stage

During the persuasion stage, an individual or agency develops a favorable or unfavorable attitude toward the change or innovation (Rogers, 1995). Characteristics of an innovation that determine the probability and speed of its adoption include relative advantage, compatibility, complexity, trialability, and observability (see Fig. 13-1). *Relative advantage* is the extent to which the innovation is perceived to be better than current practice. *Compatibility* is the degree to which the innovation is perceived to be consistent with current values, past experience, and priority of needs. *Complexity* is the degree to which the innovation is perceived to be difficult to understand or use. If the innovation requires the development of new skills, complexity increases. *Trialability* is the extent to which an individual or agency can try out the idea on a limited basis with the option of returning to previous practices. *Observability* is the extent to which the results of an innovation are visible to others. An innovation with highly visible, beneficial results will probably be rapidly adopted. Innovations that have great relative advantage, are compatible within the agency, are not complex, have trialability, and are observable will be adopted more quickly than those that do not meet these criteria.

In the persuasion stage, the proposed change is best communicated in small groups or one-to-one interactions. You will be attempting to convince others that they need to make changes in their practice based on research. You will be asked many questions about the change, such as: Have you used this intervention in your practice? How do you feel about it? What are the consequences of using it? What are the advantages and disadvantages of using it in my situation? Would you advise me to use it? Will I still be approved of and accepted if I use it? Extensive, honest communication will increase the likelihood of adoption.

Decision Stage

At the decision stage, the innovation is either adopted or rejected (see Fig. 13-1). *Adoption* involves full acceptance and the implementation of the innovation in practice. Adoption can be continued indefinitely or can be discontinued based on evaluation of the innovation's effectiveness for patients or the agency. *Rejection* of an innovation can be active or passive. *Active rejection* indicates that the innovation was examined and a decision was made not to adopt it. *Passive rejection* indicates that the innovation was never seriously considered. Over time, the agency might adhere to the decision to reject or might initiate adoption later.

Implementation Stage

In the implementation stage, the innovation is put to use by an individual, a unit, or an agency. A detailed plan for implementation that addresses the risks and benefits of the innovation will facilitate change. The types of implementation include direct application, reinvention, and indirect effects.

Direct application occurs when an innovation is used exactly as it was developed. In fact, some researchers would not consider an innovation to have been adopted unless its original form was kept intact. For example, if a study demonstrated that a particular intervention, conducted in specifically defined steps, was effective in achieving an outcome, adoption would require that the nurse perform the steps of the intervention in exactly the same way in which they were described in the study. This expectation reflects the narrow, precise definition of an innovation that is necessary to the scientific endeavor. However, this preciseness is not compatible with typical practice behavior, and research has indicated that maintenance of the original innovation does not always occur. A *research-based protocol* provides detailed guidelines that are documented with research sources for implementing an intervention in practice. These protocols are useful in promoting direct application of an intervention in nursing practice (Haller et al., 1979). For example, the protocol in

1. Wash hands, gather necessary equipment for the injection, and put on gloves.
2. Explain to the patient that you will position him/her to decrease the discomfort of the injection.
3. Position the patient in the prone position or lying face down.
4. Identify the ventrogluteal (VG) site. (A picture of the site would be provided in the protocol.)
5. Have the patient turn his/her toes inward ("toe in"). This internal rotation of the femur causes relaxation of the gluteal muscle, which decreases the discomfort from the injection.
6. Give the injection and reposition the patient for comfort after the injection.
7. Document how the injection was given and the patient's response or perceived level of comfort. (You might use the visual analogue scale presented in the section titled "Confirmation Stage" to document the discomfort experienced with the injection.)

Beyea, S. C., & Nicoll, L. H. (1995). Administration of medications via the intramuscular route: An integrative review of the literature and research-based protocol for the procedure. *Applied Nursing Research, 8*(1), 23–33.

Keen, M. F. (1986). Comparison of intramuscular injection techniques to reduce site discomfort and lesions. *Nursing Research, 35*(4), 207–210.

Kruszewski, A., Lang, S., & Johnson, J. (1979). Effect of positioning on discomfort from intramuscular injections in dorsogluteal site. *Nursing Research, 28*(2), 103–105.

Rettig, F. M., & Southby, J. R. (1982). Using different body positions to reduce discomfort from dorsogluteal injection. *Nursing Research, 31*(4), 219–221.

FIGURE 13-2
Protocol for positioning during IM injection.

Figure 13-2 provides direction for positioning a patient during an intramuscular (IM) injection to reduce the discomfort experienced by the patient. This protocol is brief and focuses on positioning during IM injections. Later in this chapter, a detailed research-based protocol is provided to direct you in selecting the best equipment to give an IM injection, identifying the IM injection site, positioning the patient to reduce discomfort with an injection, using appropriate techniques to give the injection, promoting absorption of the medication, and documenting the results.

Reinvention occurs when adopters modify the innovation to meet their own needs. Using this strategy, the steps of a procedure might be changed or deleted, or some of the steps might be combined with other care activities. Even with reinvention, nurses are using research findings to make changes in their practice. Nurses' use of knowledge can also have *indirect effects*. For example, practicing nurses and researchers might discuss the findings, cite them in clinical papers and textbooks, and use them to strengthen arguments. Thus, the knowledge would be incorporated into individuals' thinking and combined with their experience, education, and current values. In such instances, determining that the research knowledge was being utilized would be more difficult; thus, the use of certain nursing research findings may be underestimated.

Confirmation Stage

During the confirmation stage, nurses evaluate the effectiveness of the change in practice and decide to either continue or discontinue it. Using the example of the intervention to decrease patient discomfort during an IM injection, the nurse might evaluate the effectiveness of the injection technique by asking patients how much discomfort they felt during the injection or by having patients complete a visual analogue scale. On a 100-mm line like the one shown below, patients are asked to mark the level of discomfort they felt during the injection.

No
Discomfort ├───┤ Extreme
Discomfort

After one month of using the intervention, the data obtained from the pain scale can be analyzed and shared with other staff members. If the results indicate that the injection technique causes minimal discomfort, the intervention would probably be continued *(continuance)* and the protocol included in the procedure manual. If the injection technique (the innovation or intervention) had been started on one unit, it might then be used on all units in the hospital. If the data analysis indicates that the patients' discomfort was still moderate to severe, the intervention would probably be discontinued.

Discontinuance can be of at least two types: replacement and disenchantment. With *replacement discontinuance,* the innovation is rejected in order to adopt a better idea. Thus, innovations can occur in waves as new ideas replace outdated, impractical innovations. The computer is an excellent example; users can constantly upgrade their systems with new, more powerful interactive innovations in hardware and software. *Disenchantment discontinuance* occurs when an idea is rejected because the user is dissatisfied with its outcome.

Example of Research Utilization in Practice

After examining research utilization projects, barriers, and theory, you have some understanding of the research utilization process. Examining this information also raises questions. What research findings are ready for use in clinical practice? How can you use these findings to improve your practice? What are the most effective strategies for implementing findings in practice? We suggest that effective strategies for using research findings require a multifaceted approach, taking into consideration research findings, practicing nurses, and the organizations within which nurses practice. In this section, an example of research utilization is presented using Rogers's (1995) five-stage process: (1) knowledge, (2) persuasion, (3) decision, (4) implementation, and (5) confirmation (see Fig. 13-1). Research knowledge about the effects of heparin versus saline flush for irrigating intermittent intravenous devices (IID) is evaluated for use in nursing practice.

Knowledge Stage

The body of nursing research must be evaluated for scientific merit and clinical relevance; then the current findings must be summarized in preparation for use in practice (Massey & Loomis, 1988; Tanner, 1987; Tanner & Lindeman, 1989).

Evaluation of Studies' Scientific Merit

The scientific merit of nursing studies is evaluated by criteria such as (1) conceptualization and internal consistency, or logical links of a study; (2) methodological rigor, or the strength of the design, sample, instruments, and data collection and analysis processes; (3) generalizability of the findings, or the representativeness of the sample and setting; and (4) the number of replications of the study (Burns & Grove, 1997; Tanner & Lindeman, 1989). The critique steps discussed in Chapter 12 can be used to evaluate the scientific merit of studies. The research examining the efficacy of normal saline versus heparinized saline for the maintenance of IIDs has been extensive and conducted over several years (Epperson, 1984; Geritz, 1992; Shoaf & Oliver, 1992). In addition, two meta-analyses have been conducted to synthesize the findings from these numerous studies (Goode et al., 1991; Peterson & Kirchhoff, 1991). The finding that normal saline is as effective as heparinized saline in maintaining an IID has been consistently supported by replication studies and the meta-analyses.

Evaluation of Studies' Clinical Relevance

Research-based knowledge can be used to solve practice problems, enhance clinical judgment, or measure phenomena in clinical practice. The scope of utilization might be a single patient-care unit, a hospital, or all hospitals in a corporation or community. For example, Shively, Riegel, Waterhouse, Burns, Templin, and Thomason (1997) conducted a community-level research utilization project to promote the change from heparinized to saline flushes for IIDs of adult patients in three acute care facilities in one community. The change to saline flushes was successful in all three hospitals and has been maintained for 2 years. Research findings may also be used in primary care clinics and practitioners' offices, depending on the knowledge to be used in practice. The nurse(s) desiring to implement a change in practice must be able to assure the agency that the cost in time, energy, and money and any real or potential risks are outweighed by the benefits of the change. The study by Shively et al. (1997) did document that despite the research support for the use of saline flushes for adult IIDs, heparinized saline flushes continue to be used in several clinical agencies.

Summary of Research Knowledge

The research on a topic needs to be summarized to determine what is currently known and not known. Often you will have to review the literature in a selected area and summarize the findings for use in practice (see Chapter 4). In some areas, researchers have conducted integrative reviews of the research literature or meta-analyses, which greatly facilitate the process of summarizing current knowledge in an area. For example, Goode et al. (1991) conducted a meta-analysis "to estimate the effects of heparin flush and saline flush solutions on maintaining patency, preventing phlebitis, and increasing duration of peripheral heparin locks or IIDs" (p. 324). The meta-analysis was conducted on 17 quality studies that are described in Table 13-2. The total sample size of the 17 studies was 4,153; the settings were a variety of medical-surgical and critical care units. Goode et al. summarized the current knowledge as follows.

> ". . . It can be concluded that saline is as effective as heparin in maintaining patency, preventing phlebitis, and increasing duration in peripheral intravenous locks. Quality of care can be enhanced by using saline as the flush solution, thereby eliminating problems associated with anticoagulant effects and drug incompatibilities. In addition, an estimated yearly savings of $109,100,000 to $218,200,000 U.S. health care dollars could be attained." (p. 324)

The meta-analysis provides a sound scientific basis for making a change in practice. The clinical relevance is evident; the use of saline to flush IIDs promotes quality care and extensive cost savings.

If you plan on making this change in your practice setting, you need to examine the following conditions: previous practice, felt needs or problems, innovativeness, and norms of the social system (Rogers, 1995). Does your institution currently use heparin, not saline, to irrigate IIDs? Do the nurses believe this is a problem? You need to highlight problems with heparin that have been identified in the research literature. Are the nurses innovative and willing to change or are they resistant to change? Which nurses might be most helpful in assisting with the change? You also need to talk with your administrator about the change. Is the administration in your agency open or resistant to change?

Persuasion Stage

During the persuasion stage, you need to convince the administration and other nurses to change their current practice. Persuasion might be accomplished by demonstrating the relative advantage, compatibility, complexity, trialability,

TABLE 13-2. Studies Included in the Meta-Analysis

Study	N	Subjects	Assignment	Heparin Dose	Clotting Effect Size (d_c)	Phlebitis Effect Size (d_p)	Duration Effect Size (d_d)
Ashton et al., 1990	16 exp$_c$ 16 con$_c$ 13 exp$_p$ 14 con$_p$	Adult critical care	Random double blind	10/u/cc	.3590	−.1230	
Barrett et al., 1990	59 experimental 50 control	Adult Med-Surg patients	Nonrandom double blind crossover	10/u/cc	−.1068	−.4718	
Craig & Anderson, 1991	129 exp 145 con	Adult Med-Surg patients	Random double blind crossover	10/u/cc	.0095	−.0586	
Cyganski et al., 1987	225 exp 196 con	Adult Med-Surg patients	Nonrandom	100/u/cc	.2510		
Donham & Denning, 1987	8 exp$_c$ 4 con$_c$ 7 exp$_p$ 5 con$_p$	Adult critical care	Random double blind	10/u/cc	.0000	.0548	
Dunn & Lenihan, 1987	61 experimental 51 control	Adult patients	Nonrandom	50/u/cc	−.2057	−.2258	
Epperson, 1984	138 exp 120 con 138 exp 154 con	Adult Med-Surg patients	Random double blind	10/u/cc 100/u/cc			−.1176 −.1232

Study	Sample	Population	Design	Concentration			
Garrelts et al., 1989	131 exp 173 con	Adult Med-Surg patients	Random double blind	10/u/cc	−.1773	−.1057	.2753
Hamilton et al., 1988	137 exp 170 con	Adult patients	Random double blind	100/u/cc	.0850	−.1819	−.0604
Holford et al., 1977	39 experimental 140 control	Young adult volunteers	Nonrandom double blind	3.3, 10, 16.5 100, 132/u/cc	.6545		
Kasparek et al., 1988	49 exp 50 con	Adult Med patients	Random double blind	10/u/cc	.3670	−.5430	
Lombardi et al., 1988	34 experimental 40 control	Pediatric patients (4 wks to 18 yrs)	Nonrandom sequential double blind	10/u/cc		−.2324	.0000
Miracle et al., 1989	167 exp 441 con	Adult Med-Surg patients	Nonrandom	100/u/cc	−.0042		
Shearer, 1987	87 exp 73 con	Med-Surg patients	Nonrandom	10/u/cc	−.1170	−.0977	
Spann, 1988	15 experimental 19 control	Adult telemetry step down	Nonrandom double blind	10/u/cc	−.3163	−.3252	
Taylor et al., 1989	369 exp 356 con	Adult Med-Surg patients	Nonrandom time series	10/u/cc	.0308	.0288	−.1472
Tuten & Gueldner, 1991	42 exp 71 con	Adult Med-Surg patients	Nonrandom	100/u/cc	.0000	.1662	

From Goode, C. J., Titler, M., Rakel, B., Ones, D. S., Kleiber, C., Small, S., & Triolo, P. K. (1991). A meta-analysis of effects of heparin flush and saline flush: Quality and cost implications. *Nursing Research, 40*(6), p. 325. Copyright 1991, The American Journal of Nursing Company. Used with permission. All rights reserved.

TABLE 13-3. Annual Cost Savings from Changing to Saline		
Study	*Cost Savings*	*Hospital*
Craig & Anderson, 1991	$40,000/yr	525-bed tertiary care hospital
Dunn & Lenihan, 1987	$19,000/yr	530-bed private hospital
Goode et al., 1991 (this study)	$38,000/yr	879-bed tertiary care hospital
Kasparek et al., 1988	$19,000/yr	350-bed private hospital
Lombardi et al., 1988	$20,000–$25,000/yr	52-bed pediatric unit
Schustek, 1984	$20,000/yr	391-bed private hospital
Taylor et al., 1989	$30,000–$40,000/yr	216-bed private hospital

From Goode, C. J., Titler, M., Rakel, B., Ones, D. S., Kleiber, C., Small, S., & Triolo, P. K. (1991). A meta-analysis of effects of heparin flush and saline flush: Quality and cost implications. *Nursing Research, 40*(6), p. 325. Copyright 1991, The American Journal of Nursing Company. Used with permission. All rights reserved.

and observability of changing from heparin to saline as a flush solution (see Fig. 13-1). The relative advantages of using saline are the improved quality of care and cost savings that are clearly documented in the research literature (Geritz, 1992; Goode et al., 1991; Shoaf & Oliver, 1992). The cost savings for hospitals of different sizes are summarized in Table 13-3. The compatibility of the change can be determined by identifying the changes that will have to occur in your agency. What changes will the nurses have to make in irrigating IIDs with saline? What changes will have to occur in the pharmacy to provide the saline flush? Are the physicians aware of the research in this area? Are they willing to order the use of saline to flush the IIDs?

The change of peripheral IID irrigant from heparin flush to saline flush is not complex. Only the flush is changed, so no additional skill, expertise, or time is required by the nurse to make the change. Because saline flush, unlike heparin flush, is compatible with any drug that might be administered through the IID, potential complications are decreased. The change might be started on one unit as a clinical trial and then evaluated. Once the quality of care and the cost savings become observable to the nurses, physicians, and hospital administrators, the change will probably spread rapidly throughout the institution. Persuasion is likely to result in changing the irrigant from heparin flush to saline flush because the advantages are extensive and there are no identified disadvantages. The change is also compatible with existing nursing care and would be relatively simple to implement on a trial basis to demonstrate the positive outcomes for patients, nurses, and the health care agency.

Decision Stage

The decision to use saline flush rather than heparin flush as an irrigant requires approval by the institution, the physicians, and the nurses managing patients' IIDs. When a change requires institutional approval, decision-making may be necessary at several levels of the organization. Thus, a decision at one level may lead to contact with another official who must approve the action. In keeping with the guidelines of planned change, institutional changes are more likely to be effective if all those affected by the change have a voice in the decision. Who needs to approve the change in your institution? What steps do you need to take to get the change approved? Do the physicians support the change? Do the nurses on the units support the change? Who are the leaders in the institution? Can you get them to support the change? Try to get the nurses to make a commitment and take a public stand to make the change; this increases the likelihood that the change will occur. Contact the appropriate administrators and physicians, and detail the pros and cons of making the change to saline flush for irrigating IIDs. You need to indicate clearly to the physicians and administrators that the change is based on extensive research findings. Most physicians are positively influenced by research-based knowledge.

Implementation Stage

Implementing a research-based change can be simple or complex, depending on the change. The change might be implemented as indicated in the research literature or may be modified to meet the agency's needs. In some cases, a long time might be spent planning the implementation after the decision is made. In other cases, implementation can begin immediately. Usually, a great deal of support is needed during initial implementation of a change. As with any new activity, unexpected events often occur, and the nurse adopter frequently does not know how to interpret them. Contact with a person experienced in the change can make the difference between continuation and rejection of the innovation.

The change from heparin flush to saline flush will involve the physicians, who will have to order saline for flushing IIDs. You will need to speak with the physicians to gain their support for the change. You might convince some key physicians to support the change, and they will convince others. The pharmacy will have to package saline for use as an irrigant. The nurses will also be given information about the change and the rationale for it. It might be best to implement the change on one nursing unit and give the nurses on this unit an opportunity to design the protocol and plan for implementing the change. The nurses might develop a protocol similar to the one in Figure 13-3. This protocol directs you in preparing for irrigating an IID, irrigating the IID, and documenting your actions.

Confirmation Stage

After a change has been implemented in practice, the nurses who implemented the change need to confirm or document the effectiveness of the change. They need to document that the change improved quality of care, decreased the

1. Obtain the saline flush for irrigation from the pharmacy.
2. Wash hands, collect equipment for irrigating the IID, and put on gloves.
3. Cleanse the IID with alcohol prior to injecting with saline solution.
4. Flush the peripheral IID with 1 mL of normal saline every 8 hours.
5. If a patient is on IV medication, administer 1 mL of saline, administer the medication, and follow with 1 mL of saline.
6. Check the IID site for complications of phlebitis or loss of patency. The symptoms of phlebitis include erythema, tenderness, warmth, and a tender or palpable cord. Loss of patency is indicated by resistance to flushing, as evidenced by inability to administer 1 mL of flushing solution within 30 seconds.
7. Chart the time the IID was irrigated with saline and any complications of phlebitis or loss of patency.

Geritz, M. A. (1992). Saline versus heparin in intermittent infuser patency maintenance. *Western Journal of Nursing Research, 14*(2), 131–141.

Goode, C. J., Titler, M., Rakel, B., Ones, D. S., Kleiber, C., Small, S., & Triolo, P. K. (1991). A meta-analysis of effects of heparin flush and saline flush: Quality and cost implications. *Nursing Research, 40*(6), 324–330.

Shoaf, J., & Oliver, S. (1992). Efficacy of normal saline injection with and without heparin for maintaining intermittent intravenous site. *Applied Nursing Research, 5*(1), 9–12.

FIGURE 13-3
Protocol for irrigating IIDs.

cost of care, and/or saved nursing time. If the outcomes from the change in practice are positive, nurses, administrators, and physicians often want to continue the change. Nurses also usually seek feedback from those around them. Their peers' reactions to the change in nursing practice influence the continuation of the change. If peers approve, the nurses often adopt the change and even encourage others to do the same. If peers disapprove or provide negative feedback, the nurses often abandon the change.

You can confirm the effectiveness of the saline flush for irrigating IIDs by examining patient care outcomes and cost benefits. Patient care outcomes can be examined by determining the number of clotting and phlebitis complications with IIDs one month before and after the change is implemented. A finding of no significant difference supports the use of saline flush. The cost savings can be calculated for one month by determining the cost difference between heparin and saline flushes and multiplying by the number of saline flushes conducted in the month. This cost savings can then be multiplied by 12 months and compared with the cost savings summarized in Table 13-3. If positive patient outcomes and cost savings are demonstrated, the adoption of saline flush for irrigating peripheral IIDs will probably continue and be used by all nurses in the agency.

Using Published Research-Based Protocols in Your Practice

Using research findings in practice is facilitated by the publication of research-based protocols in research and clinical journals. A *research-based protocol* provides clearly developed steps for implementing a treatment or intervention in practice, and these steps are documented by findings from studies. These protocols are often developed by researchers who have conducted studies in a particular area requiring a change in practice. They might develop an integrated review of the research literature or conduct a meta-analysis on studies in an area of interest. Integrative reviews and meta-analyses provide a synthesis of the research literature and a basis for the development of research-based protocols. Published research-based protocols provide clear direction to clinicians for making changes in their practice.

Beyea and Nicoll (1995) conducted an integrative review of the literature on the administration of medications via the IM route and then developed a detailed research-based protocol for this procedure. Table 13-4 includes a description of the different sites for an IM injection (Beyea & Nicoll, 1995). Table 13-5 provides a detailed research-based protocol for administration of IM injections that includes equipment to use, site, position, and injection techniques (Beyea & Nicoll, 1995). Each step of the protocol is documented with research sources. This protocol provides clear direction for giving IM injections to your patients. You could adopt this protocol individually and follow the procedures outlined in Table 13-5 when giving IM injections. This protocol might also be adopted by a clinical agency and published in the policy and procedure manual to provide guidelines for all nurses giving IM injections in an agency. As the number of studies of nursing interventions increases, more researchers and expert clinicians have the opportunity to summarize research knowledge with an integrative review or a meta-analysis and to use this knowledge to develop a research-based protocol for practicing nurses. These protocols will increase the use of research findings to make changes in practice, which will improve the quality of care provided patients and families.

Clinical Practice Guidelines

The federal government has long recognized the importance of research utilization and has been concerned about the delay between the discovery of new knowledge and the use of that knowledge by society. In the early 1970s, the federal government organized a think tank of experts in the area of research utilization to examine the reasons for the lack of research utilization and to propose strategies to improve it. Through the years, the federal government has

Text continued on page 448

TABLE 13-4. What's in a Name?

Site	Landmarks	Also Described as	Target Muscle	Comments
Ventrogluteal (VG)	Place palm of hand against the greater trochanter and place the index finger on the anterior superior iliac spine. Extend the middle finger along the iliac crest toward the iliac tubercle. (Right hand to left hip; left hand to right hip.)	Ventrolateral gluteal Anterior gluteal Hip	Gluteus medius	Although Zelman (1961) discussed the VG site, he called it the "anterior lateral site." This use of conflicting terms has confused the location and perhaps limited its usage.
Dorsogluteal	Draw an imaginary line between the superior iliac spine and the greater trochanter. Give the injection in an area above the imaginary line.	Upper outer quadrant of buttocks Inner aspect of the upper outer quadrant Buttocks Posterior gluteal muscle	Gluteus maximus May incidentally inject in the gluteus medius and/or gluteus minimus	This site was originally called "the buttocks." In the 1960s the description evolved to "the outer aspect of the upper outer quadrant." Previously, it had been described as "the inner aspect of the upper outer quadrant." Confusion persists.

Site	Administration technique	Location	Comments
Deltoid	Expose the entire shoulder and arm area. Administer injection 1–2 in. below the acromion process.	Upper arm Fleshy muscle of the shoulder Outer aspect of the arm	Commonly referred to as the arm; identification of the deltoid site must be precise so as to avoid nerve and/or muscle injury.
Vastus lateralis	First locate the vastus lateralis muscle along the thigh. In infants and children the site for injection lies below the greater trochanter of the femur and within the upper lateral quadrant of the thigh. For adults, the site is 4 in. below the greater trochanter and 4 in. above the knee laterally in middle third of the vastus lateralis muscle.	A hands breadth below the trochanter and a hands breadth above knee Thigh Front of the leg Anterolateral thigh	In the past many nurses were taught to use the rectus femoris muscle, which is associated with injury. The rectus femoris is part of the same muscle group as the vastus lateralis, but the rectus femoris is anterior and the vastus lateralis is lateral on the thigh.

From Beyea, S. C., & Nicoll, L. H. (1995). Administration of medications via the intramuscular route: An integrative review of the literature and research-based protocol for the procedure. *Applied Nursing Research, 8*(1), 25, with permission.

TABLE 13-5. Procedure for Administration of IM Injections

Procedure	Rationale	References
1. For adults, select a 1.5-in. needle. For children, select a 1-in. needle. Use a needle of 21–23 gauge.	The needle must be long enough to reach the muscle. Injections into the subcutaneous tissue cause pain to the patient. The VG site provides the most consistent depth of subcutaneous tissue; in adults, the adipose tissue layer over the VG muscle is less than 3.75 cm (1.47 in.) in depth. Using a smaller gauge needle minimizes tissue injury and subcutaneous leakage.	Hick, Charboneau, Brakke, & Goergen, 1989; Johnson & Raptou, 1965; Michaels & Poole, 1970; Shaffer, 1929; Talbert, Haslam, & Haller, 1967
2. The maximum volume to be administered in one injection should not exceed 4 mL in adults with well-developed muscles such as the ventrogluteal. Children and individuals with less well developed muscles should receive no more than 1 to 2 mL. Children under the age of 2 years should not receive more than 1 mL. If using the deltoid, do not exceed a volume of 0.5 to 1 mL. The size of the syringe is determined by the volume to be administered and the size of the syringe should correspond as closely as possible to the amount to be administered. Volumes less than 0.5 mL require a low-dose syringe such as tuberculin syringe.	High volume injections cause more pain. Finely graduated syringes such as tuberculin syringes ensure administration of the correct dose.	Farley, Joyce, Long, & Roberts, 1986; Losek & Gyuro, 1992; Zenk, 1982
3. Use a filter needle to draw up medication from a glass ampule or vial. Hold the vial or ampule down and do not draw up the last drop in the container. After drawing the medication into the syringe, change the needle prior to administration. If using a pre-filled syringe, such as Tubex® or Carpuject®, and drawing from a vial or ampule, instill the medication into another syringe and ensure the use of a clean needle prior to injection. If using a pre-filled unit-dose medication, take caution to avoid dripping medication on the needle prior to injection. If this does occur, wipe the medication off the needle with a sterile gauze.	Glass and rubber particulate has been found in medications withdrawn with a regular needle. Holding the vial or ampule down will allow particulate matter to precipitate out of the solution, and leaving the last drops reduces the chance of withdrawing foreign particles. Changing the needle will prevent tracking the medication through the subcutaneous tissue during insertion of the needle, which can cause pain. Similarly, medication should be wiped from the needle, as this can also cause pain when it is tracked through the subcutaneous tissue.	Hahn, 1990; Keen, 1986; McConnell, 1982
4. Do not use an air bubble.	An air bubble affects the dose administered, causing an overdose of medication of at least 5% and as great as 100%, depending on the dose administered.	Chaplin, Shull, & Welk, 1985; Zenk, 1982, 1993
5. Select the ventrogluteal (VG) site as the injection site for children over 7 months and adults unless there is a strict contraindication. Strict contraindications would include preexisting tissue injury and administration of hepatitis-B vac-	The VG site is free of nerves and blood vessels. There are no documented reports of complications from IM injections administered at this site. The VG muscle is a well-developed muscle in infants, children, and adults.	Beecroft & Redick, 1990; Brandt, Smith, Ashburn, & Graves, 1972; Centers for Disease Control, 1990; Daly, Johnston, & Chung, 1992; Hochstetter, 1954, 1955, 1956

Protocol	Rationale	Supporting references
cine, which should only be administered in the deltoid. In infants less than 7 mo, the vastus lateralis should be used for administration of hepatitis-B vaccine.		
6. Prior to the administration of any IM injection, carefully assess the site for evidence of induration, abscesses or other contraindications for use of the site.	Injections are contraindicated in previously injured muscles or tissues.	Stokes, Beerman, & Ingraham, 1944
7. Position the patient to relax the muscle. Prone: Have the patient "toe in" to internally rotate the femur. Side-lying: Have the patient flex upper leg at 20°. Supine: Have the patient flex both knees, if possible, or if not possible, flex the knee on the side where the medication will be administered.	There is reduced pain with a relaxed muscle.	Keen, 1986; Kruszewski, Lang, & Johnson, 1979; Rettig & Southby, 1982
8. Identify the site by placing the palm of the hand on the greater trochanter, with the index finger toward the anterior superior iliac spine and the middle finger spread away to form a "V." Use the right hand on the left VG site; left hand on the right VG site.	The landmarks are described by Hochstetter.	Hochstetter, 1954, 1955, 1956; Zelman, 1961
9. Pull the skin down so as to administer the injection in a Z-track manner at a 90 degree angle to the iliac crest in the middle of the "V."	Z-track technique reduces discomfort and incidence of lesions.	Keen, 1983, 1986, 1990
10. Cleanse the skin in a circular fashion in an area of approximately 5–8 cm (2–3 in.) and allow the alcohol to dry.	Deep tissues can be infected with skin contaminants injected via the needle; the skin is the first line of defense. Alcohol is irritating to the subcutaneous tissue and causes pain.	Berger & Williams, 1992; Murphy, 1991
11. Insert the needle with a steady pressure and then aspirate for at least 5–10 s. Inject the medication slowly at a rate of approximately 10 s/mL.	Aspirating for 5–10 s is adequate to ensure that the needle is not in a small, low-flow blood vessel. A slow, steady injection rate promotes comfort and minimizes tissue damage.	Stokes, Beerman, & Ingraham, 1944; Zelman, 1961
12. Wait 10 s after injecting the medication before withdrawing the needle.	Waiting 10 s allows the medication to be deposited in the muscle and begin to diffuse through the muscle.	Belanger-Annable, 1985; Hahn, 1990, 1991; Keen, 1990
13. Smoothly and steadily withdraw the needle and apply gentle pressure at the site with a dry sponge.	This minimizes tissue injury. Massaging the site can result in tissue irritation.	Newton, Newton, & Fudin, 1992
14. Encourage leg exercises.	Leg exercises will promote the absorption of the medication.	Stokes, Beerman, & Ingraham, 1944
15. Whenever possible, assess the site 2–4 h after injection and as needed to identify any side effects.	Given the number of complications reported in the literature, it is important to assess the site for any signs of redness, swelling, pain, or other iatrogenic effects from the injection.	Beecroft & Redick, 1989, 1990

From Beyea, S. C., & Nicoll, L. H. (1995). Administration of medication via the intramuscular route: An integrative review of the literature and research-based protocol for the procedure, *Applied Nursing Research, 8*(1): 28–29, with permission.

supported a variety of research utilization activities, including the WICHE and CURN projects. In 1992, the Agency for Health Care Policy and Research (AHCPR), within the U.S. Department of Health and Human Services (DHHS), convened panels of expert health care providers and researchers to summarize research and develop clinical practice guidelines. These guidelines include a summary of the current research literature, mechanisms for assessing the clinical problem in practice, strategies for managing the clinical problem, and methods to evaluate patient and family outcomes. These panels summarized research findings and developed guidelines for practice in several areas. Three of these guidelines that are extremely relevant to you in your nursing practice are acute pain management in infants, children, and adolescents (Acute Pain Management Guideline Panel, 1992); prediction and prevention of pressure ulcers in adults (Panel for the Prediction and Prevention of Pressure Ulcers in Adults, 1992); and identification and treatment of urinary incontinence in adults (Urinary Incontinence Guideline Panel, 1992). The AHCPR clinical practice guidelines that are currently available can be downloaded free from the Internet at the following address: http://www.ahcpr.gov/. These clinical practice guidelines have also been published in books that can be obtained for a minimal fee from the DHHS at the following address.

Department of Health and Human Services
Public Health Service
Agency for Health Care Policy and Research
Executive Office Center
2101 East Jefferson Street, Suite 501
Rockville, MD 20852

In the future, accrediting agencies for health care organizations will require that protocols for nursing interventions be documented with research. The procedure manuals, standards of care, and nursing care plans will need to reflect current nursing research. Many progressive nurse executives realize the importance of research and are encouraging their nursing staffs to use research findings in practice. However, to improve nursing practice effectively with research knowledge, research utilization must become a priority for all nurses.

SUMMARY

The preceding chapters of this textbook describe the steps of the research process, present guidelines for critiquing studies, and provide direction for summarizing the research literature. Reading, critiquing, and summarizing research literature are essential steps for determining if findings are ready for use in practice. Many quality clinical studies were conducted and replicated in the 1980s and 1990s, providing research findings that are ready for use in practice. However, only a limited amount of this knowledge is being used to improve practice. Thus, the purpose of this chapter is to assist you in using research findings in your practice.

Research utilization is the process of communicating and using research-generated knowledge to make an impact on or a change in the existing practices in the health care system. The main elements of research utilization include summarizing knowledge generated through research; communicating the research knowledge to nurses, other health care professionals, policy makers, and consumers; and achieving desired outcomes for patients, nurses, and health care agencies. Research or empirical knowledge is generated through quality studies. Communication of research findings includes developing a research report and disseminating that report through presentations and publications to audiences of nurses, health care professionals, policy makers, and health care consumers. The desired outcomes of research utilization include providing quality nursing care, increasing positive patient outcomes, and decreasing costs for health care agencies.

Two major federally funded projects developed to increase utilization of nursing research findings are discussed: the WICHE project and the CURN project. The WICHE project focused on critiquing research and using research findings to improve practice. The CURN project was implemented to increase the utilization of research findings in the following ways: communicating findings, facilitating organizational modifications necessary for implementation, and encouraging collaborative research that is directly transferable to clinical practice. Clinical studies were critiqued, research-based protocols were developed from the findings, and implementation was initiated on test units within hospitals.

Many research findings are not being used in practice, and the barriers to research utilization are examined in this chapter. These barriers are related to the quality of the research findings, the characteristics of the nurses who need to use the findings in practice, and the characteristics of the organizations in which the research should be utilized. The barriers related to the quality of the research findings include the following: studies are not focused on relevant clinical problems, the studies conducted lack replication, and findings are not expressed in terms understood by practicing nurses. Some barriers are related to nurses; for example, they do not value research, are unaware of or are unwilling to read research reports, have inadequate education related to the research process, and do not know how to apply research findings in practice. Some organizations create barriers to research utilization in that they are traditional and oppose change.

Rogers's theory of research utilization is presented to direct your use of research findings in practice. Rogers proposes a five-stage process for research utilization: (1) knowledge, (2) persuasion, (3) decision, (4) implementation, and (5) confirmation. The knowledge stage is the first awareness of the existence of an innovation or new idea for practice. During the persuasion stage, nurses form an attitude toward the innovation. A decision is then made to adopt or reject the innovation. The implementation stage involves using the innovation to change practice. During the final stage, confirmation, nurses seek reinforcement of their decision and continue to adopt or reject the change in their practice. An example of research utilization is presented using Rogers's five stages. The research knowledge about the effects of heparin versus saline flush for irrigating IIDs is presented for use in practice.

The chapter concludes with a discussion of the research-based protocols published in professional journals and the clinical practice guidelines developed by the federal government. The research-based protocols published in research and clinical journals are often developed by researchers who have conducted studies in these areas. They might develop an integrated review of the research literature or conduct a meta-analysis on the studies in an area of interest. These integrative reviews and meta-analyses provide a synthesis of the research literature and a basis for development of research-based protocols. The clinical practice guidelines are being developed by the AHCPR of the

DHHS. In 1992, the DHHS convened panels of expert health care providers and researchers to summarize research and develop clinical practice guidelines. The guidelines are available on the Internet and from the DHHS.

These clinical practice guidelines and the research-based protocols published in the professional journals provide clear direction to clinicians for making changes in their practice.

REFERENCES

Acute Pain Management Guideline Panel. (1992, February). *Acute pain management: Operative or medical procedures and trauma. Clinical practice guideline.* AHCPR Pub. No. 92-0032. Rockville, MD: Agency for Health Care Policy and Research, Public Health Service, U.S. Department of Health and Human Services.

Ashton, J., Gibson, V., & Summers, S. (1990). Effects of heparin versus saline solution on intermittent infusion device irrigations. *Heart & Lung, 19*(6), 608–612.

Axford, R., & Cutchen, L. (1977). Using nursing research to improve preoperative care. *Journal of Nursing Administration, 7*(10), 16–20.

Barrett, P. J., & Lester, R. L. (1990). Heparin versus saline flush solutions in a small community hospital. *Hospital Pharmacy, 25*(2), 115–118.

Beecroft, P. C., & Redick, S. A. (1989). Possible complications of intramuscular injections on the pediatric unit. *Pediatric Nursing, 15*(4), 333–336, 376.

Beecroft, P. C., & Redick, S. A. (1990). Intramuscular injection practices of pediatric nurses: Site selection. *Nurse Educator, 15*(4), 23–28.

Belanger-Annable, M. C. (1985). Long acting neuroleptics: Technique for intramuscular injection. *The Canadian Nurse, 81*(8), 41–44.

Berger, K. J., & Williams, M. B. (1992). *Fundamentals of nursing: Collaborating for optimal health.* Norwalk, CT: Appleton & Lange.

Beyea, S. C., & Nicoll, L. H. (1995). Administration of medications via the intramuscular route: An integrative review of the literature and research-based protocol for the procedure. *Applied Nursing Research, 8*(1), 23–33.

Blegen, M. A., Goode, C. J., & Reed, L. (1998). Nurse staffing and patient outcomes. *Nursing Research, 47*(1), 43–50.

Bock, L. R. (1990). From research to utilization: Bridging the gap. *Nursing Management, 21*(3), 50–51.

Brandt, P. A., Smith, M. E., Asburn, S. S., & Graves, J. (1972). IM injections in children. *American Journal of Nursing, 72*(7), 1402–1406.

Brett, J. L. (1987). Use of nursing practice research findings. *Nursing Research, 36*(6), 344–349.

Bueno, M. M. (1998). Promoting nursing research through newsletters. *Applied Nursing Research, 11*(1), 41–44.

Burns, N., & Grove, S. K. (1997). *The practice of nursing research: Conduct, critique, and utilization* (3rd ed.). Philadelphia: Saunders.

Centers for Disease Control. (1990). Recommendation of the Immunization Practices Advisory Committee. Diphtheria, Tetanus, and Pertussis: Guidelines for vaccine prophylaxis and other preventive measures. *Morbidity and Mortality Weekly Report, 34*(27), 405–426.

Chaplin, G., Shull, H., & Welk, P. C. (1985). How safe is the air-bubble technique for IM injections? *Nursing85, 15*(9), 59.

Clinton, H. R. (1993). Nurses in the front lines. *Nursing & Health Care, 14*(6), 286–288.

Coyle, L. A., & Sokop, A. G. (1990). Innovation adoption behavior among nurses. *Nursing Research, 39*(3), 176–180.

Craig, F. D., & Anderson, S. R. (1991). *A comparison of normal saline versus heparinized normal saline in the maintenance of intermittent infusion devices.* Manuscript submitted for publication.

CURN Project. *Using research to improve nursing practice.* Series of Clinical Protocols: *Clean intermittent catheterization* (1982), *Closed urinary drainage systems* (1981), *Distress reduction through sensory preparation* (1981), *Intravenous cannula change* (1981), *Mutual goal setting in patient care* (1982), *Pain: Deliberative nursing interventions* (1982), *Preventing decubitus ulcers* (1981), *Reducing diarrhea in tube-fed patients* (1981), *Structured preoperative teaching* (1981). New York: Grune & Stratton.

Cyganski, J. M., Donahue, J. M., & Heaton, J. S. (1987). The case for the heparin flush. *American Journal of Nursing, 87*(6), 796–797.

Daly, J. M., Johnston, W., & Chung, Y. (1992). Injection sites utilized for DPT immunizations in infants. *Journal of Community Health Nursing, 9*(2), 87–94.

Donham, J., & Denning, V. (1987). Heparin vs. saline in maintaining patency in intermittent infusion devices: Pilot study. *The Kansas Nurse, 62*(11), 6–7.

Dracup, K. A., & Breu, C. S. (1978). Using nursing research findings to meet the needs of grieving spouses. *Nursing Research, 27*(4), 212–216.

Dunn, D. L., & Lenihan, S. F. (1987). The case for the saline flush. *American Journal of Nursing, 87*(6), 798–799.

Epperson, E. L. (1984). Efficacy of 0.9% sodium chloride injection with and without heparin for maintaining indwelling intermittent injection sites. *Clinical Pharmacy, 3*(6), 626–629.

Farley, F., Joyce, N., Long, B., & Roberts, R. (1986). Will that IM needle reach the muscle? *American Journal of Nursing, 86*(12), 1327–1328.

Fitzgerald, S. T., Hill, M. N., Santamaria, B., Howard, C., & Jadack, R. (1997). Nurses' perceptions of consensus reports containing recommendations for practice. *Nursing Outlook, 45*(5), 229–235.

Foss-Durant, A. M., & McAfee, A. (1997). A comparison of three oral care products commonly used in practice. *Clinical Nursing Research, 6*(1), 90–104.

Garrelts, J., LaRocca, J., Ast, D., Smith, D. F., & Sweet, D. E. (1989). Comparison of heparin and 0.9% sodium chloride injection in the maintenance of indwelling intermittent I.V. devices. *Clinical Pharmacy, 8*(1), 34–39.

Geritz, M. A. (1992). Saline versus heparin in intermittent infuser patency maintenance. *Western Journal of Nursing Research, 14*(2), 131–141.

Goldberg, H. I., Cummings, M. A., Steinberg, E. P., Ricci, E. M., Shannon, T., Soumerai, S. B., Mittman, B. S., Eisenberg, J., Heck, D. A., Kaplan, S., Kenzora, J. E., Vargus, A. M., Mulley, A. G., & Rimer, B. K. (1994). Deliberations on the dissemination of PORT products: Translating research findings into improved patient outcomes. *Medical Care, 32*(7), JS90–JS110.

Goode, C. J., Titler, M., Rakel, B., Ones, D. S., Kleiber, C., Small, S., & Triolo, P. K. (1991). A meta-analysis of effects of heparin flush and saline flush: Quality and cost implications. *Nursing Research, 40*(6), 324–330.

Gould, D. (1986). Pressure sore prevention and treatment: An example of nurses' failure to implement research findings. *Journal of Advanced Nursing, 11*(4), 389–394.

Hahn, K. (1990). Brush up on your injection technique. *Nursing90, 20*(9), 54–58.

Hahn, K. (1991). Extra points on injections (letter). *Nursing91, 21*(1), 6.

Haller, K. B., Reynolds, M. A., & Horsley, J. A. (1979). Developing research-based innovation protocols: Process, criteria, and issues. *Research in Nursing & Health, 2*(1), 45–51.

Hamilton, R. A., Plis, J. M., Clay, C., & Sylvan, L. (1988). Heparin sodium versus 0.9% sodium chloride injection for maintaining patency of indwelling intermittent infusion devices. *Clinical Pharmacy, 7*(6), 439–443.

Harrison, M. B., Wells, G., Fisher, A., & Prince, M. (1996). Practice guidelines for the prediction and prevention of pressure ulcers: Evaluating the evidence. *Applied Nursing Research, 9*(1), 9–17.

Hester, N. O. (1993). Pain in children. In J. J. Fitzpatrick & J. S. Stevenson (Eds.), *Annual review of nursing research* (Vol. 11, pp. 105–142). New York: Springer.

Hick, J. F., Charboneau, J. W., Brakke, D. M., & Goergen, B. (1989). Optimum needle length for DPT inoculation of infants. *Pediatrics, 84*(1), 136–137.

Hochstetter, V. A. V. (1954). Über die intraglutäale Injektion, ihre Komplikationen und deren Verhütung. *Schweizerische Medizinische Wochenschrift, 84,* 1226–1227.

Hochstetter, V. A. V. (1955). Über Probleme und Technik der intraglutäalen injektion, Teil I. Der Einfluß des Medikamentes und der Individualität des Patienten auf die Ent-

stehung von Spritzenschäden. *Schweizerische Medizinische Wochenschrift, 85,* 1138–1144.

Hochstetter, V. A. V. (1956). Über probleme und Technik der intraglutäalen Injektion, Teil II. Der Einfluß der Injektionstechnick auf die Entstehung von Spritzenschäden. *Schweizerische Medizinische Wochenschrift, 86,* 69–76.

Holford, N. H. G., Vozeh, S., Coates, P., Porvell, J. R., Thiercelin, J. F., & Upton, R. (1977). More on heparin lock. *New England Journal of Medicine, 296,* 1300–1301.

Horsley, J. A., Crane, J., & Bingle, J. D. (1978). Research utilization as an organizational process. *Journal of Nursing Administration, 8*(7), 4–6.

Horsley, J. A., Crane, J., Crabtree, M. K., & Wood, D. J. (1983). *Using research to improve nursing practice: A guide.* New York: Grune & Stratton.

Hunt, M. (1987). The process of translating research findings into nursing practice. *Journal of Advanced Nursing, 12*(1), 101–110.

Johnson, E. W., & Raptou, A. D. (1965). A study of intragluteal injections. *Archives of Physical Medicine and Rehabilitation, 46,* 167–177.

Kasparek, A., Wenger, J., & Feldt, R. (1988). *Comparison of normal versus heparinized saline for flushing of intermittent intravenous infusion devices.* Unpublished manuscript. Mercy Medical Center, Cedar Rapids, IA, pp. 1–18.

Keen, M. F. (1983). Adverse effects of frequent intramuscular injections. *Research Review, 10*(4), 15–16.

Keen, M. F. (1986). Comparison of intramuscular injection techniques to reduce site discomfort and lesions. *Nursing Research, 35*(4), 207–210.

Keen, M. F. (1990). Get on the right track with Z-track injections. *Nursing90, 20*(8), 59.

Krueger, J. C. (1978). Utilization of nursing research: The planning process. *Journal of Nursing Administration, 8*(1), 6–9.

Krueger, J. C., Nelson, A. H., & Wolanin, M. O. (1978). *Nursing research: Development, collaboration, and utilization.* Germantown, MD: Aspen.

Kruszewski, A., Lang, S., & Johnson, J. (1979). Effect of positioning on discomfort from intramuscular injections in the dorsogluteal site. *Nursing Research, 28*(2), 103–105.

Liehr, P., & Houston, S. (1993). Critiquing and using nursing research: Guidelines for the critical care nurse. *American Journal of Critical Care, 2*(5), 407–412.

Lombardi, T. P., Gunderson, B., Zammett, L. O., Walters, J. K., & Morris, B. A. (1988). Efficacy of 0.9% sodium chloride injection with or without heparin sodium for maintaining patency of intravenous catheters in children. *Children Pharmacy, 7*(11), 832–836.

Losek, J. D., & Gyuro, J. (1992). Pediatric intramuscular injections: Do you know the procedure and complications? *Pediatric Emergency Care, 8*(2), 79–81.

MacGuire, J. M. (1990). Putting nursing research findings into practice: Research utilization as an aspect of the management of change. *Journal of Advanced Nursing, 15*(5), 614–620.

Massey, J., & Loomis, M. (1988). When should nurses use research findings? *Applied Nursing Research, 1*(1),32–40.

McConnell, E. A. (1982), The subtle art of really good injections. *RN, 45*(2), 25–35.

Michaels, L., & Poole, R. W. (1970). Injection granuloma of the buttock. *Canadian Medical Association Journal, 102*, 626–628.

Michel, Y., & Sneed, N. V. (1995). Dissemination and use of research findings in nursing practice. *Journal of Professional Nursing, 11*(5), 306–311.

Miracle, V., Fangman, B., Kayrouz, P., Kederis, K., & Pursell, L. (1989). Normal saline vs. heparin lock flush solution: One institution's findings. *The Kentucky Nurse, 37*(4), 1, 6–7.

Morse, J. M. (1993). Nursing research on patient falls in health care institutions. In J. J. Fitzpatrick & J. S. Stevenson (Eds.), *Annual review of nursing research* (Vol. 11, pp. 299–316). New York: Springer.

Murphy, J. I. (1991). Reducing the pain of intramuscular (IM) injections. *Advancing Clinical Care, 6*(4), 35.

Newton, M., Newton, D., & Fudin, J. (1992). Reviewing the "big three" injection techniques. *Nursing92, 22*(2), 34–41.

Panel for the Prediction and Prevention of Pressure Ulcers in Adults. (1992, May). *Pressure ulcers in adults: Prediction and preventions. Clinical practice guideline.* AHCPR Pub. No. 92-0047. Rockville, MD: Agency for Health Care Policy and Research, Public Health Service, U.S. Department of Health and Human Services.

Pelz, D., & Horsley, J. (1981). Measuring utilization of nursing research. In J. Ciarlo (Ed.), *Utilizing evaluation.* Beverly Hills, CA: Sage.

Peterson, F. Y., & Kirchhoff, K. T. (1991). Analysis of the research about heparinized versus nonheparinized intravascular lines. *Heart & Lung, 20*(6), 631–642.

Phillips, L. R. F. (1986). *A clinician's guide to the critique and utilization of nursing research.* Norwalk, CT: Appleton-Century-Crofts.

Rettig, F. M., & Southby, J. R. (1982). Using different body positions to reduce discomfort from dorsogluteal injection. *Nursing Research, 31*(4), 219–221.

Rogers, E. M. (1995). *Diffusion of innovations* (4th ed.). New York: Free Press.

Schustek, M. (1984). The cost effective approach to PRN device maintenance. *Journal of National Intravenous Therapy Associates, 7*, 527.

Shaffer, L. W. (1929). The fate in intragluteal injections. *Archives of Dermatology and Syphilology, 19*, 347–363.

Shearer, J. (1987). Normal saline flush versus dilute heparin flush patency in heparin locks. *National Intravenous Therapy Association, 10*(6), 425–427.

Shively, M., Riegel, B., Waterhouse, D., Burns, D., Templin,

K., & Thomason, T. (1997). Testing a community level research utilization intervention. *Applied Nursing Research, 10*(3), 121–127.

Shoaf, J., & Oliver, S. (1992). Efficacy of normal saline injection with and without heparin for maintaining intermittent intravenous site. *Applied Nursing Research, 5*(1), 9–12.

Smith, M. C., & Stullenbarger, E. (1991). A prototype for integrative review and meta-analysis of nursing research. *Journal of Advanced Nursing, 16*(11), 1272–1283.

Spann, J. M. (1988). Efficacy of two flush solutions to maintain catheter patency in heparin locks. *Dissertation Abstracts, 28*(01)1337125, 1–58.

Stokes, J. H., Beerman, H., & Ingraham, N. R. (1944). *Modern clinical syphilology: Diagnosis, treatment, case study* (3rd ed.). Philadelphia: Saunders.

Talbert, J. L., Haslam, R. H. A., & Haller, J. A. (1967). Gangrene of the foot following intramuscular injection in the lateral thigh: A case report with recommendations for prevention. *Journal of Pediatrics, 70*(1), 110–117.

Tanner, C. A. (1987). Evaluating research for use in practice: Guidelines for the clinician. *Heart & Lung, 16*(4), 424–431.

Tanner, C. A., & Lindeman, C. A. (1989). *Using nursing research.* Pub. No. 15-2232. New York: National League for Nursing.

Taylor, N., Hutchinson, E., Milliken, W., & Larson, E. (1989). Comparison of normal versus heparinized saline for flushing infusion devices. *Journal of Nursing Quality Assurance, 3*(4), 49–55.

Tuten, S. H., & Gueldner, S. H. (1991). Efficacy of sodium chloride versus dilute heparin for maintenance of peripheral intermittent intravenous devices. *Applied Nursing Research, 4*(2), 63–71.

Urinary Incontinence Guideline Panel. (1992, March). *Urinary incontinence in adults: Clinical practice guideline.* AHCPR Pub. No. 92-0038. Rockville, MD: Agency for Health Care Policy and Research, Public Health Service, U.S. Department of Health and Human Services.

Walczak, J. R., McGuire, D. B., Haisfield, M. E., & Beezley, A. (1994). A survey of research-related activities and perceived barriers to research utilization among professional oncology nurses. *Oncology Nursing Forum, 21*(4), 710–715.

Wichita, C. (1977). Treating and preventing constipation in nursing home residents. *Journal of Gerontological Nursing, 3*(6), 35–39.

Zelman, S. (1961). Notes on the techniques of intramuscular injections. *The American Journal of Medical Science, 241*(5), 47–58.

Zenk, K. E. (1982). Improving the accuracy of mini-volume injections. *Infusion, 6*(1), 7–12.

Zenk, K. E. (1993). Beware of overdose. *Nursing93, 23*(3), 28–29.

Glossary

Abstract (adjective)   Expressed without reference to any specific instance.

Abstract (noun)   Clear, concise summary of a study, usually limited to 100 to 250 words.

Abstract thinking   Thinking that is oriented to the development of an idea, without application to or association with a particular instance; independent of time and space. Abstract thinkers tend to look for meaning, patterns, relationships, and philosophical implications.

Academic library   Library located within an institution of higher learning; contains numerous reports in journals and books.

Accessible population   Portion of the target population to which the researcher has reasonable access.

Across-method triangulation   Combining research methods or strategies from two or more research traditions in the same study.

Action application of research   Using research findings to support the need for change, as an impetus for evaluation of services, and/or a model for practice.

Active rejection   Decision not to adopt an innovation that was examined.

Adoption   Full acceptance and implementation of an innovation in practice.

Alpha (α)   Cutoff point used to determine whether the samples being tested are members of the same population or of different populations; alpha is commonly set at .05, .01, or .001.

Alternate forms reliability   Comparison of the equivalence of two versions of the same paper-and-pencil instrument.

Analysis of covariance (ANCOVA)   Statistical procedure designed to reduce the variance within groups by partialing out the variance due to a confounding variable by performing regression analysis prior to performing ANOVA.

Analysis of variance (ANOVA)   Statistical test used to examine differences among two or more groups by comparing the variability between groups with the variability within groups.

Analysis phase   Phase of a critique in which the reader determines the strengths and limitations of the logical links connecting one study element with another.

Analytic induction   Qualitative research technique that includes enumerative induction, in which a number and variety of instances are collected that verify the model, and eliminative induction, which requires that the hypothesis be tested against alternatives.

Analytical preciseness   Performing a series of transformations during which concrete data are transformed across several levels of abstraction to develop a theoretical schema that imparts meaning to the phenomenon under study.

Analyzing a research report   Critical thinking skill that involves determining the value of a study by breaking the contents of a study report into parts and examining the parts in depth for accuracy, completeness, uniqueness of information, and organization.

Anonymity   Conditions in which the subject's identity cannot be linked, even by the researcher, with his or her individual responses.

Applied research   Scientific investigations conducted to generate knowledge that will directly influence clinical practice.

Approximate replication   Operational replication that involves repeating the original study under similar conditions, following the original methods as closely as possible.

Ascendance to an open context   Ability to see depth and complexity within the phenomenon examined and a greater capacity for insight than with the sedimented view. Requires deconstructing sedimented views and reconstructing another view.

Associative hypothesis   Hypothesis that identifies variables that occur or exist together in the real world, such that when one variable changes, the other changes.

Associative relationship   Relationship in which variables or concepts that occur or exist together in the real world are identified; thus, when one variable changes, the other changes. Hypotheses can be developed to identify associative relationships.

Assumptions   Statements taken for granted or considered true, even though they have not been scientifically tested.

Asymmetrical relationship   Relationship in which, if A occurs or changes, then B will occur or change, but there may be no indication that if B occurs or changes, A will occur or change (A → B).

Auditability   Rigorous development of a decision trail that is reported in sufficient detail to allow a second researcher to use the original data and the decision trail to arrive at conclusions similar to those of the original researcher.

Authority   Person with expertise and power who is able to influence the opinions and behavior of others.

Autonomous agents   Prospective subjects who are informed about a proposed study and who can voluntarily choose to participate or not participate.

Basic research Scientific investigations for the pursuit of "knowledge for knowledge's sake" or for the pleasure of learning and finding truth.

Beneficence, principle of Principle that encourages the researcher to do good and "above all, do no harm."

Benefit-risk ratio Ratio considered by researchers and reviewers of research as they weigh potential benefits (positive outcomes) and risks (negative outcomes) of a study to promote the conduct of ethical research.

Bias Any influence or action in a study that distorts the findings or slants them away from the true or expected.

Bibliography A list of publications for a specific topic or specialty area.

Bivariate analysis Statistical procedures that involve the comparison of summary values from two groups on the same variable or of two variables within a group.

Bivariate correlation Measure of the extent of the linear relationship between two variables.

Blocking System used in randomized block design in which subjects are included with various levels of an extraneous variable in the sample, and the number of subjects are controlled at each level of the variable and are randomly assigned to groups within the study.

Body of knowledge Information, principles, and theories that are organized by the beliefs accepted in a discipline at a given time.

Borrowing Appropriation and use of knowledge from other disciplines to guide nursing practice.

Box-and-whisker plots Exploratory data analysis technique to provide fast visualization of some of the major characteristics of the data, such as the spread, symmetry, and outliers.

Bracketing Qualitative research technique of suspending or setting aside what is known about an experience being studied.

Breach of confidentiality Accidental or direct action that allows an unauthorized person to have access to raw study data.

Byte Computer space for storing a single character, such as a number or a letter of the alphabet.

Canonical correlation Extension of multiple regression with more than one dependent variable.

Carryover effect Application of one treatment can influence the response to following treatments.

Case study In-depth analysis and systematic description of one patient or a group of similar patients to promote understanding of nursing interventions.

Case study design Intensive exploration of a single unit of study, such as a person, a family, a group, a community, or an institution.

Catalog System for identifying what is contained in the library.

Causal hypothesis Hypothesis that states the relationship between two variables, in which one variable (independent variable) is thought to cause or determine the presence of the other variable (dependent variable).

Causality   Relationship that includes three conditions: (1) there must be a strong correlation between the proposed cause and effect, (2) the proposed cause must precede the effect in time, and (3) the cause must be present whenever the effect occurs.

Cell   Intersection between the row and column in a table where a specific numerical value is inserted.

Central processing unit (CPU)   Device that controls computer operations and includes the internal memory, control unit, and arithmetic and logic unit.

Centralized diffusion system   System that involves group decision-making within an organization and usually a change agent to promote utilization of research-based innovations.

Change agent   A professional outside a social system who enters the system to promote adoption of a research-based innovation.

Chi-square test of independence   Used to analyze nominal data to determine significant differences between observed frequencies within the data and frequencies that were expected.

Cleaning data   Checking raw data to determine errors in data recording, coding, or entry.

Clinical significance   Importance (significance) of research findings in answering a clinical problem.

Cluster sampling   Sampling in which a frame is developed that includes a list of all the states, cities, institutions, or organizations (clusters) that could be used in a study; a randomized sample is drawn from this list.

Cochran Q test   Nonparametric test that is an extension of the McNemar test for two related samples.

Code   A symbol or abbreviation used to classify words or phrases in qualitative data.

Codebook   Record that documents the location or the column(s) that represent each variable and other information entered in a computer file.

Coding   A way of indexing or identifying categories in qualitative data.

Coercion   An overt threat of harm or excessive reward intentionally presented by one person to another in order to obtain compliance, such as offering prospective subjects a large sum of money to participate in a dangerous research project.

Cognitive application of research   Research-based knowledge used to affect a person's way of thinking, approaching, and/or observing situations.

Cognitive clustering   Comprehensive, scholarly synthesis of scientifically sound research that is evident in integrative reviews of research and meta-analyses.

Cohorts   Samples in time-dimensional studies within the field of epidemiology.

Coinvestigators   Two or more professionals conducting a study, whose salaries may be paid partially or in full by grant funding.

Communication of research findings   Developing a research report and disseminating it through presentations and publications to a variety of audiences.

Comparative descriptive design   Design used to describe differences in variables in two or more groups in a natural setting.

Comparison group   The group of subjects in a study not receiving a treatment when nonrandom methods are used for sample selection.

Comparison phase   Phase or step of a critique in which the reader compares the ideal for each step of the research process with the real steps in a study.

Compatibility   Degree to which an innovation is perceived to be consistent with current values, past experience, and priority of needs.

Complete observer   Researcher who is passive and has no direct social interaction in the setting.

Complete participation   Situation in which the researcher becomes a member of the group and conceals the researcher role.

Complete review   The review process for studies with risks that are greater than minimal.

Complex hypothesis   Hypothesis that predicts the relationship (associative or causal) among three or more variables; thus, the hypothesis can include two (or more) independent and/or two (or more) dependent variables.

Complexity   Degree to which an innovation is perceived to be difficult to understand or use.

Comprehending a research report   Critical thinking process used in reading a research report that involves focusing on understanding the major concepts and the logical flow of ideas within a study.

Comprehension phase   Step of a critique during which the reader gains understanding of the terms in a research report; identifies the study elements; and grasps the nature, significance, and meaning of these elements.

Computer search   A function conducted to scan the citations in different databases and identify sources relevant to a selected topic.

Computerized database   A structured compilation of information that can be scanned, retrieved, and analyzed by computer and can be used for decisions, reports, and research.

Concept   Term that abstractly describes and names an object or phenomenon, thus providing it with a separate identity or meaning.

Concept analysis   Strategy through which a set of attributes or characteristics essential to the connotative meaning or conceptual definition of a concept is identified.

Concept derivation   Process of extracting and defining concepts from theories in other disciplines.

Concept synthesis   Process of describing and naming a previously unrecognized concept.

Conceptual clustering step of critique   Step in which current knowledge in an area of study is carefully analyzed, summarized, and organized theoretically to maximize the meaning attached to research findings, highlight gaps in the knowledge base, generate research questions, and provide knowledge for use in practice.

Conceptual definition   Definition that provides a variable or concept with connotative (abstract, comprehensive, theoretical) meaning; established through concept analysis, concept derivation, or concept synthesis.

Conceptual map   Strategy for expressing a framework of a study that diagrammatically shows the interrelationships of concepts and statements.

Conceptual model   A set of highly abstract, related constructs that broadly explains phenomena of interest, expresses assumptions, and reflects a philosophical stance.

Conclusion   Synthesis and clarification of the meaning of study findings.

Concrete thinking   Thinking that is oriented to and limited by tangible things or events observed and experienced in reality.

Concurrent relationship   Relationship in which variables or concepts occur simultaneously.

Concurrent replication   Internal replication that involves the collection of data for the original study and its replication simultaneously to provide a check of the reliability of the original study findings.

Confidence interval   Range in which the value of the parameter is estimated to exist.

Confidentiality   Management of private data in research in such a way that subjects' identities are not linked with their responses.

Confirmation stage   Stage in Rogers's theory of research utilization in which nurses evaluate the effectiveness of the change in practice and decide to either continue or discontinue the change.

Confirmatory analysis   Analysis performed to confirm expectations regarding data that are expressed as hypotheses, questions, or objectives.

Confounding variables   Variables recognized before the study is initiated but cannot be controlled, or variables not recognized until the study is in process.

Consent form   Written form, tape recording, or videotape used to document a subject's agreement to participate in a study.

Constant comparison   A methodological technique in grounded theory research in which every piece of data is compared with every other piece.

Construct validity   Process with which the researcher examines the fit between conceptual and operational definitions of variables and determines whether the instrument actually measures the theoretical construct it purports to measure.

Constructs   Concepts at very high levels of abstraction that have general meanings.

Consultants   People hired for specific tasks during a study.

Content analysis   Qualitative analysis technique used to classify words in a text into a few categories chosen because of their theoretical importance.

Content-related validity   Examines the extent to which the method of measurement includes all the major elements relevant to the construct being measured.

Contingency tables   Cross-tabulation tables that allow visual comparison of summary data output related to two variables within a sample.

Contingent relationship   Relationship that occurs only when a third variable or concept is present.

Continuance   Decision to continue the use of an innovation and include the protocol in the procedure manual.

Control   Imposing of rules by the researcher to decrease the possibility of error and increase the probability that the study's findings are an accurate reflection of reality.

Control group   The group of elements or subjects not exposed to the experimental treatment.

Convenience sampling   Including subjects in the study because they happened to be in the right place at the right time; entering available subjects into the study until the desired sample size is reached.

Correlational analysis   Statistical procedure conducted to determine the direction (positive or negative) and magnitude or strength ($+1$ to -1) of the relationship between two variables.

Correlational coefficient   Statistical term used to indicate the degree of relationship between two variables; the coefficients range in value from $+1.00$ (perfect positive relationship) to 0.00 (no relationship) to -1.00 (perfect negative or inverse relationship).

Correlational research   Systematic investigation of relationships between two or more variables to explain the nature of relationships in the world, not to examine cause and effect.

Covert data collection   Data collection that occurs without subjects' knowledge or awareness.

Cramer's V   Analysis technique for nominal data; a modification of phi for contingency tables.

Criterion-referenced testing   Comparison of a subject's score with a criterion of achievement that includes the definitions of target behaviors. When the behaviors are mastered, the subject is considered proficient in these behaviors.

Critical analysis of studies   Examination of the strengths, weaknesses, meaning, and significance of nursing studies using four steps: comprehension, comparison, analysis, and evaluation.

Critique   Careful examination of all aspects of a study to judge its strengths, limitations, meaning, and significance.

Cross-sectional designs   Designs used to examine groups of subjects in various stages of development simultaneously, with the intent of inferring trends over time.

Cultural immersion   Strategy used in ethnographic research for gaining increased familiarity with aspects of a culture such as language, sociocultural norms, and traditions.

Culture   A way of life belonging to a designated group of people.

Curvilinear relationship   Relationship between two variables that varies depending on the relative values of the variables.

Data   Pieces of information that are collected during a study.

Data analysis   Techniques used to reduce, organize, and give meaning to data.

Data coding sheet   A sheet for organizing and recording data for rapid entry into a computer.

Data collection   Identification of subjects and the precise, systematic gathering of information (data) relevant to the research purpose or the specific objectives, questions, or hypotheses of a study.

Data storage and retrieval   The computer's ability to store vast amounts of data and rapidly retrieve these data for examination and analyses.

Data triangulation   Collection of data from multiple sources in the same study.

Database   See Computerized database.

Debriefing   Complete disclosure of the study purpose and results at the end of a study.

Debugging   Identifying and replacing errors in a computer program with accurate information.

Decentralized diffusion system   System involving one-to-one communication and individual decisions regarding the use of research-based innovations.

Deception   Misinforming subjects for research purposes. After a study is completed, subjects must be informed of the true purpose and outcomes of a study so that areas of deception are clarified.

Decision stage   Stage in Rogers's theory of research utilization in which nurse(s) either adopt(s) or reject(s) an innovation or change in practice.

Decision theory   Theory based on assumptions associated with the theoretical normal curve; used in testing for differences between groups, with the expectation that all of the groups are members of the same population. The expectation is expressed as a null hypothesis, and the level of significance (alpha) is set prior to data collection.

Decision trail   See Auditability.

Declaration of Helsinki   Ethical code based on the Nuremberg Code that differentiated therapeutic from nontherapeutic research.

Deductive reasoning   Reasoning from the general to the specific or from a general premise to a particular situation.

Degrees of freedom (df)   The freedom of a score's value to vary given the other existing scores' values and the established sum of these scores ($df = N - 1$).

Delphi technique   Method of measuring the judgments of a group of experts for assessing priorities or making forecasts.

Demographic variables   Characteristics or attributes of subjects that are collected to describe the sample.

Dependent groups   Subjects or observations selected for data collection that are in some way related to the selection of other subjects or observations. For example, when subjects in the control group are matched for age or gender with the subjects in the experimental group, these groups are dependent groups.

Dependent variable   The response, behavior, or outcome that is predicted or explained in research; changes in the dependent variable are presumed to be caused by the independent variable.

Description Identification of the characteristics of nursing phenomena and sometimes the relationships among these phenomena.

Descriptive codes Terms used to organize and classify qualitative data.

Descriptive correlational design Design used to describe variables and examine relationships that exist in a situation.

Descriptive design Design used to identify a phenomenon of interest, identify variables within the phenomenon, develop conceptual and operational definitions of variables, and describe variables.

Descriptive research Research that provides an accurate portrayal or account of characteristics of a particular individual, event, or group in real-life situations for the purpose of discovering new meaning, describing what exists, determining the frequency with which something occurs, and categorizing information.

Descriptive statistics Statistics that allow the researcher to organize the data in ways that give meaning and facilitate insight, such as frequency distributions and measures of central tendency and dispersion.

Descriptive vividness Description of the site, subjects, experience of collecting data, and the researcher's thoughts during the qualitative research process presented clearly enough that the reader has the sense of personally experiencing the event.

Design Blueprint for conducting a study; maximizes control over factors that could interfere with the validity of the findings.

Design validity Quality of the study design and the ability of the design to generate accurate findings. Types of design validity include statistical conclusion validity, internal validity, construct validity, and external validity.

Deterministic relationships Statements of what always occurs in a particular situation, such as a scientific law.

Developmental grant proposals Proposals written to obtain funding for the development of a new program in a discipline.

Dialectic reasoning Reasoning that involves a holistic perspective, in which the whole is greater than the sum of the parts; examining factors that are opposites and making sense of them by merging them into a single unit or idea greater than either alone.

Diary Record of events kept by a subject over time that is collected and analyzed by a researcher.

Difference scores Deviation scores obtained by subtracting the mean from each raw score; measure of dispersion.

Diffusion Process of communicating research findings (innovations) through certain channels over time among the members of a discipline.

Diminished autonomy Condition of subjects whose ability to give informed consent voluntarily is decreased because of legal or mental incompetence, terminal illness, or confinement to an institution.

Direct application   The use of an innovation exactly as it was developed.

Direct measure   A concrete variable that can be measured objectively with a specific measurement strategy, such as using a scale to measure weight.

Directional hypothesis   Hypothesis stating the specific nature of the interaction or relationship between two or more variables.

Discomfort and harm from a study   Phrase used to describe the degree of risk for a subject participating in a study. These levels of risk include no anticipated effects, temporary discomfort, unusual levels of temporary discomfort, risk of permanent damage, or certainty of permanent damage.

Discontinuance   Decision to discontinue the use of an innovation.

Discriminant analysis   Analysis that allows the researcher to identify characteristics associated with group membership and to predict group membership.

Disenchantment discontinuance   Decision to discontinue the use of an innovation because the user is dissatisfied with its outcome.

Dissemination of research findings   The diffusion or communication of research findings.

Dissertation   An extensive, usually original research project that is completed by a doctoral student as part of the requirements for a doctoral degree.

Distribution   The spread of scores in a sample; includes the frequency and range of scores in the sample.

Effect size   The degree to which the phenomenon studied is present in the population or to which the null hypothesis is false.

Electronic mail   Computer networking system that allows a user to rapidly exchange messages, files, data, and research reports using satellite networks.

Element   A person (subject), event, behavior, or any other single unit of a study.

Embodied   The belief that the person is a self within a body.

Emic approach   Anthropological research approach to studying behaviors from within a culture.

Empirical generalizations   Statements that have been repeatedly tested through research and have not been disproven (scientific theories have empirical generalizations).

Empirical literature   Relevant studies published in journals and books; also includes unpublished studies such as masters theses and doctorate dissertations.

Empirical world   The world we experience through our senses; the concrete portion of our existence.

Environmental variable   A type of extraneous variable composing the setting in which a study is conducted.

Equivalence   Focuses on comparing measurements made by two or more observers measuring the same event; referred to as interrater reliability.

Error score   Amount of random error in the measurement process.

Ethical inquiry   Intellectual analysis of ethical problems related to obligation, rights, duty, right and wrong, conscience, choice, intention, and responsibility to obtain desirable, rational ends.

Ethical principles   Principles of respect for persons, beneficence, and justice that are relevant to the conduct of research.

Ethnographic research   Qualitative research methodology for investigating cultures that involves collection, description, and analysis of data to develop a theory of cultural behavior.

Ethnonursing research   Type of research that emerged from Leininger's Theory of Transcultural Nursing; focuses mainly on observing and documenting interactions with people to determine how daily life conditions and patterns influence human care, health, and nursing care practices.

Etic approach   Anthropological research approach to studying behavior from outside the culture and examining similarities and differences across cultures.

Evaluation phase   Step of a critique in which the reader examines the meaning and significance of a study according to set criteria and compares it with previous studies conducted in the area.

Event partitioning designs   Merger of the longitudinal and trend designs to increase sample size and avoid the effects of history on the validity of findings.

Event-time matrix   Qualitative analysis technique that can facilitate comparisons of the events occurring in different sites during particular time periods.

Exact replication   Precise or exact duplication of the initial researcher's study to confirm the original findings.

Exempt from review   Designation given to studies that have no apparent risks for the research subjects and thus do not require institutional review.

Existence statement   Declaration that a given concept exists or a given relationship occurs.

Expedited review   Review process for studies that have some risks, but the risks are minimal or no greater than those ordinarily encountered in daily life or during the performance of routine physical or psychological examinations.

Experimental designs   Designs that provide the greatest amount of control possible in order to examine causality more closely.

Experimental group   The group of subjects receiving the experimental treatment.

Experimental research   Objective, systematic, controlled investigation to examine probability and causality among selected variables for the purpose of predicting and controlling phenomena.

Explanation   Clarification of relationships among variables and identification of reasons why certain events occur.

Explanatory codes   Codes that are developed late in the data collection process after theoretical ideas from the qualitative study have begun to emerge.

Explanatory effects matrix   Qualitative analysis technique that can assist in answering questions such as why an outcome was achieved or what caused the outcome.

Exploratory analysis   Examining the data descriptively so as to become as familiar as possible with the data.

External criticism   Method for determining the validity of source materials in historical research; involves knowing where, when, why, and by whom a document was written.

External storage device   Mechanism for permanently storing data and programs outside a computer.

External validity   Extent to which study findings can be generalized beyond the sample used in the study.

Extraneous variables   Variables that exist in all studies and can affect the measurement of study variables and the relationships among these variables.

Face validity   Verification that the instrument appeared to measure the content desired.

Factor analysis   Analysis that examines interrelationships among large numbers of variables and disentangles those relationships to identify clusters of variables that are most closely linked. Two types of factor analysis are exploratory and confirmatory.

Factorial analysis of variance   Analysis technique that is mathematically a specialized version of multiple regression; various types of factorial ANOVAs have been developed to analyze data from specific experimental designs.

Fatigue effect   Effect that occurs when a subject becomes tired or bored with a study.

Feasibility of a study   A study's suitability; determined by examining the time and money commitment; the researcher's expertise; availability of subjects, facility, and equipment; cooperation of others; and the study's ethical considerations.

Findings   The translated and interpreted results from a study.

Foundational inquiry   Research on the foundations for a science, such as studies that provide analyses of the structure of a science and the process of thinking about and valuing certain phenomena held in common by the science. Debates related to quantitative and qualitative research methods emerged from foundational inquiries.

Framework   The abstract, logical structure of meaning that guides the development of the study and enables the researcher to link the findings to nursing's body of knowledge.

Fraudulent publications   Publications that do not reflect what was actually done; indicated by documentation or testimony from coauthors.

Frequency distribution   Statistical procedure that involves listing all possible measures of a variable and tallying each datum on the listing.

Friedman two-way analysis of variance by ranks   Nonparametric test used with matched samples or in repeated measures.

Generalization   Extension of the implications of the findings from the sample that was studied to the larger population or from the situation studied to a larger situation.

Gestalt   Organization of knowledge about a particular phenomenon into a cluster of linked ideas; the clustering and interrelatedness enhance the meaning of the ideas.

Grant   Proposal developed to seek research funding from private or public institutions.

Grounded   A theory that has its roots in the qualitative data from which it was derived.

Grounded theory research   Inductive research technique based on symbolic interaction theory; conducted to discover the problems that exist in a social scene and the process that persons involved use to handle them; involves formulation, testing, and redevelopment of propositions until a theory is developed.

Grouped frequency distribution   A means of grouping continuous measures of data into categories.

Hardware, computer   Machinery or physical equipment of the computer, including the input device, central processing unit, output device, and external storage device.

Hawthorne effect   Psychological response in which subjects change their behavior simply because they are subjects in a study, not because of the research treatment.

Heterogeneity   Degree to which subjects have a wide variety of characteristics, thus reducing the risk of bias in studies not using random sampling.

Heuristic relevance   Standard for evaluating a qualitative study, in which the study's intuitive recognition, relationship to the existing body of knowledge, and applicability are examined.

Hierarchical statement set   A specific proposition and a hypothesis or research question. If a conceptual model is included in the framework, the set may also include a general proposition.

Highly controlled setting   Artificially constructed environment that is developed for the sole purpose of conducting research, such as a laboratory, research or experimental center, or test unit.

Historical research   Narrative description or analysis of events that occurred in the remote or recent past.

History effect   Event that is not related to the planned study but occurs during the time of the study and could influence the responses of subjects to the treatment.

Homogeneity in design   Degree to which objects are similar or share a form of equivalence, such as limiting subjects to only one level of an extraneous variable to reduce its impact on the study findings.

Homogeneity in instruments   The correlation of various items within an instrument that is calculated for paper-and-pencil tests using the Cronbach alpha coefficient.

Homoscedastic   Term describing data that are evenly dispersed above and below the regression line, indicating a linear relationship on a scatter diagram (plot).

Human rights   Claims and demands that have been justified in the eyes of an individual or by the consensus of a group of individuals and are protected in research.

Hypothesis   Formal statement of the expected relationship between two or more variables in a specified population.

Implementation stage   Stage in Rogers's theory of research utilization in which an individual or agency puts to use a research-based change. The types of implementation include direct application, reinvention, and indirect effects.

Implication   The meaning of research conclusions for the body of knowledge, theory, and practice.

Incomplete disclosure   Failure to inform subjects completely about the purpose of a study because that knowledge might alter the subjects' actions; subjects must be debriefed when the study is finished.

Independent groups   Study groups selected such that the selection of one subject is totally unrelated to the selection of other subjects. For example, if subjects are randomly assigned to a treatment group or a control group, the groups are independent.

Independent variable   The treatment or experimental activity that is manipulated or varied by the researcher to create an effect on the dependent variable.

Index   Library resource that provides assistance in identifying journal articles and other publications relevant to a topic.

Indirect effects   Use of research findings by citing them in clinical papers and textbooks and incorporating them to strengthen arguments.

Indirect measure   Method used with abstract concepts when the concepts are not measured directly; rather, indicators or attributes of the concepts are used to represent the abstraction and are measured in the study.

Inductive reasoning   Reasoning from the specific to the general, in which particular instances are observed and then combined into a larger whole or general statement.

Inference   Generalization from a specific case to a general truth, from a part to the whole, from the concrete to the abstract, or from the known to the unknown.

Inferential statistics   Statistics designed to allow inference from a sample statistic to a population parameter; commonly used to test hypotheses of similarities and differences in subsets of the sample under study.

Informed consent   Agreement by a prospective subject to participate voluntarily in a study after he or she has assimilated essential information about the study.

Inherent variability   Variability in which a few random observations can be naturally expected in the data in the extreme ends of the tail.

Innovation   Idea, practice, or object that is perceived as new by an individual, a nursing unit, an entire agency, or another decision-making unit.

Innovation-decision process   Process that includes the steps of knowledge, persuasion, decision, implementation, and confirmation to promote diffusion or communication of research findings to members of a discipline.

Innovators   Individuals who actively seek out new ideas.

Input device   Device that enables the user to enter data and instructions into the computer system.

Institutional review   Process of examining studies for ethical concerns by a committee of peers.

Instrument validity   Extent to which an instrument actually reflects the abstract construct being examined.

Instrumentation   Component of measurement that involves the application of specific rules to develop a measurement device or instrument.

Integrative review of research   Review conducted to identify, analyze, and synthesize the results from independent studies to determine the current knowledge (what is known and not known) in a particular area.

Intellectual research critique   Careful examination of all aspects of a study to judge the strengths, weaknesses, meaning, and significance of the study based on previous research experience and knowledge of the topic.

Interlibrary loan department   Department that locates books and articles in other libraries and provides the sources within a designated time.

Internal computer memory   The part of a computer that stores operating programs and monitors, tracks, and temporarily stores data.

Internal criticism   Criticism involving examination of the reliability of historical documents.

Internal validity   Extent to which the effects detected in a study are a true reflection of reality rather than being the result of the effects of extraneous variables.

Internet   A worldwide network that connects computers together.

Interpretation of research outcomes   Examining the results from data analysis, forming conclusions, considering the implications for nursing, exploring the significance of the findings, generalizing the findings, and suggesting further studies.

Interpretive codes   Organizational system developed late in the qualitative data collection and analysis process as the researcher gains insight into the existing processes.

Interpretive reliability   Extent to which each judge assigns the same category to a given unit of data.

Interrater reliability   Degree of consistency between two raters who are independently assigning ratings to a variable or attribute being investigated; also referred to as equivalence.

Interrupted time series designs   Designs similar to descriptive time designs, except that a treatment is applied at some point in the observations.

Interval estimate   Range of values (identified by the researcher) on a number line where the population parameter is thought to be.

Interval-scale measurement   Use of interval scales or methods of measurement with equal numerical distances between intervals of the scale; follows the rules of mutually exclusive categories, exhaustive categories, and rank ordering, such as temperature.

Interview Structured or unstructured oral communication between the researcher and subject, during which information is obtained for a study.

Introspection Process of turning one's attention inward toward one's own thoughts, providing increased awareness and understanding of the flow and interplay of feelings and ideas.

Intuiting Process of actually looking at the phenomenon in qualitative research; all awareness and energy are focused on the subject of interest.

Intuition Insight or understanding of a situation or an event as a whole that usually cannot be logically explained.

Intuitive recognition Theoretical schema derived from the data of a qualitative study that has meaning within an individual's personal knowledge base.

Invasion of privacy Sharing private information with others without an individual's knowledge or against his or her will.

Investigator triangulation Phenomenon that occurs when two or more research-trained investigators with divergent backgrounds explore the same phenomenon.

Iterative operations Series of fixed functions performed numerous times by the computer.

Justice, principle of Principle stating that human subjects should be treated fairly.

Kendall's tau Nonparametric test used to determine correlations among variables that have been measured at the ordinal level.

Knowledge Information that is acquired in a variety of ways, is expected to be an accurate reflection of reality, and is incorporated and used to direct a person's actions.

Knowledge stage Stage of Rogers's theory of research utilization in which nurses become aware of the existence of an innovation or new idea for use in practice.

Kolmogorov-Smirnov two-sample test Nonparametric test used to determine whether two independent samples have been drawn from the same population.

Kurtosis Degree of peakedness (platykurtic, mesokurtic, or leptokurtic) of the curve that is related to the spread or variance of scores.

Lambda Analysis technique that measures the degree of association (or relationship) between two nominal-level variables.

Landmark study Major project generating knowledge that influences a discipline and sometimes society in general.

Level of significance See Alpha.

Levels of measurement Organized set of rules for assigning numbers to objects so that a hierarchy in measurement from low to high is established. The levels of measurement are nominal, ordinal, interval, and ratio.

Library resources Library personnel, interlibrary loan department, circulation department, reference department, audiovisual department, computer search department, and photocopy services.

Library sources Sources for research, including journals, books, monographs, master's theses, dissertations, government documents, and other publications of research findings.

Likert scale   Instrument designed to determine the opinion on or attitude toward a subject; contains a number of declarative statements with a scale after each statement.

Limitations   Theoretical and methodological restrictions in a study that may decrease the generalizability of the findings.

Linear relationship   Relationship between two variables or concepts that remain consistent regardless of the values of each variable or concept.

Literature review   Summary of theoretical and empirical sources to generate a picture of what is known and not known about a particular problem.

Logic   A science that involves valid ways of relating ideas to promote human understanding; includes abstract and concrete thinking and logistic, inductive, and deductive reasoning.

Logistic reasoning   Reasoning used to break the whole into parts that can be carefully examined, as can the relationships among the parts.

Longitudinal designs   Designs used to examine changes in the same subjects over an extended period.

Mainframe computer   Computer with the largest memory and greatest speed; used in universities and large companies.

Manipulation   Moving around or controlling the movement of, as in the manipulation of a treatment.

Mann-Whitney U test   Test used to analyze ordinal data (with 95% of the power of the t-test) to detect differences between groups of normally distributed populations.

Manual search   Examination of catalogs, indexes, abstracts, and bibliographies for relevant sources.

Map   See Conceptual map.

Matching   Selecting subjects in the control group who are equivalent to subjects in the experimental group in relation to important extraneous variables.

Maturation effect   Unplanned and unrecognized changes subjects experience during a study, such as growing older, wiser, stronger, hungrier, or more tired, that can influence the findings of the study.

McNemar test   Nonparametric test used to analyze the changes that occur in dichotomous variables.

Mean   The value obtained by summing all the scores and dividing the total by the number of scores being summed.

Measurement   Process of assigning numbers to objects, events, or situations in accord with some rule.

Measurement error   Difference between what exists in reality and what is measured by a research instrument.

Measures of central tendency   Statistical procedures (mode, median, and mean) for determining the center of a distribution of scores.

Measures of dispersion   Statistical procedures (range, difference scores, sum of squares, variance, and standard deviation) for examining how scores vary or are dispersed around the mean.

Median The score at the exact center of the ungrouped frequency distribution.

Memoing A way of recording insights or ideas related to notes, transcripts, or codes during qualitative data analysis that is developed by the researcher.

Mentor An individual who provides information, advice, and emotional support to a protégé.

Mentorship Intense form of role-modeling in which an expert nurse serves as a teacher, sponsor, guide, exemplar, and counselor for the novice nurse.

Meta-analysis Merging of findings from several studies to determine what is known about a particular phenomenon.

Methodological congruence Standard for evaluating qualitative research, in which documentation rigor, procedural rigor, ethical rigor, and auditability of the study are examined.

Methodological designs Designs used to develop the validity and reliability of instruments to measure research concepts and variables.

Methodological limitations Restrictions in the study design that limit the credibility of the findings and the population to which the findings can be generalized.

Methodological triangulation The use of two or more research methods or procedures in a study (such as different designs, instruments, and data collection procedures).

Microcomputer Personal computer that fits on a person's lap or desktop and is usually used by one individual.

Minicomputer Computer of intermediate size, memory capabilities, and speed.

Minimal risk Risk of harm anticipated in the proposed research that is not greater, considering probability and magnitude, than that ordinarily encountered in daily life or during the performance of routine physical or psychological examinations.

Modal percentage Percentage appropriate for nominal data; indicates the relationship of the number of data scores represented by the mode to the total number of data scores.

Modality Characteristic of distributions; symmetrical distributions are usually unimodal.

Mode Numerical value or score that occurs with the greatest frequency in a distribution but does not necessarily indicate the center of the data set.

Model testing designs Designs used to test the accuracy of a hypothesized causal model or map.

Monographs Sources that are usually written once, such as books, booklets of conference proceedings, or pamphlets, and may be updated with a new edition.

Mono-method bias Bias that occurs when more than one measure of a variable is used in a study, but all measures use the same method of recording.

Mono-operation bias Bias that occurs when only one method of measurement is used to measure a construct.

Mortality   Subjects dropping out of a study before completion, creating a threat to the internal validity of the study.

Multicausality   Recognition that a number of interrelating variables can be involved in causing a particular effect.

Multicollinearity   Phenomenon that occurs when the independent variables in a regression equation are strongly correlated.

Multimethod-multitrait technique   Technique involving the use of a variety of data collection methods, such as interview and observation; the same measurement methods are used for each concept.

Multiple regression   Extension of simple linear regression, with more than one independent variable entered into the analysis.

Multiple triangulation   The use of two or more types of triangulation (theoretical, data, methodological, investigator, and analysis) in a study.

Multivariate analysis techniques   Techniques used to analyze data from complex, multivariate research projects; they include multiple regression, factorial analysis of variance, analysis of covariance, factor analysis, discriminant analysis, canonical correlation, structural equation modeling, time series analysis, and survival analysis.

Natural setting   Field setting or uncontrolled, real-life situation examined in research.

Necessary relationship   Relationship in which one variable or concept must occur for the second variable or concept to occur.

Negative linear relationship   Relationship in which one variable or concept changes (its value increases or decreases), and the other variable or concept changes in the opposite direction.

Network sampling   Snowballing technique that takes advantage of social networks and the fact that friends tend to have characteristics in common; subjects meeting the sample criteria are asked to assist in locating others with similar characteristics.

Networking   Process of developing channels of communication among people with common interests.

Nominal-scale measurement   Lowest level of measurement used when data can be organized into categories that are exclusive and exhaustive, but the categories cannot be compared, such as gender, race, marital status, and nursing diagnoses.

Nondirectional hypothesis   Hypothesis that states that a relationship exists but does not predict the exact nature of the relationship.

Nonequivalent control group designs   Designs in which the control group is not selected by random means, such as the one-group posttest-only design, the posttest-only design with nonequivalent groups, and the one-group pretest-posttest design.

Nonparametric statistics   Statistical techniques used when the assumptions of parametric statistics are not met; most commonly used to analyze nominal and ordinal data.

Nonprobability sampling   Sampling in which not every element of the population has an opportunity for selection, such as convenience sampling, quota sampling, purposive sampling, and network sampling.

Nonsignificant results   Negative results or results contrary to the researcher's hypotheses that can be an accurate reflection of reality or can be caused by study weaknesses.

Nontherapeutic research   Research conducted to generate knowledge for a discipline; the results might benefit future patients but will probably not benefit the research subjects.

Norm-referenced   Term describing test performance standards that have been carefully developed over years with large, representative samples, using standardized tests with extensive reliability and validity.

Normal curve   Symmetrical, unimodal, bell-shaped curve that is a theoretical distribution of all possible scores; no real distribution exactly fits the normal curve.

Null hypothesis   Hypothesis stating that no relationship exists between the variables being studied; a statistical hypothesis used for statistical testing and for interpreting statistical outcomes.

Nuremberg code   Ethical code of conduct to guide investigators in conducting research ethically.

Nursing process   Subset of the problem-solving process. Steps include assessment, diagnosis, plan, implementation, evaluation, and modification.

Nursing research   Scientific process that validates and refines existing knowledge and generates new knowledge that directly and indirectly influences clinical nursing practice.

Observability   Extent to which the results of an innovation are visible to others.

Observational measurement   Use of structured and unstructured observation to measure study variables.

Observed score   Actual score or value obtained for a subject on a measurement tool.

Observer-as-participant   Researcher whose time is spent observing and interviewing subjects, with less time spent in the participant role.

One-tailed test of significance   Analysis used with directional hypotheses, in which extreme statistical values of interest are thought to occur in a single tail of the curve.

Open context   Condition that requires deconstructing a sedimented view, allowing one to see the depth and complexity within the phenomenon being examined in qualitative research.

Operational definition   Description of how variables or concepts will be measured or manipulated in a study.

Operational reasoning   Identification and discrimination of many alternatives or viewpoints; focuses on the process of debating alternatives.

Ordinal-scale measurement   Measurement yielding data that can be ranked, but the intervals between the ranked data are not necessarily equal, such as levels of coping.

Outcomes research.   Important scientific methodology that was developed to examine the end results of patient care. The strategies used in outcomes research are a departure from the traditional scientific endeavors and incorporate evaluation research, epidemiology, and economic theory perspectives.

Outliers   Extreme scores or values that occur because of inherent variability, measurement error, execution error, or error in identifying the variables important in explaining the nature of the phenomenon under study.

Output devices   Devices used to display, print, or store information generated from a computer.

Parallel forms reliability   See Alternate forms reliability.

Parameter   Measure or numerical value of a population.

Parametric statistical analyses   Statistical techniques used when three assumptions are met: (1) the sample was drawn from a population for which the variance can be calculated, and the distribution is expected to be normal or approximately normal; (2) the level of measurement should be interval, with an approximately normal distribution; and (3) the data can be treated as random samples.

Paraphrase   Express clearly and concisely the ideas of an author in your own words.

Partially controlled setting   Environment that is manipulated or modified in some way by the researcher.

Participant observation   Special form of observation in which researchers immerse themselves in the setting so that they can hear, see, and experience the reality as the participants do; the participants are aware of the dual role of the researcher (participant and observer).

Passive rejection   Decision not to adopt an innovation that was never seriously considered.

Pearson's product-moment correlation   Parametric test used to determine relationships among variables.

Periodicals   Sources that are published over time and are numbered sequentially for the years published, such as journals.

Personal experience   Gaining knowledge by being personally involved in an event, situation, or circumstance. Benner (1984) described five levels of experience in the development of clinical knowledge and expertise: (1) novice, (2) advanced beginner, (3) competent, (4) proficient, and (5) expert.

Persuasion stage   Stage of Rogers's theory of research utilization in which an individual or agency develops a favorable or unfavorable attitude toward the change or innovation to be used in practice.

Phenomenological research   Inductive, descriptive qualitative methodology developed from phenomenological philosophy for the purpose of describing experiences as they are lived by the study participants.

Phi coefficient   Analysis technique used to determine relationships in dichotomous, nominal data.

Philosophical analysis   Use of concept or linguistic analyses to examine meaning and develop theories of meaning in philosophical inquiry.

Philosophical inquiry Research using intellectual analyses to clarify meanings, make values manifest, identify ethics, and study the nature of knowledge. Types of philosophical inquiry include foundational inquiry, philosophical analyses, and ethical analyses.

Physiologic measurement Techniques used to measure physiologic variables either directly or indirectly, such as techniques to measure heart rate or mean arterial pressure.

Pilot study Smaller version of a proposed study conducted to develop and/or refine the methodology, such as the treatment, instruments, or data collection process to be used in the larger study.

Pink sheet Letter rejecting a research grant proposal, with a critique by the scientific committee that reviewed the proposal.

Point estimate Single figure that estimates a related figure in the population of interest.

Population All elements (individuals, objects, events, or substances) that meet the sample criteria for inclusion in a study; sometimes referred to as a target population.

Positive linear relationship Relationship in which one variable changes (its value increases or decreases) and the second variable changes in the same direction.

Poster session Visual presentation of a study, with tables and illustrations on a display board.

Post-hoc analyses Statistical techniques performed in studies with more than two groups, in which the analysis indicates that the groups are significantly different but does not identify which groups are different.

Power Probability that a statistical test will detect a significant difference that exists; power analysis is used to determine the power of a study.

Power analysis Technique used to determine the risk of a Type II error so that the study can be modified to decrease the risk if necessary.

Practice effect Effect that occurs when subjects improve as they become more familiar with the experimental protocol.

Precision Accuracy with which the population parameters have been estimated within a study; also used to describe the degree of consistency or reproducibility of measurements with physiologic instruments.

Prediction Ability to estimate the probability of a specific outcome in a given situation that can be achieved through research.

Prediction equation Outcome of regression analysis.

Predictive correlational design Design developed to predict the value of one variable based on values obtained for other variables; an approach to examining causal relationships between variables.

Premise Statement of the proposed relationship between two or more concepts.

Preproposal Short document (four pages plus appendices) written to explore the funding possibilities for a research project.

Primary source Source whose author originated or is responsible for generating the ideas published.

Principal investigator   Individual who will have primary responsibility for administering a research grant and interacting with the funding agency.

Privacy   Freedom of an individual to determine the time, extent, and general circumstances under which private information will be shared with or withheld from others.

Probability   Addresses the relative rather than the absolute causality and is the chance that a given event will occur in a situation.

Probability sampling   Random sampling technique in which every member (element) of the population has a probability higher than zero of being selected for the sample; examples include simple random sampling, stratified random sampling, cluster sampling, and systematic sampling.

Probability statement   Statement expressing the likelihood that something will happen in a given situation; addresses relative rather than absolute causality.

Probability theory   Theory addressing statistical analysis from the perspective of the extent of a relationship or the probability of accurately predicting an event.

Problematic reasoning   Reasoning that involves identifying a problem, selecting solutions to the problem, and resolving the problem.

Problem-solving process   Systematic identification of a problem, determination of goals related to the problem, identification of possible approaches to achieve those goals, implementation of selected approaches, and evaluation of goal achievement.

Process   Purpose, series of actions, and goal.

Process-outcome matrix   Qualitative analysis technique that allows the researcher to trace the processes that led to differing outcomes.

Projective techniques   Techniques for measuring individuals' responses to unstructured or ambiguous situations as a means of describing attitudes, personality characteristics, and motives of the individuals (e.g., the Rorschach inkblot test).

Proposition   Abstract statement that further clarifies the relationship between two concepts.

Public library   Library that serves the needs of the community in which it is located; usually contains few research reports.

Purposive sampling   Judgmental sampling that involves the conscious selection by the researcher of certain subjects or elements to include in a study.

Q-plots   Exploratory data analysis technique in which the scores or data are displayed in a distribution by quartile.

Q-sort   Technique for comparative rating, in which a subject sorts cards with statements into designated piles (usually 7 to 10 piles in the distribution of a normal curve) that might range from best to worst.

Qualitative research   Systematic, subjective approach used to describe life experiences and give them meaning.

Quantitative research   Formal, objective, systematic process used to describe, test relationships, and examine cause-and-effect interactions among variables.

Quantitative research process Conceptualizing planning, implementing, and communicating the findings of a research project.

Quasi-experimental research Type of quantitative research conducted to explain relationships, clarify why certain events happen, and examine causality between selected independent and dependent variables.

Query letter Letter sent to an editor of a journal to determine interest in publishing an article or to a funding agency to determine interest in providing funds for a study.

Questionnaire Printed self-report form designed to elicit information that can be obtained through written or verbal responses of the subject.

Quota sampling Convenience sampling technique with an added strategy to ensure the inclusion of subjects who are likely to be underrepresented in the convenience sample, such as women, minority groups, and undereducated persons.

Random assignment Procedure used to assign subjects randomly to treatment or control groups; subjects have an equal opportunity to be assigned to either group.

Random error Error that causes individuals' observed scores to vary haphazardly around their true scores.

Random sampling Technique in which every member (element) of the population has a probability higher than zero for being selected for a sample.

Random variation The expected difference in values that occurs when one examines different subjects from the same sample.

Range Simplest measure of dispersion; obtained by subtracting the lowest score from the highest score.

Rating scale Scale that lists an ordered series of categories of a variable and is assumed to be based on an underlying continuum.

Ratio-scale measurement Highest measurement form; meets all the rules of other forms of measure: mutually exclusive categories, exhaustive categories, rank ordering, equal spacing between intervals, and a continuum of values and has an absolute zero, such as weight.

Reading research reports Involves skills of skimming, comprehending, and analyzing the content of the report.

Reasoning Processing and organizing ideas in order to reach conclusions; types of reasoning include problematic, operational, dialectic, and logistic.

Refereed journal Journal that uses referees or expert reviewers to determine whether a manuscript will be accepted for publication.

Referencing Comparing a subject's score against a standard; used in norm-referenced and criterion-referenced testing.

Reflexive thought A process in which a qualitative researcher explores personal feelings and experiences that may influence the study and integrates this understanding into the study.

Regression analysis Statistical procedure used to predict the value of one variable using known values of one or more other variables.

Regression line The line that best represents the values of the raw scores plotted on a scatter diagram; the procedure for developing the line of best fit is the method of least squares.

Reinvention   Modification of an innovation by its adopters to meet their own needs.

Rejection   Decision not to use an innovation; can be active or passive. See Active rejection, Passive rejection.

Relational statement   Declaration that a relationship of some kind exists between two or more concepts.

Relative advantage   Extent to which an innovation is perceived to be better than current practice.

Relevant literature   Sources that are pertinent or highly important in providing the in-depth knowledge needed to make changes in practice or to study a selected problem.

Reliability   Extent to which an instrument consistently measures the concept of interest; three types of reliability are stability, equivalence, and homogeneity.

Reliability testing   Measure of the amount of random error in the measurement technique.

Replacement discontinuance   Decision to discontinue the use of an innovation in order to adopt a better idea.

Replication study   Reproducing or repeating a study to determine whether similar findings will be obtained.

Representative sample   Sample that is like the population in as many ways as possible.

Representativeness   The sample, accessible population, and target population being alike in as many ways as possible.

Research   Diligent, systematic inquiry or investigation to validate and refine existing knowledge and generate new knowledge.

Research-based protocol   Document providing clearly developed steps for implementing a treatment or intervention in practice that is based on findings from studies.

Research design   Blueprint for conducting a study; maximizes control over factors that could interfere with the validity of the findings; guides the planning and implementation of a study in a way that is most likely to achieve the intended goal.

Research hypothesis   Alternative hypothesis to the null hypothesis; states that a relationship exists between two or more variables.

Research objective   Clear, concise, declarative statement expressed to direct a study; focuses on identification and description of variables and/or determination of the relationships among variables.

Research outcomes   Conclusions or findings, generalization of findings, implications of findings for nursing, and suggestions for further study presented in the discussion section of the research report.

Research problem   Situation in need of solution, improvement, or alteration or a discrepancy between the way things are and the way they ought to be.

Research process   Process that requires an understanding of a unique language and involves rigorous application of a variety of research methods.

Research proposal   Written plan identifying the major elements of a study (such as the problem, purpose, and framework) and outlining the methods that will be used to conduct the study.

Research purpose   Concise, clear statement of the specific goal or aim of the study that is generated from the problem.

Research question   Concise interrogative statement developed to direct a study; focuses on description of variables, examination of relationships among variables, and determination of differences between two or more groups.

Research report   Report summarizing the major elements of a study and identifying the contributions of that study to nursing knowledge.

Research topic   Concept or broad problem area that provides the basis for generating numerous questions and research problems.

Research utilization   Process by which research knowledge is communicated to members of a social system to achieve a desired outcome.

Research variables or concepts   The qualities, properties, or characteristics identified in the research purpose and objectives that are observed or measured in a study.

Researcher-participant relationships   Relationships between the researcher and the individuals being studied in qualitative research.

Respect for persons, principle of   Principle indicating that persons have the right to self-determination and the freedom to participate or not participate in research.

Results   Outcomes from data analysis that are generated for each research objective, question, or hypothesis; results can be mixed, nonsignificant, significant and not predicted, significant and predicted, or unexpected.

Review of literature   Summary of current theoretical and empirical sources to generate a picture of what is known and not known about a particular problem.

Review of relevant research literature   Review of current studies conducted to generate what is known and not known about a problem and to determine whether the knowledge is ready for use in practice.

Rigor   Striving for excellence in research through the use of discipline, scrupulous adherence to detail, and strict accuracy.

Robust   Term describing an analysis procedure that will yield accurate results even if some of the assumptions are violated by the data being analyzed.

Rogers's Theory of Research Utilization   Theory to direct the use of research findings in practice that includes the stages of knowledge, persuasion, decision, implementation, and confirmation.

Role-modeling   Learning by imitating the behaviors of an exemplar or role model.

Sample   Subset of the population that is selected for a study.

Sample characteristics   Demographic data analyzed to provide a picture of the sample.

Sample size   The number of subjects, events, behaviors, or situations that are examined in a study.

Sampling   The process of selecting a group of people, events, behaviors, or other elements that are representative of the population being studied.

Sampling criteria   List of the characteristics essential for membership in the target population.

Sampling distribution   Table of statistical values (such as the mean) of many samples obtained from the same population.

Sampling error   Difference between a sample statistic used to estimate a parameter and the actual but unknown value of the parameter.

Sampling frame   List of every member of the population; the sampling criteria are used to define membership.

Sampling method   Strategies used to obtain a sample, including probability and nonprobability sampling techniques; also referred to as a sampling plan.

Sampling plan   Process for making selections of subjects for inclusion in a study.

Scale   Self-report form of measurement composed of several items thought to measure the construct being studied; the subject responds to each item on the continuum or scale provided.

Science   Coherent body of knowledge composed of research findings, tested theories, scientific principles, and laws for a discipline.

Scientific community   Cohesive group of scholars within a discipline who stimulate the creation of new research ideas and the development of innovative methodologies to conduct research.

Scientific method   All procedures that scientists have used, currently use, or may use in the future to pursue knowledge; examples include quantitative research, qualitative research, outcomes research, and triangulation.

Scientific misconduct   Practices such as fabrication, falsification, or forging of data; dishonest manipulation of the study design or methods; and plagiarism.

Scientific theory   Theory with valid and reliable methods of measuring each concept and relational statement that have been repeatedly tested through research and demonstrated to be valid.

Secondary analysis design   Design for studying data previously collected in another study; data are reexamined using different organizations of the data and different statistical analyses.

Secondary source   Source whose author summarizes or quotes content from primary sources.

Sedimented view   View from the perspective of a specific frame of reference, worldview, or theory that gives a sense of certainty, security, and control.

Seeking approval to conduct a study   Submitting a research proposal to a selected group for review and often verbally defending that proposal.

Semantic differential scale   Two opposite adjectives with a 7-point scale between them; the subject selects a point on the scale that best describes his or her view of the concept being examined.

Sensitivity of physiologic measures   Amount of change of a parameter that can be measured precisely.

Serendipity   Accidental discovery of something valuable or useful during the conduct of a study.

Setting   Location for conducting research; can be natural, partially controlled, or highly controlled.

Significant results   Results that are in keeping with those identified by the researcher.

Simple hypothesis   Hypothesis stating the relationship (associative or causal) between two variables.

Simple linear regression   Parametric analysis technique that provides a means to estimate the value of a dependent variable based on the value of an independent variable.

Simple random sampling   Random selection of elements from the sampling frame for inclusion in a study.

Situated   The belief that the person is shaped by the language, culture, history, purposes, and values of his or her world and is constrained by that shaping in the ability to establish meanings.

Skewness   Asymmetrical (positively or negatively skewed) curve developed from an asymmetrical distribution of scores.

Skimming research reports   Quickly reviewing a source to gain a broad overview of the content by reading the title, the author's name, the abstract or introduction, headings, one or two sentences under each heading, and the discussion section.

Social system   Set of interrelated individuals (such as the nurses on a specific hospital unit, in one hospital, or in a corporation of hospitals) engaged in joint problem-solving to accomplish a common goal or outcome.

Software, computer   Instructions or programs that direct the operations of the computer hardware.

Special library   Library that contains a collection of material on a specific topic or specialty area.

Split-half reliability   Technique used to determine the homogeneity of an instrument's items, in which the items are split in half and a correlational procedure is performed between the two halves.

Stability   Type of measurement reliability that is concerned with the consistency of repeated measures; usually referred to as test-retest reliability.

Standard deviation   Measure of dispersion that is calculated by taking the square root of the variance.

Standardized scores   Scores used to express deviations from the mean (difference scores) in terms of standard deviation units, such as Z-scores, in which the mean is 0 and the standard deviation is 1.

Statement   Expresses a claim that is important to a theory; theories include existence and relational statements.

Statistic Numerical value obtained from a sample; it is used to estimate the parameters of a population.

Statistical conclusion validity Extent to which the conclusions about relationships and differences drawn from statistical analyses are an accurate reflection of reality.

Statistical regression Movement or regression of extreme scores toward the mean in studies using a pretest-posttest design.

Statistical significance Extent to which the results are probably not due to chance.

Stem-and-leaf displays Type of exploratory data analysis in which scores are visually presented to obtain insights.

Story A time-bound event shared orally with others.

Storytakers People listening to a story.

Storytellers People sharing a story.

Storytelling The process used to share stories.

Stratification Design strategy used to distribute subjects evenly throughout the sample.

Stratified random sampling Technique used when the researcher knows some of the variables in the population that are critical to achieving representativeness; the sample is divided into strata or groups using these identified variables.

Structural equation modeling Analysis technique designed to test theories.

Structured interview Interview in which strategies are used that give the researcher increasing control over the content, such as a questionnaire with structured responses.

Structured observation Clear identification of what is to be observed and precise definition of how the observations are to be made, recorded, and coded.

Subjects Individuals participating in a study (those being studied).

Substantive theory Theory recognized within a discipline as useful for explaining important phenomena.

Substitutable relationship Relationship in which a similar concept can be substituted for the first concept and the second concept will occur.

Sufficient relationship Relationship in which, when the first variable or concept occurs, the second will occur, regardless of the presence or absence of other factors.

Summary statistics See Descriptive statistics.

Survey design Design used to describe a phenomenon by collecting data using questionnaires or personal interviews.

Survival analysis Set of techniques designed to analyze repeated measures from a given time (e.g., beginning of the study, onset of a disease, beginning of a treatment) until a certain attribute (e.g., death, treatment failure, recurrence of the phenomenon) occurs.

Symbolic interaction theory Explores how people define reality and how their beliefs are related to their actions.

Symmetrical relationship Relationship in which, if A occurs or changes, B will occur or change, and if B occurs or changes, A will occur or change (A ⟷ B).

Symmetry plot   Exploratory data analysis technique designed to determine the presence of skewness in the data.

Synthesis of sources   Clustering and interrelating ideas from several sources to form a gestalt or a new, complete picture of what is known and not known in an area.

Systematic bias   Phenomenon that occurs when the selected subjects' measurement values vary in some way from those of the population.

Systematic error   Measurement error that is not random but occurs consistently in the same direction, such as a scale that inaccurately weighs subjects 3 pounds heavier than their actual weight.

Systematic extension replication   Constructive replication performed under distinctly new conditions, in which the researchers conducting the replication do not follow the design or methods of the original researchers; rather, the second investigative team begins with a similar problem statement but formulates new means to verify the first investigator's findings.

Systematic sampling   Selecting every *k*th individual from an ordered list of all members of a population, using a randomly selected starting point.

Systematic variation   See Systematic bias.

Tails   Extremes of the normal curve, on which the significant statistical values fall.

Target population   The population determined by the sampling criteria.

Tendency statement   Deterministic relationship that describes what always happens if there are no interfering conditions.

Tentative theory   Theory that is newly proposed, has had minimal exposure to critique by scholars in the discipline, and has had little testing.

Testable hypothesis   Hypothesis containing variables that are measurable or manipulatable in the real world.

Test-retest reliability   Determination of the stability or consistency of a measurement technique by correlating the scores obtained from repeated measures.

Theoretical connectedness   Theoretical schema developed from a qualitative study; is clearly expressed, logically consistent, reflective of the data, and compatible with nursing's knowledge base.

Theoretical limitations   Weaknesses in the study framework and conceptual and operational definitions that restrict the abstract generalization of the findings.

Theoretical literature   Concept analyses, maps, theories, and conceptual frameworks that support a selected research problem and purpose.

Theoretical triangulation   Use of two or more frameworks or theoretical perspectives in the same study; the hypotheses are developed based on the different theoretical perspectives and are tested using the same data set.

Theory   Integrated set of defined concepts, existence statements, and relational statements that present a view of a phenomenon and can be used to describe, explain, predict, and/or control that phenomenon.

Therapeutic research Research that provides a patient with an opportunity to receive an experimental treatment that might have beneficial results.

Thesis A research project completed by a student as part of the requirements for a master's degree

Time-dimensional designs Designs used to examine the sequence and patterns of change, growth, or trends across time.

Time lag Time span between the generation of new knowledge through research and the use of this knowledge in practice.

Time-series analysis Technique designed to analyze changes in a variable across time and thus uncover patterns in the data.

Traditions Truths or beliefs that are based on customs and past trends.

Trend designs Designs used to examine changes in the general population in relation to a particular phenomenon.

Trial and error Approach with unknown outcomes used in an uncertain situation when other sources of knowledge are unavailable.

Trialability Extent to which the results of an individual or agency allow an idea to be tried out on a limited basis, with the option of returning to previous practices.

Triangulation Use of two or more theories, methods, data sources, investigators, or analysis methods in a study.

True score Score that would be obtained if there were no error in measurement (but there is always some measurement error).

t-Test Parametric analysis technique used to determine significant differences between measures of two samples.

Two-tailed test of significance Analysis technique used for a nondirectional hypothesis when the researcher assumes that an extreme score can occur in either tail of the curve.

Type I error Error that occurs when the researcher concludes that the samples tested are from different populations (a significant difference exists between groups) when, in fact, the samples are from the same population (no significant difference exists between groups); the null hypothesis is rejected when it is true.

Type II error Error that occurs when the researcher concludes that no significant difference exists between the samples examined when, in fact, a difference exists; the null hypothesis is regarded as true when it is false.

Ungrouped frequency distribution A means of identifying and displaying all numerical values obtained for a particular variable from the subjects studied.

Unitizing reliability Extent to which each judge (data collector, coder, researcher) consistently identifies the same units within the data as appropriate for coding.

Unstructured interview Interview that is initiated with a broad question; subjects are usually encouraged to elaborate further on particular dimensions of a topic and often control the content of the interview.

Unstructured observations Spontaneous observation and recording of what is seen; planning is minimal.

Utilization of research findings   The use of knowledge generated through research to guide nursing practice.

Validity   Determination of the extent to which an instrument actually reflects the abstract construct (or concept) being examined.

Variables   Qualities, properties, or characteristics of persons, things, or situations that change or vary and are manipulated or measured in research.

Virus, computer   Program developed to alter and/or destroy information stored in a computer.

Visual analogue scale   A line 100 mm long, with right angle stops at either end, on which subjects are asked to record their response to a study variable.

Voluntary consent   Decision made by a prospective subject, of his or her own volition, without coercion or any undue influence, to participate in a research study.

Wald-Wolfowitz runs test   Nonparametric analysis technique used to determine differences between two populations.

Wilcoxon matched-pairs signed-ranks test   Nonparametric analysis technique used to examine changes that occur in pretest-posttest measures or matched-pairs measures.

World Wide Web (WWW)   An information service for access to the Internet resources by content rather than file names.

Z-Score   Standardized score of the normal curve that is equivalent to the standard deviations of the normal curve.

Using the Internet (or World Wide Web) to Increase Your Understanding of Nursing Research*

Learning about the Internet

The Internet (Web) contains invaluable sources of information to assist you in gaining a better understanding of nursing research. This appendix will provide you with initial guidelines for using the Internet related to nursing research. Access to the Web requires a computer and a modem or connection through a network at the university or job site. If you are inexperienced in using the Internet, the following sources may be helpful to you. Please note that because Web sites may be moved or discontinued, some of these Web "addresses" may have worked at the time our text was written but not work when you try to access them. The Internet sources included in this appendix are only a sample of what is available.

> Learning About the Internet
> University of Chicago
> **http://www.uchicago.edu/inet/about.html**
>
> Beginners Luck: Helpful Resources for Internet Novices
> **http://www.execpc.com/~wmhogg/beginner.html**

Searching for Information in the Internet

The Internet is chaotic. The content within it is unorganized and constantly changing. "Search engines" have been designed to locate information for you on a particular topic. Each search engine is unique, and some are more complete in the information they gather on a topic than others. The methods used to conduct a search vary from one search engine to another. Each search engine provides instructions for how to conduct a search using the engine. Search engines continue to evolve. Using a search engine, you could, for example, search for information related to pediatric nursing research, power analysis, or

---

*Although used synonymously in this appendix, the terms "Internet" and "World Wide Web" do not technically refer to the same thing. The World Wide Web is a part of the Internet. Simplistically, one can think of the Web as the sum total of web sites and web pages, whereas on the Internet one can also send and receive electronic messages ("e-mail"), transfer files, participate in discussion groups or "chat rooms," and register for "listservs." From a technical standpoint, these latter applications are not part of the Web, though they can be accessed through software programs called "web browsers."

coping measures. Sometimes, the results of a search will yield thousands of sites. Most search engines rank the sites and list those first that are closest to the search terms used. However, sometimes it is necessary to narrow the search to limit the number of sites identified. Search engines are not yet effective in searching the entire Web. Therefore, a search using one engine may yield very little information. Conducting the same search using another engine may provide you with better information. You may be amazed by the information you can locate on the Web on a topic that you have difficulty understanding. You might find it fun to try out some searches related to nursing research just to see what you can find. If you locate an interesting site, you can save the address for future easy access by "bookmarking" the site or saving it as a favorite site. The following address introduces you to search engines and explains how to use them. If you find a great site that we have not listed, please share it with us. You may e-mail **Burns@uta.edu**

> Researching with the Web—How to find exactly what you are looking for on the Internet—Lickity split. By Jeff Prosise, PC Magazine, June 11, 1996. **http://www.zdnet.com/pcmag/issues/1511/pcmg0081.htm**

Information Validity

It is important to be cautious about the information you obtain at a Web site. When you access the Web site, look for information on the author of the site. Some sites have been developed by very reputable scholars or universities. Other sites provide information that is inaccurate or is a biased opinion of the person who developed the site. Other sites provide information that has not been regularly updated by the author. Check for information on when the site was last updated.

Using Internet Information

Teachers frequently require that you seek Internet sources in developing papers or reports. In many cases, the information you obtain on the Internet is more current than that found in published sources. Information obtained from the Web should be cited as you cite references such as journal articles. Otherwise, you are plagiarizing the information. The fourth edition of the American Psychological Association Referencing Style Manual provides guidance in citing an Internet source. An example of citing a source from the Internet is in Chapter 4 on Literature Review. The following sections indicate Web sites you might find interesting or useful in learning nursing research.

Online Nursing Journals

Online journals may publish their articles only on the Web. Some Online journals may require that you subscribe to them to access their articles. Others have printed versions of the journal and may provide only a few articles that can be accessed on the Web. Current online journals are listed at the following Web sites:

Nursing Links (Online Journals, Nursing Schools, Organizations)
http://www.wfubmc.edu/nursing/links/index.htm

Online Journals in Nursing
http://www.uiowa.edu/~libsci/courses/246/prev-sem1/journals.html

Academic Journal Directory
http://www.son.utmb.edu/catalog/catalog.htm

Abstracts of Nursing Studies

Many nursing organizations are now including abstracts of nursing research presented at their conferences at the organization's Web site. This provides you access to the latest studies conducted on a topic, well in advance of the published report of the study. Some organizations may limit their abstracts to those presented at the most recent conference, while others provide an archive of previous year's abstracts.

Southern Nursing Research Society Abstracts
http://www.uams.edu/nursing/snrs/conference96.htm

Research Centers at Schools of Nursing

Many nursing research centers provide information about research, and about the researchers at their school. Many of these sites include the researchers' photographs, their e-mail addresses, and their current research activities. To access these centers, search for the name of the university.

Duke University Nursing Research Center
http://son3.mc.duke.edu/Research/nrcMain.htm

Creighton University Nursing Research Center
http://nursing.creighton.edu/special/isong2/Research/Index.htm

Research Activities of Nursing Organizations

Many nursing organizations now have a Web site. If the organization has a research arm or focus, you may find interesting information available. The following Web sites provide lists of nursing organizations with their Web links.

MedNet: Nursing Connections—provides links to Web pages of nursing organizations   **http://www.sermed.com/nursing.htm**

BROWNson's nursing notes: Nursing Organizations
http://members.tripod.com/~DianneBrownson/organizations.html

Midwest Alliance in Nursing   **http://www.main-nursing.org/**

Navy Nurse Corp Nursing Research
http://www-nmcsd.med.navy.mil/support/nursingresearch/index.html

National Student Nurses Association   **http://www.nsna.org/**

Southern Nursing Research Society
http://www.uams.edu/nursing/snrs/mainmenu.htm

Sigma Theta Tau International Honor Society of Nursing
http://stti-web.iupui.edu/

Health Web—Nursing Research
http://www.lib.umich.edu/hw/nursing/research.html

World Health Organization   **http://www.who.org/**

Information about Nurse Researchers

A good source of information about nurse researchers is the Sigma Theta Tau International Registry of Nursing Research. Additional information can be found by searching the Web by the researcher's name.

Sigma Theta Tau International Registry of Nursing Research
http://www.stti.iupui.edu/rnr/

Handouts from Nursing Research Instructors across the World

Increasing numbers of faculty who teach nursing research include content for their students on the Web. These sites can vary from a treasure trove of information to a few handouts or slides. Finding good information requires the patience to rummage around in various sites. These sites change as the teacher changes and good content provided at the site may sometimes just disappear from the Web. Following are some examples of these sites.

Journal Articles: The Role of Nursing Research
http://jan.ucc.nau.edu/~mezza/nur390/Mod1/role/journal.html

Research Methods in Nursing: Virtual Handouts
http://www.missouri.edu/~nursgede/n390links.html

Research Methods in Nursing: Reading List
http://www.missouri.edu/~nursgede/n390bib.html

Recommended Readings: Utilizing Research in Nursing Practice
http://jan.ucc.nau.edu/~mezza/nur390/Mod1/utilizing/reading.html

Nursing Lecture Notes
http://128.248.32.78/NUSC218/lec/lec-1/index.htm

Research Resources   **http://www.slu.edu/services/research/resources/**

Health Web: Nursing Research Information
http://www.lib.umich.edu/hw/nursing/research.html

Information about Various Research Methodologies or Research Foci

Researchers with a particular interest will sometimes develop a Web site related to their research to allow easy communication of their work and to maintain connections across the world. Some are centers that have funding for their work. Following are some examples.

Centre for Evidence Based Medicine   **http://163.1.212.5/**

Center for Research on Chronic Illness   **http://www.unc.edu/depts/crci/**

Minimal Nursing Data
http://www.kuleuven.ac.be/facdep/medicine/maat/czv/md/nmds/index.htm

Worldwide Nurse: Nursing Research
http://www.wwnurse.com/nursing/research.html

QualPage: Resources for Qualitative Research
http://www.ualberta.ca/~jrnorris/qual.html

Information about Statistical Procedures

Statistical information that clearly explains a concept you need to know more about are sometimes hard to find. An increasing number of Internet sources on statistics are beginning to appear on the Web. Just search by the statistical term or procedure you need to know about. Examples are:

Stat Concepts: A Visual of Statistical Ideas
http://www-cba.bgsu.edu/asor/facstaff/jharvil/anaheim/index.htm

Introduction to Biobehavioral Statistics
http://wsup03.psy.twsu.edu/Stat15/index.htm

Online Bookstores through which You Can Purchase Books Related to Nursing Research

Books on nursing research topics are often difficult to get at the local bookstore. Books can now be easily ordered on the Web. Some example sites follow.

Amazon Books   **http://www.amazon.com/**

Barnes & Noble Books   **http://www.barnesandnoble.com/**

Borders Books   **http://152.160.1.39/**

"Listservs" That Use E-mail to Facilitate Sharing of Research Information

Listservs send e-mail messages to all who are registered users. There is usually a dialogue back and forth about a topic. One can query those on a listserv seeking information about a particular topic.

NURSERES   Discussion list for nurse researchers

mail the command

subscribe nurseres yourfirstname yourlastname

to **LISTSERV@LISTSERV.KENT.EDU**

Government Agencies Providing Research Information

Government agencies are easily accessible on the Web and provide considerable information. Many agencies have information about research, research findings, and health policy issues that are related to research. Two examples follow. Others are easily located by searching the Web by the title of the agency.

National Institute of Nursing Research   **http://www.nih.gov/ninr/**

Agency for Health Care Policy and Research   **http://www.ahcpr.gov/**

Sources for Further Exploration of the Use of the Internet for Nursing Research

Anonymous (1998). Guide to the Internet. *Lancet, 351* (Suppl) SI1–7.

Bachman, J. A., & Panzarine, S. (1998). Enabling student nurses to use the information superhighway. *Journal of Nursing Education, 37*(4), 155–161.

Balas, J. (1998). Online treasures. Copyright in the digital era. *Computers in Libraries, 18*(6), 38–40.

DeLorenzo, L. (1997). Information superhighway leads to grants. *Nursing Spectrum, 9A*(7), 7.

Fawcett, J., & Buhle, E. L. Jr. (1995). Using the Internet for data collection. An innovative electronic strategy. *Computers in Nursing, 13*(6), 273–279.

Fleitas, J. (1998). Computer monitor. Spinning tales from the World Wide Web: Qualitative research in an electronic environment. *Qualitative Health Research, 8*(2), 283–292.

Flower, J. (1997). Log on. The opportunity in the Internet gap. *Healthcare Forum Journal, 40*(4), 50–51, 53.

Gagliardi, A. (1996). Building partnerships, promoting evidence . . . Ontario Health Care Evaluation Network. *Registered Nurse Journal, 8*(5), 13–14.

Houston, J. D., & Fiore, D. C. (1998). Online medical surveys: Using the Internet as a research tool. *MD Computing, 15*(2), 116–120.

Jenkins, J., & Erdman, K. (1998). Web-based documentation systems. *Home Health Care Management & Practice, 19*(2), 52–61.

Lakeman, R. (1997). Using the Internet for data collection in nursing research . . . presented as a paper at a qualitative research conference for health researchers held at the Eastern Institute of Technology, Taradale, New Zealand, January 1997, *Computers in Nursing, 15*(5), 269–275.

Land, T. (1998). Web extension to American Psychological Association Style (WEAPAS). Todd Land, AKA Beads Land ** 1998. **Webmaster@beads land.com.**

LaPerriere, B., Edwards, P., Romeder, J., Maxwell-Young, L. (1998). Internet travels. Using the Internet to support self-care. *Canadian Nursing, 94*(5), 47–48.

McGarry, N. (1998). So what exactly is the Internet. *World of Irish Nursing, 5*(8), 24.

Murray, P. J. (1996). Research and the Internet: Some practical and ethical issues. *Nursing Standard. 10(28 NURS STAND ONLINE)*: 1–4 Apr 3.

Nicoll, L. H. (1998). *Computers in Nursing's nurses' guide to the Internet,* 2nd ed. Philadelphia: Lippincott-Raven.

Rogers, B. (1997). Research corner: Research and the Internet. *AAOHN Journal, 45*(4), 204–205. (American Association of Occupational Health Nursing)

Szabo, A., & Frenkl, R. (1996). From the field. Consideration of research on Internet: Guidelines and implications for human movement studies. *Clinical Kinesiology: Journal of the American Kinesiotherapy Association, 50*(3), 58–65.

Schnugh, L. (1997). The Internet is alive and well in South Africa. *Cyberskeptic's Guide to Internet Research, 2*(4), 4.

Sibbald, B. (1998). Nursing informatics for beginners. *Canadian Nurse, 94*(4), 22–30.

Sparks, S. M., & Rizzolo, M. A. (1998). World Wide Web search tools. *Image: Journal of Nursing Scholarship, 30*(2), 167–171.

Yentsen, J. (1998). Connecting points: Electronic nursing resources. Systematic, fast, comprehensive search strategies in nursing. *Computers in Nursing, 16*(1), 23–29.

Yerks, A. M., (1996). The Internet and pediatric nursing: Guide to the Information Superhighway. *Pediatric Nursing, 22*(1), 11–15, 26–27.

Text Credits

Selected passages from the following sources have been used with permission throughout the text.

Alexy, B., Nichols, B., Heverly, M. A., & Garzon, L. (1997). Prenatal factors and birth outcomes in the Public Health Service: A rural/urban comparison. *Research in Nursing & Health, 20*(1), 60–70. ©1997. Reprinted by permission of John Wiley and Sons, Inc.

Algase, D. L., Kupferschmid, B., Beel-Bates, C. A., & Beattie, E. R. (1997). Estimates of stability of daily wandering behavior among cognitively impaired long-term care residents. *Nursing Research, 46*(3), 172–178.

Armstrong, M. L. (1991). Career-oriented women with tattoos. *Image: Journal of Nursing Scholarship, 23*(4), 215–220.

Bailey, B. J. (1996). Mediators of depression in adults with diabetes. *Clinical Nursing Research, 5*(1), 28–42. ©1996. Reprinted by permission of Sage Publications, Inc.

Baker, C. F., Garvin, B. J., Kennedy, C. W., & Polivka, B. J. (1993). The effect of environmental sound and communication on CCU patients' heart rate and blood pressure. *Research in Nursing & Health, 16*(6), 415–421. ©1993. Reprinted by permission of John Wiley and Sons, Inc.

Baker, H. M. (1997). Rules outside the rules for administration of medication: A study in New South Wales, Australia. *Image: Journal of Nursing Scholarship, 29*(2), 155–158.

Bayley, E. W., Richmond, T., Noroian, E. L., & Allen, L. R. (1994). A delphi study on research priorities for trauma nursing. *American Journal of Critical Care, 3*(3), 208–216. Reprinted with permission of American Journal of Critical Care.

Beach, E. K., Smith, A., Luthringer, L., Utz, S. K., Aherns, S., & Whitmire, V. (1996). Self-care limitations of persons after acute myocardial infarction. *Applied Nursing Research, 9*(1), 24–28.

Becker, P. T., Engelhardt, K. F., Steinmann, M. F., & Kane, J. (1997). Infant age, context, and family system influences on the interactive behavior of mothers of infants with mental delay. *Research in Nursing & Health, 20*(1), 39–50. ©1997. Reprinted by permission of John Wiley and Sons, Inc.

Benner, P. (1984). *From novice to expert: Excellence and power in clinical nursing practice.* ©1984 by Addison-Wesley Publishing Company. Reprinted by permission.

Berg J., Dunbar-Jacob, J., & Sereika, S. M. (1997). An evaluation of a self-management program for adults with asthma. *Clinical Nursing Research, 6*(3), 225–238. ©1997. Reprinted by permission of Sage Publications, Inc.

Bloch, D. (1990). Strategies for setting and implementing the National Center for Nursing Research priorities. *Applied Nursing Research, 3*(1), 2–6.

Bostrom, J. Mechanic, J., Lazar, N., Michelson, S., Grant, L., & Nomura, L. (1996). Preventing skin breakdown: Nursing practices, costs, and outcomes. *Applied Nursing Research, 9*(4), 184–188.

Bournaki, M. (1997). Correlates of pain-related responses to venipunctures in school-age children. *Nursing Research, 46*(3), 147–154.

Brandt, B., DePalma, J., Irwin, M., Shogan, J., & Lucke, J. F. (1996). Comparison of central venous catheter dressings in bone marrow transplant recipients. *Oncology Nursing Forum, 23*(5), 829–836.

Brown, S. C. (1997). Chest pain and cocaine use in 18 to 40 year-old persons: A retrospective study. *Applied Nursing Research, 10*(3), 136–142.

Carson, M. A. (1996). The impact of relaxation technique on the lipid profile. *Nursing Research, 45*(5), 271–276.

Carty, E. M., Bradley, C., & Winslow, W. (1996). Women's perceptions of fatigue during pregnancy and postpartum: The impact of length of hospital stay. *Clinical Nursing Research, 5*(1), 67–80. ©1996. Reprinted by permission of Sage Publications, Inc.

Cason, C. L., & Grissom, N. L. (1997). Ameliorating adults' acute pain during phlebotomy with a distraction intervention. *Applied Nursing Research, 10*(4), 168–173.

Chang, S. B., & Hill, M. N. (1996). HIV/AIDS related knowledge, attitudes, and preventive behavior of pregnant Korean women. *Image: Journal of Nursing Scholarship, 28*(4), 321–324.

Coffey, A., & Atkinson, P. (1996). *Making sense of qualitative data.* ©1996. Reprinted by permission of Sage Publications, Inc.

Corff, K. E., Seiderman, R., Venkataraman, P. S., Lutes, L., & Yates, B. (1995). Facilitated tucking: A nonpharmacologic comfort measure for pain in preterm neonates. *Obstetric Gynecologic & Neonatal Nursing, 24*(2), 143–147. ©AWHONN.

Coyne, M. L., & Hoskins, L. (1997). Improving eating behaviors in dementia using behavioral strategies. *Clinical Nursing Research, 6*(3), 275–290.

Craft, M. J., & Moss, J. (1996). Accuracy of infant emesis volume assessment. *Applied Nursing Research, 9*(1), 2–8.

Czar, M. L., & Engler, M. M. (1997). Perceived learning needs of patients with coronary artery disease using a questionnaire assessment tool. *Heart & Lung, 26*(2), 109–117.

Dansky, K. H., Dellasaga, C., Schellenbarger, T., & Russo, P. C. (1996). After hospitalization: Home health care for elderly persons. *Clinical Nursing Research, 5*(2), 185–198. ©1996. Reprinted by permission of Sage Publications, Inc.

Deiriggi, P. M. (1990). Effects of waterbed floatation on indicators of energy expenditure in preterm infants. *Nursing Research, 39*(3), 140–146.

Dildy, S. P. (1996). Suffering in people with rheumatoid arthritis. *Applied Nursing Research, 9*(4), 177–183.

Dodd, M. J., Larson, P. J., Dibble, S. L., Miakowski, C., Greenspan, D., MacPhail, P., Hauch, W. W., Paul, St., M., Ignoffo, R., & Shiba, G. (1996). Randomized clinical trial of chlorhexidine versus placebo for prevention of oral mucositis in patients receiving chemotherapy. *Oncology Nursing Forum, 23*(6), 921–927.

Drew, N. (1989). The interviewer's experience as data in phenomenological research. *Western Journal of Nursing Research, 11*(4), 431–439. ©1989. Reprinted by permission of Sage Publications, Inc.

Fagerhaugh, S., & Strauss, A. (1977). *Politics of pain management: Staff-patient interaction.* ©1977 by Addison-Wesley Publishing Company. Reprinted by permission.

Fahs, P. S. S., & Kinney, M. R. (1991). The abdomen, thigh, and arm as sites for subcutaneous sodium heparin injections. *Nursing Research, 40*(4), 204–207.

Fitzpatrick, M. L. (Ed.). *Historical Studies in Nursing* (New York: Teachers College Press, ©1978 by Teachers College, Columbia University. All rights reserved.), pp. 3–11, 15-20. Reprinted by permission of the publisher.

Froman, R. D., & Owens, S. V. (1997). Further validation of the AIDS Attitude Scale. *Research in Nursing & Health, 20*(2), 161–167. ©1997. Reprinted by permission of John Wiley and Sons, Inc.

Goode, C. J., Titler, M., Rakel, B., Ones, D. S., Kleiber, C., Small, S., & Triolo, P. K. (1991). A meta-anaylsis of effects of heparin flush and saline flush: Quality and cost implications. *Nursing Research, 40*(6), 324–330.

Harrison, M. B., Wells, G., Fisher, A., & Prince, M. (1996). Practice guidelines for the prediction and prevention of pressure ulcers: Evaluating the evidence. *Applied Nursing Research, 9*(1), 9–17.

Hastings-Tolsma, M. T., Yucha, C. B., Tompkins, J., Robson, L., & Szeverenyi, N. (1993). Effect of warm and cold applications on the resolution of IV infiltrations. *Research in Nursing & Health, 16*(3), 171–178. ©1993. Reprinted by permission of John Wiley and Sons, Inc.

Hatton, D. C. (1997). Managing health problems among homeless women with children in a transitional shelter. *Image: Journal of Nursing Scholarship, 29*(1), 33–37.

Heater, B. S., Becker, A. M., & Olson, R. K. (1988). Nursing interventions and patient outcomes: A meta-analysis of studies. *Nursing Research, 37*(5), 303–307.

Hulme, P. A., & Grove, S. K. (1994). Symptoms of female survivors of child sexual abuse. *Issues in Mental Health Nursing, 15*(5), 519–532.

Jadack, R. A., Hyde, J. S., & Keller, M. L., (1995). Gender and knowledge about HIV, risky sexual behaviors, and safer sex practices. *Research in Nursing & Health, 18*(4), 313–324. ©1995. Reprinted by permission of John Wiley and Sons, Inc.

Jemmot, L. S., & Jemmott, J. B., III (1991). Applying the theory of reasoned action to AIDS risk behavior: Condom use among black women. *Nursing Reasearch, 40*(4), 228–234.

Johnson, J. E. (1996). Social support and physical health in the rural elderly. *Applied Nursing Research, 9*(2), 61–66.

Johnson, J. E., Fieler, V. K., Wlasowicz, G. S., Mitchell, M. L., & Jones, L. S. (1997). The effects of nursing care guided by self-regulation theory on coping with radiation therapy. *Oncology Nursing Forum, 24*(6), 1041–1050.

Koetzer, A. M. (1990). Creative strategies for pediatric nursing research: Data collection. *Journal of Pediatric Nursing, 5*(1), 50–53.

Koniak, D. (1985). Autotutorial and lecture-demonstration instruction: A comparative analysis of the effects upon students' learning of a developmental assessment skill. *Western Journal of Nursing Research, 7*(1), 80–100. ©1985. Reprinted by permission of Sage Publications, Inc.

Lanza, M. L., Kayne, H. L., Pattison, I., Hicks, C., & Islam, S. (1996). The relationship of behavioral cues to assaultive behaviors. *Clinical Nursing Research, 5*(1), 6–27. ©1996. Reprinted by permission of Sage Publications, Inc.

Levine, R. J. (1986). *Ethics and regulation of clinical research* (2nd ed.). Baltimore and Munich: Urban & Schwarzenberg.

Lillard, J., & McFann, C. L. (1990). A marital crisis: For better or worse . . . hospice involvement. *Hospice Journal—Physical, Psychosocial & Pastoral Care of the Dying, 6*(2), 95–109. ©1990 Haworth Press, Inc.

Lindquist, R., Banasik, J., Barnsteiner, J., Beecroft, P. C., Prevost, S., Riegel, B., Sechrist, K., Strzelecki, C., & Titler M. (1993). Determining AACN's research priorities for the 90s. *American Journal of Critical Care, 2*(2), 110–117. Reprinted with permission of American Journal of Critical Care.

LoBiondo-Wood, G., Williams, L., Wood, R. P., & Shaw, B. W. (1997). Impact of liver transplantation on quality of life: A longitudinal perspective. *Applied Nursing Research, 10*(1), 27–32.

Logan, J., & Jenny, J. (1997). Qualitative analysis of patients' work during mechanical ventilation and weaning. *Heart & Lung, 26*(2), 140–147.

Lusk, B. (1997). Historical methodology for nursing research. *Image: Journal of Nursing Scholarship, 29*(4), 355–359.

Marsh, G. W. (1990). Refining an emergent lifestyle-change theory through matrix analysis. *Advances in Nursing Science, 12*(3), 41–52.

Medoff-Cooper, B., & Gennaro, S. (1996). The correlation of sucking behaviors and Bayley Scales of Infant Development at six months of age in VLBW infants. *Nursing Research, 45*(5), 291–297.

Menzel, L. K. (1997). A comparison of patients' communication-related responses during intubation and after extubation. *Heart & Lung, 26*(5), 363–371.

Metheny, N., Eisenberg, P., & McSweeney, M. (1988). Effect of feeding tube properties and three irrigants on clogging rates. *Nursing Research, 37*(3), 165–169.

Milligan, R. A., Flenniken, P. M., & Pugh, L. C. (1996). Positioning intervention to minimize fatigue in breastfeeding women. *Applied Nursing Research, 9*(2), 67–70.

Morse, J. M., & Field, P. A. (1995). *Qualitative research methods for health professionals* (2nd ed.). Thousand Oaks, CA. ©1995. Reprinted by permission of Sage Publications, Inc.

Morse, J. M., Solberg, S. M., Neander, W. L., Bottoroff, J. L., & Johnson, J. L. (1990). Concepts of caring and caring as a concept. *Advances in Nursing Science, 13*(1), 1–14. ©1990 Aspen Publishers, Inc.

Mullins, I. L. (1996). Nurse caring behaviors for persons with acquired immunodeficiency syndrome/human immunodeficiency virus. *Applied Nursing Research, 9*(1), 18–23.

Neuberger, G. B., Press, A. N., Lindsley, H. B., Hinton, R., Cagle, P. E., Carlson, K., Scott, S., Dahl, J., & Kramer, B. (1997). Effects of exercise on fatigue, aerobic fitness, and disease activity measures in persons with rheumatoid arthritis. *Research in Nursing & Health, 20*(3), 195–204. ©1997. Reprinted by permission of John Wiley and Sons, Inc.

Newton, M. E. (1965). The case for historical research. *Nursing Research, 14*(1), 20–26.

O'Brien, M. T. (1993). Multiple sclerosis: The relationship among self-esteem, social support, and coping behavior. *Applied Nursing Research, 44*(1), 14–19.

O'Brien, S., Dalton, J. A., Konsler, G., & Carlson, J. (1996). The knowledge and attitudes of experienced oncology nurses regarding the management of cancer-related pain. *Oncology Nursing Forum, 23*(3), 515–521.

Palmer, M. H., Myers, A. H., & Fedenko, K. M. (1997). Urinary continence changes after hip-fracture repair. *Clinical Nursing Research, 6*(1), 8–24. ©1997. Reprinted by permission of Sage Publications, Inc.

Pellino, T. A. (1987). Relationships between patient attitudes, subjective norms, perceived control, and analgesic use following elective orthopedic surgery. *Research in Nursing & Health, 20*(2), 97–105. ©1987. Reprinted by permission of John Wiley and Sons, Inc.

Prescott, P. A., & Soeken, K. L. (1989). Methodology corner: The potential uses of pilot work. *Nursing Research, 38*(1), 60–62.

Redeker, N. S., Mason, D. J., Wykpisz, E., & Glica, B. (1996). Sleep patterns in women after coronary artery bypass surgery. *Applied Nursing Research, 9*(3), 115–122.

Reese, J. L., Means, M. E., Hanrahan, K., Clearman, B., Colwill, M., & Dawson, C. (1996). Diarrhea associated with nasogastric feedings. *Oncology Nursing Forum, 23*(1), 59–68.

Rogers, B. (1989). Establishing research priorities in occupational health nursing. *American Association of Occupational Health Nurses Journal, 37*(12), 493–500. Reprinted by permission of AAOHN.

Ropka, M. E. (1996). Commentary [on Diarrhea associated with nasogastric feedings by Reese, Means, Hanrahan, Clearman, Colwill, & Dawson]. *Oncology Nursing Forum, 23*(1), 66–68.

Russell, K. M., & Champion, V. L. (1996). Health beliefs and social influence in home safety practices of mothers with preschool children. *Image: Journal of Nursing Scholarship, 28*(1), 59–64.

Scherer, Y. K., & Schmeider, L. E. (1996). The role of self-efficacy in assisting patients with chronic obstructive pulmonary disease to manage breathing difficulty. *Clinical Nursing Research, 5*(3), 343–355. ©1996. Reprinted by permission of Sage Publications, Inc.

Timmerman, G. M., & Stevenson, J. S. (1996). The relationship between binge eating severity and body fat in nonpurge binge eating women. *Research in Nursing & Health, 19*(5), 389–398. ©1996. Reprinted by permission of John Wiley and Sons, Inc.

Topp, R. Estes, P. K., Dayhoff, N., & Suhrheinrich, J. (1997). Postural control and strength and mood among older adults. *Applied Nursing Research, 19*(1), 80–86.

Troy, N. W., & Dalgas-Pelish, P. (1997). The natural evolution of postpartum fatigue among a group of primiparous women. *Clinical Nursing Research, 6*(2), 126–141. ©1997. Reprinted by permission of Sage Publications, Inc.

Tulman, L., & Fawcett, J. (1990). A framework for studying functional status after diagnosis of breast cancer. *Cancer Nursing, 13*(2), 95–99.

VandenBosch, T., Montoye, C., Satwicz, M., Durkee-Leonard, K, & Boylan-Lewis, B. (1996). Predictive validity of the Braden Scale and nurse perception in identifying pressure ulcer risk. *Applied Nursing Research, 9*(2), 80–86.

Vyhildal, S. K., Moxness, D., Bosak, K. S., Van Meter, F. G., & Bergstrom, N. (1997). Mattress replacement or foam overlay? Prospective study on the incidence of pressure ulcers. *Applied Nursing Research, 10*(3), 111–120.

Williams, M. A. (1980). Editorial: Assumptions in research. *Research in Nursing & Health, 3*(2), 47–48. ©1980. Reprinted by permission of John Wiley and Sons, Inc.

Wineman, N. M., Schwartz, K. M., Goodkin, D. E., & Rudick, R. A. (1996). Relationships among illness uncertainty, stress, coping, and emotional well-being at entry into a clinical drug trial. *Applied Nursing Research, 9*(2), 53–60.

Winslow, E. H., Lane, L. D., & Gaffney, F. A. (1984). Oxygen uptake and cardiovascular response in patients and normal adults during in-bed and out-of-bed toileting. *Journal of Cardiac Rehabilitation, 4*(8), 348–354.

Index

Note: Page numbers in *italics* refer to figures; those followed by t refer to tables.